T0206299

Clinical Trial Optimization Using R

Chapman & Hall/CRC Biostatistics Series

Published Titles

Adaptive Design Methods in Clinical Trials, Second Edition
Shein-Chung Chow and Mark Chang

Adaptive Designs for Sequential Treatment Allocation
Alessandro Baldi Antognini
and Alessandra Giovagnoli

Adaptive Design Theory and Implementation Using SAS and R, Second Edition
Mark Chang

Advanced Bayesian Methods for Medical Test Accuracy
Lyle D. Broemeling

Analyzing Longitudinal Clinical Trial Data: A Practical Guide
Craig Mallinckrodt and Ilya Lipkovich

Applied Biclustering Methods for Big and High-Dimensional Data Using R
Adetayo Kasim, Ziv Shkedy,
Sebastian Kaiser, Sepp Hochreiter,
and Willem Talloen

Applied Meta-Analysis with R
Ding-Geng (Din) Chen and Karl E. Peace

Applied Surrogate Endpoint Evaluation Methods with SAS and R
Ariel Alonso, Theophile Bigirumurame,
Tomasz Burzykowski, Marc Buyse,
Geert Molenberghs, Leacky Muchene,
Nolen Joy Perualila, Ziv Shkedy,
and Wim Van der Elst

Basic Statistics and Pharmaceutical Statistical Applications, Second Edition
James E. De Muth

Bayesian Adaptive Methods for Clinical Trials
Scott M. Berry, Bradley P. Carlin,
J. Jack Lee, and Peter Muller

Bayesian Analysis Made Simple: An Excel GUI for WinBUGS
Phil Woodward

Bayesian Designs for Phase I–II Clinical Trials
Ying Yuan, Hoang Q. Nguyen,
and Peter F. Thall

Bayesian Methods for Measures of Agreement
Lyle D. Broemeling

Bayesian Methods for Repeated Measures
Lyle D. Broemeling

Bayesian Methods in Epidemiology
Lyle D. Broemeling

Bayesian Methods in Health Economics
Gianluca Baio

Bayesian Missing Data Problems: EM, Data Augmentation and Noniterative Computation
Ming T. Tan, Guo-Liang Tian,
and Kai Wang Ng

Published Titles

Bayesian Modeling in Bioinformatics
Dipak K. Dey, Samiran Ghosh,
and Bani K. Mallick

**Benefit-Risk Assessment in
Pharmaceutical Research and
Development**
Andreas Sashegyi, James Felli,
and Rebecca Noel

**Benefit-Risk Assessment Methods in
Medical Product Development: Bridging
Qualitative and Quantitative Assessments**
Qi Jiang and Weili He

**Bioequivalence and Statistics in Clinical
Pharmacology, Second Edition**
Scott Patterson and Byron Jones

**Biosimilar Clinical Development:
Scientific Considerations and New
Methodologies**
Kerry B. Barker, Sandeep M. Menon,
Ralph B. D'Agostino, Sr., Siyan Xu, and Bo Jin

**Biosimilars: Design and Analysis of
Follow-on Biologics**
Shein-Chung Chow

Biostatistics: A Computing Approach
Stewart J. Anderson

**Cancer Clinical Trials: Current and
Controversial Issues in Design and
Analysis**
Stephen L. George, Xiaofei Wang,
and Herbert Pang

**Causal Analysis in Biomedicine and
Epidemiology: Based on Minimal
Sufficient Causation**
Mikel Aickin

**Clinical and Statistical Considerations in
Personalized Medicine**
Claudio Carini, Sandeep Menon, and Mark Chang

Clinical Trial Data Analysis Using R
Ding-Geng (Din) Chen and Karl E. Peace

**Clinical Trial Data Analysis Using R and SAS,
Second Edition**
Ding-Geng (Din) Chen, Karl E. Peace,
and Pinggao Zhang

Clinical Trial Methodology
Karl E. Peace and Ding-Geng (Din) Chen

Clinical Trial Optimization Using R
Alex Dmitrienko and Erik Pulkstenis

**Computational Methods in Biomedical
Research**
Ravindra Khattree and Dayanand N. Naik

Computational Pharmacokinetics
Anders Källén

**Confidence Intervals for Proportions
and Related Measures of Effect Size**
Robert G. Newcombe

**Controversial Statistical Issues in
Clinical Trials**
Shein-Chung Chow

**Data Analysis with Competing Risks
and Intermediate States**
Ronald B. Geskus

**Data and Safety Monitoring Committees
in Clinical Trials, Second Edition**
Jay Herson

**Design and Analysis of Animal Studies
in Pharmaceutical Development**
Shein-Chung Chow and Jen-pei Liu

**Design and Analysis of Bioavailability
and Bioequivalence Studies, Third Edition**
Shein-Chung Chow and Jen-pei Liu

Design and Analysis of Bridging Studies
Jen-pei Liu, Shein-Chung Chow,
and Chin-Fu Hsiao

**Design & Analysis of Clinical Trials for
Economic Evaluation & Reimbursement:
An Applied Approach Using SAS & STATA**
Iftekhar Khan

**Design and Analysis of Clinical Trials
for Predictive Medicine**
Shigeyuki Matsui, Marc Buyse,
and Richard Simon

**Design and Analysis of Clinical Trials with
Time-to-Event Endpoints**
Karl E. Peace

Design and Analysis of Non-Inferiority Trials
Mark D. Rothmann, Brian L. Wiens,
and Ivan S. F. Chan

**Difference Equations with Public Health
Applications**
Lemuel A. Moyé and Asha Seth Kapadia

Published Titles

DNA Methylation Microarrays: Experimental Design and Statistical Analysis
Sun-Chong Wang and Arturas Petronis

DNA Microarrays and Related Genomics Techniques: Design, Analysis, and Interpretation of Experiments
David B. Allison, Grier P. Page,
T. Mark Beasley, and Jode W. Edwards

Dose Finding by the Continual Reassessment Method
Ying Kuen Cheung

Dynamical Biostatistical Models
Daniel Commenges and
Hélène Jacqmin-Gadda

Elementary Bayesian Biostatistics
Lemuel A. Moyé

Emerging Non-Clinical Biostatistics in Biopharmaceutical Development and Manufacturing
Harry Yang

Empirical Likelihood Method in Survival Analysis
Mai Zhou

Essentials of a Successful Biostatistical Collaboration
Arul Earnest

Exposure–Response Modeling: Methods and Practical Implementation
Jixian Wang

Frailty Models in Survival Analysis
Andreas Wienke

Fundamental Concepts for New Clinical Trialists
Scott Evans and Naitee Ting

Generalized Linear Models: A Bayesian Perspective
Dipak K. Dey, Sujit K. Ghosh, and
Bani K. Mallick

Handbook of Regression and Modeling: Applications for the Clinical and Pharmaceutical Industries
Daryl S. Paulson

Inference Principles for Biostatisticians
Ian C. Marschner

Interval-Censored Time-to-Event Data: Methods and Applications
Ding-Geng (Din) Chen, Jianguo Sun,
and Karl E. Peace

Introductory Adaptive Trial Designs: A Practical Guide with R
Mark Chang

Joint Models for Longitudinal and Time-to-Event Data: With Applications in R
Dimitris Rizopoulos

Measures of Interobserver Agreement and Reliability, Second Edition
Mohamed M. Shoukri

Medical Biostatistics, Third Edition
A. Indrayan

Meta-Analysis in Medicine and Health Policy
Dalene Stangl and Donald A. Berry

Methods in Comparative Effectiveness Research
Constantine Gatsonis and Sally C. Morton

Mixed Effects Models for the Population Approach: Models, Tasks, Methods and Tools
Marc Lavielle

Modeling to Inform Infectious Disease Control
Niels G. Becker

Modern Adaptive Randomized Clinical Trials: Statistical and Practical Aspects
Oleksandr Sverdlov

Monte Carlo Simulation for the Pharmaceutical Industry: Concepts, Algorithms, and Case Studies
Mark Chang

Multiregional Clinical Trials for Simultaneous Global New Drug Development
Joshua Chen and Hui Quan

Multiple Testing Problems in Pharmaceutical Statistics
Alex Dmitrienko, Ajit C. Tamhane,
and Frank Bretz

Published Titles

Noninferiority Testing in Clinical Trials: Issues and Challenges
Tie-Hua Ng

Optimal Design for Nonlinear Response Models
Valerii V. Fedorov and Sergei L. Leonov

Patient-Reported Outcomes: Measurement, Implementation and Interpretation
Joseph C. Cappelleri, Kelly H. Zou, Andrew G. Bushmakin, Jose Ma. J. Alvir, Demissie Alemayehu, and Tara Symonds

Quantitative Evaluation of Safety in Drug Development: Design, Analysis and Reporting
Qi Jiang and H. Amy Xia

Quantitative Methods for Traditional Chinese Medicine Development
Shein-Chung Chow

Randomized Clinical Trials of Nonpharmacological Treatments
Isabelle Boutron, Philippe Ravaud, and David Moher

Randomized Phase II Cancer Clinical Trials
Sin-Ho Jung

Repeated Measures Design with Generalized Linear Mixed Models for Randomized Controlled Trials
Toshiro Tango

Sample Size Calculations for Clustered and Longitudinal Outcomes in Clinical Research
Chul Ahn, Moonseong Heo, and Song Zhang

Sample Size Calculations in Clinical Research, Second Edition
Shein-Chung Chow, Jun Shao, and Hansheng Wang

Statistical Analysis of Human Growth and Development
Yin Bun Cheung

Statistical Design and Analysis of Clinical Trials: Principles and Methods
Weichung Joe Shih and Joseph Aisner

Statistical Design and Analysis of Stability Studies
Shein-Chung Chow

Statistical Evaluation of Diagnostic Performance: Topics in ROC Analysis
Kelly H. Zou, Aiyi Liu, Andriy Bandos, Lucila Ohno-Machado, and Howard Rockette

Statistical Methods for Clinical Trials
Mark X. Norleans

Statistical Methods for Drug Safety
Robert D. Gibbons and Anup K. Amatya

Statistical Methods for Healthcare Performance Monitoring
Alex Bottle and Paul Aylin

Statistical Methods for Immunogenicity Assessment
Harry Yang, Jianchun Zhang, Binbing Yu, and Wei Zhao

Statistical Methods in Drug Combination Studies
Wei Zhao and Harry Yang

Statistical Testing Strategies in the Health Sciences
Albert Vexler, Alan D. Hutson, and Xiwei Chen

Statistics in Drug Research: Methodologies and Recent Developments
Shein-Chung Chow and Jun Shao

Statistics in the Pharmaceutical Industry, Third Edition
Ralph Buncher and Jia-Yeong Tsay

Survival Analysis in Medicine and Genetics
Jialiang Li and Shuangge Ma

Theory of Drug Development
Eric B. Holmgren

Translational Medicine: Strategies and Statistical Methods
Dennis Cosmatos and Shein-Chung Chow

Chapman & Hall/CRC Biostatistics Series

Clinical Trial Optimization Using R

Edited by

Alex Dmitrienko
Erik Pulkstenis

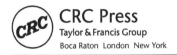

CRC Press
Taylor & Francis Group
Boca Raton London New York

CRC Press is an imprint of the
Taylor & Francis Group, an **informa** business
A CHAPMAN & HALL BOOK

CRC Press
Taylor & Francis Group
6000 Broken Sound Parkway NW, Suite 300
Boca Raton, FL 33487-2742

First issued in paperback 2019

ISBN-13: 978-1-4987-3507-0 (hbk)
ISBN-13: 978-0-367-26125-2 (pbk)

Library of Congress Cataloging-in-Publication Data

Names: Dmitrienko, Alex. | Pulkstenis, Erik.
Title: Clinical trial optimization using R / Alex Dmitrienko, Erik Pulkstenis.
Description: Boca Raton : CRC Press, 2017. | Includes bibliographical
references and index.
Identifiers: LCCN 2016057709 | ISBN 9781498735070 (hardback : alk. paper)
Subjects: LCSH: Clinical trials--Statistical methods. | R (Computer program language)
Classification: LCC R853.C55 D6525 2017 | DDC 610.72/7--dc23
LC record available at https://lccn.loc.gov/2016057709

Visit the Taylor & Francis Web site at
http://www.taylorandfrancis.com

and the CRC Press Web site at
http://www.crcpress.com

Contents

Preface   xiii

List of Contributors   xvii

1   Clinical Scenario Evaluation and Clinical Trial Optimization   1
    Alex Dmitrienko and Gautier Paux
   1.1   Introduction   1
   1.2   Clinical Scenario Evaluation   2
       1.2.1   Components of Clinical Scenario Evaluation   2
       1.2.2   Software implementation   4
       1.2.3   Case study 1.1: Clinical trial with a normally distributed
            endpoint   16
       1.2.4   Case study 1.2: Clinical trial with two time-to-event
            endpoints   20
   1.3   Clinical trial optimization   28
       1.3.1   Optimization strategies   30
       1.3.2   Optimization algorithm   33
       1.3.3   Sensitivity assessments   34
   1.4   Direct optimization   38
       1.4.1   Case study 1.3: Clinical trial with two patient popula-
            tions   38
       1.4.2   Qualitative sensitivity assessment   43
       1.4.3   Quantitative sensitivity assessment   44
       1.4.4   Optimal selection of the target parameter   53
   1.5   Tradeoff-based optimization   59
       1.5.1   Case study 1.4: Clinical trial with an adaptive design   59
       1.5.2   Optimal selection of the target parameter   67

2   Clinical Trials with Multiple Objectives   71
    Alex Dmitrienko and Gautier Paux
   2.1   Introduction   71
   2.2   Clinical Scenario Evaluation framework   73
       2.2.1   Data models   74
       2.2.2   Analysis models   74
       2.2.3   Evaluation models   85
   2.3   Case study 2.1: Optimal selection of a multiplicity adjustment   91

ix

	2.3.1	Clinical trial	92
	2.3.2	Qualitative sensitivity assessment	99
	2.3.3	Quantitative sensitivity assessment	107
	2.3.4	Software implementation	114
	2.3.5	Conclusions and extensions	120
2.4		Case study 2.2: Direct selection of optimal procedure parameters	121
	2.4.1	Clinical trial	121
	2.4.2	Optimal selection of the target parameter in Procedure B1	133
	2.4.3	Optimal selection of the target parameters in Procedure B2	140
	2.4.4	Sensitivity assessments	145
	2.4.5	Software implementation	149
	2.4.6	Conclusions and extensions	154
2.5		Case study 2.3: Tradeoff-based selection of optimal procedure parameters	156
	2.5.1	Clinical trial	156
	2.5.2	Optimal selection of the target parameter in Procedure H	161
	2.5.3	Software implementation	168
	2.5.4	Conclusions and extensions	172

3 Subgroup Analysis in Clinical Trials   173

Alex Dmitrienko and Gautier Paux

3.1		Introduction	173
3.2		Clinical Scenario Evaluation in confirmatory subgroup analysis	175
	3.2.1	Clinical Scenario Evaluation framework	175
	3.2.2	Multiplicity adjustments	181
	3.2.3	Decision-making framework	184
3.3		Case study 3.1: Optimal selection of a multiplicity adjustment	188
	3.3.1	Clinical trial	189
	3.3.2	Direct optimization based on disjunctive power	194
	3.3.3	Direct optimization based on weighted power	196
	3.3.4	Qualitative sensitivity assessment	199
	3.3.5	Quantitative sensitivity assessment	203
	3.3.6	Software implementation	208
	3.3.7	Conclusions and extensions	213
3.4		Case study 3.2: Optimal selection of decision rules to support two potential claims	215
	3.4.1	Clinical trial	215
	3.4.2	Influence condition	215
	3.4.3	Optimal selection of the influence threshold	219
	3.4.4	Software implementation	225
	3.4.5	Conclusions and extensions	228

3.5 Case study 3.3: Optimal selection of decision rules to support
three potential claims 228
3.5.1 Clinical trial 228
3.5.2 Interaction condition 233
3.5.3 Optimal selection of the influence and interaction thresholds 238
3.5.4 Software implementation 244
3.5.5 Conclusions and extensions 249

4 Decision Making in Clinical Development **251**
*Kaushik Patra, Ming-Dauh Wang, Jianliang Zhang, Aaron Dane, Paul
Metcalfe, Paul Frewer, and Erik Pulkstenis*
4.1 Introduction 251
4.2 Clinical Scenario Evaluation in Go/No-Go decision making and
determination of probability of success 253
4.2.1 Clinical Scenario Evaluation approach 253
4.2.2 Go/No-Go decision criteria 255
4.2.3 Probability of success 258
4.2.4 Probability of success applications 262
4.3 Motivating example 264
4.3.1 Clinical trial 265
4.3.2 Software implementation 268
4.4 Case study 4.1: Bayesian Go/No-Go decision criteria 269
4.4.1 Clinical trial 269
4.4.2 General sensitivity assessments 271
4.4.3 Bayesian Go/No-Go evaluation using informative priors 274
4.4.4 Sample size considerations 276
4.4.5 Software implementation 279
4.4.6 Conclusions and extensions 282
4.5 Case study 4.2: Bayesian Go/No-Go evaluation using an alternative decision criterion 283
4.5.1 Clinical trial 283
4.5.2 Software implementation 285
4.5.3 Conclusions and extensions 286
4.6 Case study 4.3: Bayesian Go/No-Go evaluation in a trial with
an interim analysis 286
4.6.1 Clinical trial 287
4.6.2 Software implementation 289
4.6.3 Conclusions and extensions 290
4.7 Case study 4.4: Decision criteria in Phase II trials based on
Probability of Success 290
4.7.1 Clinical trial 290
4.7.2 Software implementation 292
4.7.3 Conclusions and extensions 293

4.8 Case study 4.5: Updating POS using interim or external information 294
    4.8.1 Clinical trial 295
    4.8.2 Software implementation 298

Bibliography **301**

Index **309**

Preface

Clinical development is a strategic and operational, scientific process that involves a significant level of multidimensional decision making, often in the presence of incomplete information or considerable uncertainty. Along the way, several key questions must be answered including selection of the right dose and schedule, selection of the right patient population and selection of the right analytical strategy to provide optimal treatment options for patients with the highest probability of success. Against this backdrop, more fundamental questions loom, e.g., whether the drug is even safe or effective at all and whether the final risk-benefit profile will be acceptable.

Adding to the research burden is the desire to make correct decisions as quickly and efficiently as possible. The rise in adaptive design science over the past decade speaks to the increasing desire to learn in real time, and immediately incorporate that learning into drug development, in an attempt to eliminate or reduce the white space present in a traditional drug development paradigm. Advances in multiplicity theory support the growing pressure to definitively establish as many hypotheses/claims as possible within the constraints of Type I error rate control. At the same time clinical trial programs are changing with the lines becoming increasingly blurred between traditional phases of drug development, or individual trials that are increasing in complexity to ask more questions (e.g., platform trials). External pressures also exist, driven by the changes in reimbursement and increased expectations that medications demonstrate their value to the patient and clinical community in a more comprehensive way. The goal is simply no longer to conduct two large Phase III trials with statistically significant p-values because the bar has been raised.

Despite significant methodological advances provided by the statistical and clinical community and associated computational advances, it remains clear that development risk remains high, and that decision making has not yet been universally optimized within clinical development. This can be seen by the accumulating evidence that Phase II results often do not translate to Phase III success (Brutti, De Santis, and Gubbiotti, 2008; Kirby et al., 2012; Kola and Landis, 2004; Chuang-Stein and Kirby, 2014). One review of 253 published Phase III oncology trials found that 62% of the trials failed to establish a statistically significant treatment effect, mostly due to the fact that observed treatment effects were simply smaller than expected based on previous data (Gan et al., 2012).

This combination of increasing clinical trial complexity/options, coupled with increasing scrutiny on the risk-benefit profile that new treatments bring to the table, against a backdrop of lackluster industry development performance introduces both financial constraints, and a heightened level of urgency around strategic drug development decision making in order to stop development of inferior compounds early and accelerate development of promising compounds (Arrowsmith and Miller, 2013; Paul et al., 2010). As a result, clinical trial optimization is an absolute necessity in support of these objectives, though quantitative methods to this end are frequently not part of the drug development process.

Clinical trial optimization can be thought of at the trial level, or the development plan level as clinical research designed to most efficiently and with least risk answer the most important research questions to the developer. Historically the process has been fairly empiric, though the increasing availability of computational resources and methods, along with the generally low success rates, is driving an opportunity to marry clinical trial modeling and simulation with decision making in a more comprehensive and holistic fashion, resulting in evidence-based development which examines the operating characteristics of development decisions themselves. In this book, we explore a promising approach known as the Clinical Scenario Evaluation framework (Benda et al., 2010) which endeavors to optimize clinical development considering a set of objectives, design and analysis alternatives, underlying assumptions and, finally, quantitative metrics to facilitate decision making with better line of sight into the decision space one is dealing with. We use specific common clinical trial problems to elucidate the methodology in a case study setting. R code is provided to both demonstrate common methods while providing some preliminary tools for the practitioner. Examples include optimally spending the Type I error rate across trial objectives or patient subgroups in the presence of multiple desired claims and optimally selecting associated decision rules or analytical methods in Chapters 2 and 3. In addition, we present an evaluation of Go/No-Go decision making at the proof-of-concept stage as well as considerations for probability of success based on Bayesian principles in Chapter 4. These case studies serve to scratch the surface regarding the potential utility of modeling and simulation to optimize decision making within a complex and highly dimensional development decision space.

The Clinical Scenario Evaluation paradigm is broadly flexible and applicable to any scenario a clinical trial or researcher can envision and, as a result, may impact the overall quality of the drug development process. It is a valuable tool available to the researcher and enables a move from empirical decision making around myriads of options, to a more disciplined and evidence-based approach to how one designs clinical trials and clinical trial programs.

Acknowledgments

We would like to thank the reviewers who have provided valuable comments on selected chapters in the book: Thomas Brechenmacher (Novartis), Michael Lee (Johnson and Johnson), Christoph Muysers (Bayer), Xin Wang (AbbVie).

We would also like to thank the book's acquisitions editor, David Grubbs, for his support and his work on this book publishing project.

Alex Dmitrienko, Mediana Inc.
Erik Pulkstenis, MedImmune.

List of Contributors

This book is based on a collaborative effort of nine statisticians from the pharmaceutical industry:

Aaron Dane, Therapeutic Area Head for Infection, Biometrics and Information Sciences, AstraZeneca; Independent Consultant, DaneStat Consulting Limited.

Alex Dmitrienko, President, Mediana Inc.

Paul Frewer, Statistical Science Director, Biometrics and Information Sciences, AstraZeneca.

Paul Metcalfe, Scientific Computing Director, Advanced Analytics Centre, Biometrics and Information Sciences, AstraZeneca.

Kaushik Patra, Science Director, Biostatistics, MedImmune; Director, Biostatistics, Alexion.

Gautier Paux, Senior Statistician, Clinical Biostatistics Unit, Institut de Recherches Internationales Servier.

Erik Pulkstenis, Vice President, Clinical Biostatistics and Data Management, MedImmune.

Ming-Dauh Wang, Principal Research Scientist, Global Statistical Sciences, Eli Lilly and Company.

Jianliang Zhang, Senior Director, Statistical Methods, MedImmune.

1

Clinical Scenario Evaluation and Clinical Trial Optimization

Alex Dmitrienko

Mediana Inc.

Gautier Paux

Institut de Recherches Internationales Servier

1.1 Introduction

It was pointed out in the preface that clinical trial sponsors are actively looking for ways to develop more efficient approaches to designing, conducting and analyzing trials. This can be accomplished most effectively through a comprehensive quantitative assessment of available options, including innovative trial designs and statistical methods. Clinical Scenario Evaluation (CSE) was introduced in Benda et al. (2010), and subsequently refined in Friede et al. (2010) and other publications, as an efficient quantitative approach to evaluating trial designs and data analysis methods in individual clinical trials or, more generally, in clinical development programs.

A general CSE-based approach to designing a clinical trial incorporates a thorough assessment of multiple competing strategies which enables the trial's team to assess the pros and cons of the applicable trial designs and analysis techniques and to examine their sensitivity to potential changes in the underlying assumptions. This approach has the potential to help trial sponsors set up more robust designs that avoid overly optimistic assumptions that are still very common in Phase III trials (Gan et al., 2012) and, along the same line, improve on simplistic or suboptimal analytical methods such as inefficient multiplicity adjustments that are often employed in clinical trials; see, for example, PREVAIL trial (Beer et al., 2014) or APEX trial (Cohen et al., 2013; Cohen et al., 2014). In fact, CSE has been successfully leveraged in multiple Phase II and III clinical trials and led to tangible improvements compared to ad-hoc approaches to trial design and analysis. Examples and references can be found in Benda et al. (2010), Friede et al. (2010), as well as more recent publications, including Dmitrienko, Paux and Brechenmacher (2015) and Dmitrienko et al. (2016).

As a powerful approach to improving the probability of success and building robust trial designs and analysis strategies, the general CSE framework will play a central role in this book. The guiding principles of CSE will be introduced in Section 1.2 and will be applied in Chapters 2, 3 and 4. The discussion of CSE applications in these chapters will focus mostly on efficacy assessments in a single clinical trial. However, it is important to note that many other applications fall within the CSE domain. This includes, for example, a systematic assessment of safety signals as well as CSE-based evaluations at the program level. For a discussion of key considerations related to applying CSE techniques to multiple clinical trials within the same development program, see Benda et al. (2010).

It is important to explore the connections between CSE and clinical trial optimization. As pointed out in Benda et al. (2010), due to its emphasis on identifying best-performing designs and analysis strategies in clinical trials, CSE provides a foundation for developing a holistic approach to optimizing drug development. The key principles of CSE-based clinical trial optimization will be introduced in Section 1.3 and illustrated throughout this book. Practical and easy-to-implement clinical trial optimization strategies will be emphasized in the book. The resulting strategies provide quantitative information to support internal decision making and efficient dialog with external clinical experts and regulators. To facilitate the application of CSE and optimization methods to real-life trials, multiple case studies and R code will be provided in Chapters 2, 3 and 4.

1.2 Clinical Scenario Evaluation

This section introduces the key principles and building blocks of the general CSE approach with emphasis on the trial-level and analysis-level evaluations introduced in Benda et al. (2010). The process of setting up a CSE framework and defining its components in real clinical trials will be illustrated in Section 1.2.2 using an R package that was designed to support CSE in clinical trial applications (**Mediana** package).

1.2.1 Components of Clinical Scenario Evaluation

It is broadly recognized that evaluation of candidate trial designs and analysis methods in clinical trials is, by nature, a multidimensional process. Benda et al. (2010) proposed to decompose this complex problem into a small number of components that define the core building blocks of the overall CSE framework. These components were referred to as *assumptions*, *options* and *metrics* in the

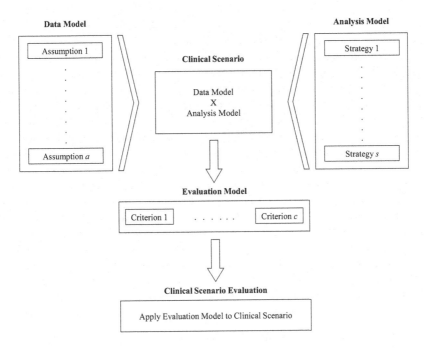

FIGURE 1.1: General Clinical Scenario Evaluation framework.

original CSE publications. Dmitrienko et al. (2016) revised this terminology to introduce more descriptive labels for each CSE component:

- *Data models*, previously known as assumptions, define the process of generating the trial data.

- *Analysis models*, previously known as options, specify the analysis strategies applied to the trial data.

- *Evaluation models*, previously known as metrics, specify the criteria for evaluating the performance of the analysis strategies applied to the trial data.

Within the data and analysis models, multiple statistical assumptions or analysis strategies can be specified and the combination of these two models represents a *clinical scenario*. CSE focuses on the application of the criteria defined in the evaluation model to the clinical scenarios of interest. A visual representation of the CSE framework is provided in Figure 1.1.

This decomposition into three independent components provides a structured framework for clinical trial simulations which enables clinical trial researchers to carry out a systematic quantitative assessment of the operating characteristics of candidate designs and statistical methods to characterize their performance in multiple settings. Ultimately, this assessment supports the selection of a robust approach to clinical trial design and analysis which demonstrates optimal performance.

It was emphasized in the introduction that, within the CSE framework, emphasis is placed on realistic assumptions as opposed to simplistic assumptions that may be introduced to streamline the process of designing a clinical trial or simplify the data analysis models. For example, when designing a trial with a time-to-event endpoint, it is quite common to assume that this endpoint follows an exponential distribution because this distribution supports the assumption of proportional hazards and leads to a straightforward closed-form expression for the required number of events in the trial. CSE encourages clinical trial sponsors to take advantage of simulation-based methods to facilitate an exhaustive performance assessment by exploring a multitude of data models and analysis strategies, as well as a wide range of sensitivity assessments to ultimately arrive at optimal and robust trial designs and data analysis methods according to the pre-defined success criteria. In general, simulation-based approaches have found numerous applications in clinical trials and have been used to construct design and analysis evaluation frameworks that are conceptually similar to CSE; see, for example, Westfall et al. (2008).

1.2.2   Software implementation

It was pointed out in Friede et al. (2010) that there may be an important gap between the general set of CSE principles and their practical implementation. This section introduces an R package (**Mediana**) that provides clinical trial statisticians and drug developers in general with a powerful set of tools to close this gap and enable CSE-based solutions in a broad range of clinical trial applications. The package was developed by Paux and Dmitrienko (2016) and is currently maintained by representatives from multiple biopharmaceutical companies.

Mediana has been built to support a general framework for CSE-based clinical trial simulations. This package is fully aligned with the CSE approach and can be used to perform a systematic and critical review of options related to candidate trial designs and statistical methods or adjustments used in the analysis. The package supports a broad class of data models, analysis strategies and commonly used evaluation criteria. A full documentation of this package can be found in the web-based manual at

`http://gpaux.github.io/Mediana`

This manual includes multiple case studies that have been created to facilitate the implementation of simulation-based CSE approaches in multiple settings and help the user understand individual features of the **Mediana** package. In addition, for more information on other software tools that support CSE and clinical trial optimization, visit the Biopharmnet web site at

`http://biopharmnet.com/mediana`

It is important to point out that this R package has been designed from the ground up to be easily extensible. All options defined in each model actually represent calls to R functions with the same name and thus users can add their own options, e.g., new statistical tests, by developing custom R functions. This important feature will be illustrated in Chapters 2 and 3.

The current version of the **Mediana** package supports the following commonly used types of trial designs:

- *Fixed designs* with a fixed follow-up period (period from a patient's enrollment to discontinuation).

- *Event-driven designs* with a variable follow-up period. This setting is common in trials with time-to-event outcomes and is characterized by the fact that a patient may reach the primary endpoint before the end of the follow-up period.

Other design options will be enabled in a future version of the package. This includes support to *adaptive designs* in early-stage and late-stage clinical trials.

This section provides a more formal description of the main components of the CSE framework implemented in the **Mediana** package, which follows a four-step process. The data, analysis and evaluation models are sequentially specified using the `DataModel`, `AnalysisModel` and `EvaluationModel` objects, respectively. The same process is used to set up each of the three models, namely, a model is initialized and then specific components of each model are added to it. Finally, Clinical Scenario Evaluation can be performed by wrapping up the data, analysis and evaluation models into the `CSE` function, along with the simulation parameters that are specified in the `SimParamaters` object. Multiple examples of setting up CSE framework in real-life clinical trials will be provided in Case studies 1.1 and 1.2.

Data model

As explained in Section 1.2.1, a data model defines the process of generating patient data in a clinical trial. In particular, this model focuses on specifying the parameters of the individual *samples* within a single trial, defined as mutually exclusive groups of patients, such as treatment arms.

The first step is to initialize the data model. This is easily accomplished by the command presented in Listing 1.1.

LISTING 1.1: Initialization of a data model

```
data.model = DataModel()
```

It is highly recommended to use this command as it simplifies the specification of the data model components, i.e., the number of patients (sample size) (`SampleSize`) or number of events (`Event`), outcome distribution

(OutcomeDist), design parameters (Design) and sample parameters (Sample). Each component is specified in a data model simply by adding it in one-by-one to the DataModel object using the + operator.

SampleSize object

This object specifies the common number of patients enrolled in each sample in a fixed-design trial with a balanced design (all samples are assumed to have the same sample size). A SampleSize object is defined with a single argument, denoted by sample.size, which specifies a list or vector of sample sizes. Alternatively, if an unbalanced design is considered in a clinical trial, the sample sizes need to be defined within each sample (see the Sample object below).

Several equivalent specifications of the SampleSize object are presented in Listing 1.2.

LISTING 1.2: Specification of SampleSize objects

```
SampleSize(c(50, 55, 60, 65, 70))
SampleSize(seq(50, 70, 5))
```

In this example, the sponsor would like to simulate a clinical trial with a broad range of sample sizes in each sample, e.g., in each treatment arm. Several sample sizes may be defined, as illustrated above, in a given sample and represent the *sample size sets* evaluated in a particular clinical scenario.

Event object

This object specifies the total number of events (or target event counts) among all samples in an event-driven clinical trial. An Event object has two arguments:

- n.events defines a vector of target event counts.

- rando.ratio defines a vector of randomization ratios for each Sample object defined in the DataModel object.

As for the number of events, several target event counts can be defined as illustrated above and represent the *number of event sets* evaluated in the current clinical scenario. Also, the specification of the randomization ratio must respect the order of the samples in the data model, i.e., the first number corresponds to the randomization ratio of the first sample included in the data model.

OutcomeDist object

This object specifies the distribution of patient outcomes in a data model. An OutcomeDist object is defined by two arguments:

- `outcome.dist` defines the outcome distribution, i.e., the distribution of the trial endpoint, or, in a more general setting, the distribution of multiple endpoints such as the primary endpoint and key secondary endpoints.

- `outcome.type` defines the outcome type (optional). There are two acceptable values for this argument: `standard` (fixed-design setting, by default) and `event` (event-driven design setting).

The **Mediana** package supports a wide variety of trial endpoints, including continuous, binary, survival-type (time-to-event) and count-type outcomes, as well as more complex settings involving simultaneous evaluation of multiple endpoints with different marginal distributions. Data models with repeated measures can be considered as well by assuming that each patient's outcome follows an appropriate multivariate distribution. Distributions supported in the current version of the **Mediana** package are listed in Table 1.1 along with the required parameters to be included in the `outcome.par` argument of the `Sample` object. Note that parameters of multivariate distributions, such as parameters of the marginal distributions and correlation matrix, need to be defined using nested lists.

TABLE 1.1: Outcome distributions supported in the current version of the **Mediana** package.

Outcome distribution	outcome.dist	outcome.par
Uniform	UniformDist	max
Normal	NormalDist	mean, sd
Exponential	ExpoDist	rate
Binomial	BinomDist	prop
Beta	BetaDist	prop
Poisson	PoissonDist	mean
Negative binomial	NegBinomDist	dispersion, mean
Multivariate normal	MVNormalDist	par, corr
Multivariate binomial	MVBinomDist	par, corr
Multivariate exponential	MVExpoDist	par, corr
Multivariate mixed	MVMixedDist	type, par, corr

The process of specifying parameters of outcome distributions in each sample will be illustrated in Case study 1.1 (see Listing 1.11) and Case study 1.2 (see Listing 1.19).

Note that the outcome's type must be defined for each endpoint if a patient's outcome follows a multivariate distribution, e.g., `c("event","event")` if a bivariate exponential distribution is specified. The specification of the `outcome.type` argument is essential to obtain censored events for time-to-event endpoints if the `SampleSize` object is used to define the number of patients instead of the number of events (`Event` object).

Finally, other outcome distributions can be enabled in a data model by writing a custom R function which implements random number generation for that particular distribution.

Design object

The `Design` object is optional and can be defined in event-driven designs if the user is interested in modeling the enrollment (or accrual) and dropout (or loss to follow up) processes. A `Design` object is defined by the following arguments:

- `enroll.period` defines the duration of the enrollment period.

- `enroll.dist` defines the enrollment distribution. Any univariate distribution included in the **Mediana** package or specified by the user can be selected. The most popular distributions include the uniform, beta and exponential distributions.

- `enroll.dist.par` defines the parameters of the enrollment distribution (optional). No parameters are needed if the enrollment distribution is assumed to be uniform over the accrual period.

- `followup.period` defines the length of the follow-up period for each patient in trial designs with a fixed follow-up period, i.e., the length of time from the enrollment to planned discontinuation is constant across patients.

- `study.duration` defines the total trial duration in trial designs with a variable follow-up period. The total trial duration is defined as the time from the enrollment of the first patient to the discontinuation of the last patient. The user must specify either `followup.period` or `study.duration`.

- `dropout.dist` defines the dropout distribution. As with the enrollment distribution, any univariate built-in or user-specified distribution can be chosen and the most popular choices include the uniform and exponential distributions.

- `dropout.dist.par` defines the parameters of the dropout distribution (optional).

Since CSE supports a thorough exploration of multiple options in a trial, the user can define several sets of design parameters by adding multiple `Design` objects to the data model. These sets are known as *design parameter sets* and enable the user to compactly define multiple scenarios that can be evaluated simultaneously. Also, the length of the enrollment period, total trial duration and follow-up periods are measured using the same time units. Note that the current version of **Mediana** supports only basic patient dropout models. More advanced modeling options, including informative dropouts, and methods for analyzing incomplete data in clinical trials (see, for example, Mallinckrodt and Lipkovich, 2017) will be supported in a future version of the package.

Listing 1.3 gives an example of design parameters in a trial with a uniform enrollment distribution and exponential dropout distribution. More information on the specification of design parameters in clinical trials will be provided in Case study 1.2 (see Listing 1.18).

LISTING 1.3: Specification of the Design object

```
Design(enroll.period = 9,
       study.duration = 21,
       enroll.dist = "UniformDist",
       dropout.dist = "ExpoDist",
       dropout.dist.par = parameters(rate = 0.0115))
```

Sample object

This object specifies parameters of a sample in a data model. As explained above, samples are defined as mutually exclusive groups of patients, for example, treatment arms. Therefore, several `Sample` objects can be added to a `DataModel` object. A `Sample` object is defined by three arguments:

- `id` defines the sample's unique ID (label). This ID is used in the specification of the trial's analysis model.

- `outcome.par` defines the parameters of the outcome distribution for the sample, including key data model parameters such as the treatment effects and additional parameters that play a supportive role, e.g., correlation coefficients. The parameters depend on the endpoint's distribution, e.g., if the primary endpoint is normally distributed (`outcome.dist = "NormalDist"`), two parameters (`mean` and `sd`) must be specified. The parameters required for each distribution are listed in Table 1.1.

- `sample.size` defines the number of patients in the sample (optional). This option is helpful for modeling unbalanced trial designs with unequal allocation of patients to the treatment arms. The sample sizes must be specified in the `SampleSize` object or in each individual `Sample` object.

Based on general CSE principles, the **Mediana** package makes it easy for the user to specify several sets of assumptions in `outcome.par`. These sets may correspond to a range of optimistic, realistic and pessimistic treatment effect assumptions that support general sensitivity assessments. The assumptions sets represent the *outcome parameter sets* that will be evaluated in the clinical scenario. In this case, each assumption can be included in the `outcome.par` argument, as illustrated in the specification of the `Sample` object in Case study 1.1 (see Listing 1.11). Further, the specification of multivariate distribution parameters will be illustrated in Chapter 2 (see Case study 2.2).

Analysis model

The analysis model defines the statistical methods (e.g., significance tests or descriptive statistics) that are applied to the trial data. As in data models, the first step in setting up an analysis model is to initialize the model as shown in Listing 1.4.

LISTING 1.4: Initialization of an analysis model

```
analysis.model = AnalysisModel()
```

After that, the specification of an analysis model's components can be accomplished by adding appropriate objects to the `AnalysisModel` object using the + operator. Components include the statistical test (`Test`), descriptive statistics (`Statistic`), a single multiplicity adjustment procedure (`MultAdjProc`), or a set of multiplicity adjustment procedures (`MultAdj`).

Test object

The `Test` object specifies a significance test that will be applied to one or more samples included in a data model. This object is defined by the following four arguments:

- `id` defines the test's unique ID (label).

- `method` defines the significance test.

- `samples` defines the IDs of the samples (defined in the data model) that the significance test is applied to.

- `par` defines the parameter(s) of the statistical test (optional).

Several commonly used significance tests are already implemented in the **Mediana** package and are listed in Table 1.2. Note that all tests are set up as one-sided tests and produce one-sided p-values. In addition, the user can easily define other significance tests by implementing a custom function for each test. If several significance tests need to be specified in an analysis model, for example, in clinical trials with multiple endpoints, several `Test` objects can be added to an `AnalysisModel` object.

TABLE 1.2: Statistical tests supported in the current version of the **Mediana** package.

Test	method	par
Two-sample t-test	TTest	
Non-inferiority t-test	TTestNI	margin
Two-sample test for proportions	PropTest	yates
Non-inferiority test for proportions	PropTestNI	yates, margin
Wilcoxon-Mann-Whitney test	WilcoxTest	
Fisher exact test	FisherTest	
Log-rank test	LogrankTest	
Poisson regression test	GLMPoissonTest	
Negative-binomial regression test	GLMNegBinomTest	

Since the significance tests listed in Table 1.2 are one-sided tests, the sample order in the `samples` argument of a test is important. In particular, the **Mediana** package assumes that a numerically larger value of the endpoint is expected in Sample 2 compared to Sample 1. Suppose, for example, that a higher treatment response indicates a beneficial effect (e.g., higher improvement rate). In this case Sample 1 should include control patients whereas Sample 2 should include patients allocated to the experimental treatment arm. The sample order needs to be reversed if a beneficial treatment effect is associated with a lower value of the endpoint (e.g., lower blood pressure).

Moreover, it is important to point out that several samples from a data model can be combined to form samples in an analysis model. For example, if the treatment and placebo groups were specified in the data model according to the status of a biomarker (i.e., positive or negative), the test of the treatment effect in the overall population can be accomplished by combining the biomarker-positive and biomarker-negative samples. This feature will be illustrated in Chapter 3 (see Case study 3.1).

Statistic object

The `Statistic` object specifies a descriptive statistic that will be computed based on one or more samples defined in a data model. Specification of this object is similar to that of the `Test` object with the same four arguments:

- `id` defines the statistic's unique ID (label).

- `method` defines the type of statistic/method for computing the statistic.

- `samples` defines the samples (pre-defined in the data model) to be used for computing the statistic.

- `par` defines the parameter(s) of the statistic method (optional).

Several built-in methods for computing descriptive statistics are implemented in the **Mediana** package (see Listing 1.3) but, as with statistical tests, the user can also define custom functions for computing other descriptive statistics. If several descriptive statistics need to be specified, several `Statistic` objects can be added to an `AnalysisModel` object.

Specification of a `Statistic` object is similar to the specification of a `Test` object and will be illustrated in Case studies 1.1 (see Listing 1.13) and 1.2 (see Listing 1.22).

MultAdjProc object

This object specifies a multiplicity adjustment procedure that will be applied to the significance tests (i.e., `Test` object) in order to protect the overall Type I error rate. A `MultAdjProc` object is defined by three arguments:

- `proc` defines a multiplicity adjustment procedure.

- `par` defines the parameter(s) of the multiplicity adjustment procedure (optional).

TABLE 1.3: Descriptive statistics supported in the current version of the **Mediana** package.

Statistic	method	par
Median	`MedianStat`	
Mean	`MeanStat`	
Standard deviation	`SdStat`	
Minimum	`MinStat`	
Maximum	`MaxStat`	
Number of events	`EventCountStat`	
Number of patients	`PatientCountStat`	
Difference of means between two samples	`DiffMeanStat`	
Difference of proportions between two samples	`DiffPropStat`	
Hazard ratio between two samples	`HazardRatioStat`	
Effect size for a continuous endpoint	`EffectSizeContStat`	
Effect size for a binary endpoint	`EffectSizePropStat`	
Effect size for a survival endpoint (log of HR)	`EffectSizeEventStat`	

- `tests` defines the specific tests (defined in the analysis model) to which the multiplicity adjustment procedure will be applied. This parameter is optional and, if no tests are defined, the multiplicity adjustment procedure will be applied to all tests defined in the `AnalysisModel` object.

Several commonly used multiplicity adjustment procedures are included in the **Mediana** package. In addition, the user can easily define custom multiplicity adjustments. The built-in multiplicity adjustments are defined in Table 1.4 along with the required parameters that need to be included in the `par` argument. More information about the multiple adjustment procedures can be found in Chapter 2.

For multiplicity adjustment procedures that support hypothesis-specific weights, the hypotheses are assumed to be equally weighted if the `weight` parameter is missing. Additionally, if a gatekeeping procedure for testing several families of hypotheses is specified, the component procedures used in the individual families must be defined (components are based on the Bonferroni, Holm, Hochberg or Hommel procedures).

It is worth noting that several `MultAdjProc` objects can be added to an `AnalysisModel` object using either the + operator or by grouping them into a `MultAdj` object. This latter object is provided mainly for convenience and its use is optional. A *multiplicity adjustment set* is then created to enable the user to evaluate the performance of several multiplicity adjustments in a clinical trial.

For more information on specifying multiplicity adjustments and their parameters in an analysis model, see Chapters 2 and 3.

TABLE 1.4: Multiplicity adjustment procedures supported in the current version of the **Mediana** package.

Multiplicity adjustment procedure	proc	par
Bonferroni procedure	BonferroniAdj	weight (optional)
Holm procedure	HolmAdj	weight (optional)
Hochberg procedure	HochbergAdj	weight (optional)
Hommel procedure	HommelAdj	weight (optional)
Fixed-sequence procedure	FixedSeqAdj	
Family of chain procedures	ChainAdj	weight, transition
Normal parametric multiple testing procedure	NormalParamAdj	weight, corr
Family of parallel gatekeeping procedures	ParallelGatekeepingAdj	family, gamma, proc
Family of multiple-sequence gatekeeping procedures	MultipleSequence GatekeepingAdj	family, gamma, proc
Family of mixture-based gatekeeping procedures	MixtureGatekeepingAdj	family, gamma, proc, serial, parallel

Evaluation model

Evaluation models are used within the **Mediana** package to specify the success criteria or metrics for evaluating the performance of the selected clinical scenario (combination of data and analysis models). An evaluation model can be initialized as shown in Listing 1.5.

LISTING 1.5: Initialization of an evaluation model

```
evaluation.model = EvaluationModel()
```

The evaluation model is specified by adding appropriate metrics using `Criterion` objects defined below.

Criterion object

This object specifies the success criteria that will be applied to a clinical scenario to evaluate the performance of selected data analysis methods. A `Criterion` object is defined by six arguments:

- `id` defines the criterion's unique ID (label).

- `method` defines the criterion.

- `tests` defines the IDs of the significance tests (defined in the analysis model) that the criterion is applied to.

- `statistics` defines the IDs of the descriptive statistics (defined in the analysis model) that the criterion is applied to.

- `par` defines the parameter(s) of the criterion (optional).

- `label` defines the label(s) of the criterion values (the label(s) will be used in the summary table).

Several commonly used success criteria are implemented in the **Mediana** package (see Table 1.5). The user can also define custom criteria based on statistical significance and/or clinical relevance. This process will be illustrated in Chapters 2 and 3.

TABLE 1.5: Evaluation criteria supported in the current version of the **Mediana** package.

Evaluation criterion	method	par
Marginal power	MarginalPower	alpha
Disjunctive power	DisjunctivePower	alpha
Conjunctive power	ConjunctivePower	alpha
Weighted power	WeightedPower	alpha, weight

Simulation-based Clinical Scenario Evaluation

After the clinical scenarios (data and analysis models) and evaluation model have been defined, the user is ready to perform Clinical Scenario Evaluation by calling the `CSE` function. To accomplish this, the simulation parameters need to be defined in a `SimParameters` object, such as the one presented in Listing 1.6.

LISTING 1.6: Specification of simulation parameters

```
sim.parameters = SimParameters(n.sims = 10000,
                               proc.load = "full",
                               seed = 42938001)
```

The `SimParameters` object is a required argument of the `CSE` function and has the following arguments:

- `n.sims` defines the number of simulations.

- `seed` defines the seed to be used in the simulations, to ensure that the simulation results will be reproducible.

- `proc.load` defines the processor load in parallel computations.

The `proc.load` argument is used to define the number of processor cores dedicated to the simulations in order to speed up the process. A numeric value can be used to define the number of cores. Alternatively, as shown in Listing 1.6, a character value can be specified which automatically detects the number of cores, i.e., `low` (1 processor core), `med` (number of available processor cores / 2), high (number of available processor cores - 1), or full (all available processor cores).

Finally, the CSE function is invoked (Listing 1.7) to run simulations under the CSE approach. This function uses four arguments:

- data defines a DataModel object.

- analysis defines an AnalysisModel object.

- evaluation defines an EvaluationModel object.

- simulation defines a SimParameters object.

LISTING 1.7: Performing Clinical Scenario Evaluation

```
results = CSE(data.model,
              analysis.model,
              evaluation.model,
              sim.parameters)
```

The simulation results are saved in an object of the class CSE (this object is named results in Listing 1.7). This object contains complete information about this particular evaluation, including the data, analysis and evaluation models specified by the user, as well as the simulation parameters. The most important component of this object is the data frame contained in the list named simulation.results (e.g., results$simulation.results). This data frame includes the values of the success criteria and metrics defined in the evaluation model for each clinical scenario. The summary of the results can be obtained using the summary function as shown in Listing 1.8.

LISTING 1.8: Creating a summary of the simulation results

```
summary(results)
```

Finally, it is worth noting that a very useful feature of the **Mediana** package is the generation of a Microsoft Word-based report to provide a summary of the simulation results. For more information on simulation reports, see the package's web-based manual.

For the purpose of illustration, two simple case studies will now be used to illustrate the process of setting up the building blocks of the CSE framework using **Mediana**. Case study 1.1 focuses on a clinical trial with a simple two-arm design and a single normally distributed endpoint. Case study 1.2 illustrates the CSE specifications for a trial that evaluates the efficacy profile of an experimental treatment on two time-to-event endpoints. More complex CSE settings and their implementation using **Mediana** will be illustrated in Chapters 2 and 3.

1.2.3   Case study 1.1: Clinical trial with a normally distributed endpoint

This case study deals with a simple setting, namely, a clinical trial with two treatment arms (experimental treatment versus placebo) and a single endpoint. Suppose that a sponsor is designing a Phase III clinical trial in patients with pulmonary arterial hypertension (PAH). The efficacy of experimental treatments for PAH is commonly evaluated using a six-minute walk test and the primary endpoint is defined as the change from baseline to the end of the 16-week treatment period in the six-minute walk distance.

Specification of the data model

After the `DataModel` object is initialized (see Listing 1.1), the sample sizes and other parameters of the two samples corresponding to the two treatment arms in this trial need to be specified. The change from baseline in the six-minute walk distance is assumed to follow a normal distribution and this distribution is defined in the `OutcomeDist` object (Listing 1.9).

LISTING 1.9: Outcome distribution specification in Case study 1.1

```
data.model = data.model +
   OutcomeDist(outcome.dist = "NormalDist")
```

The trial's sponsor would like to perform power evaluation over a broad range of sample sizes in each treatment arm (50, 60 and 70 patients per arm). The sample sizes are specified in the `SampleSize` object as shown in Listing 1.10.

LISTING 1.10: Sample size specification in Case study 1.1

```
data.model = data.model +
   SampleSize(c(50, 60, 70))
```

In the spirit of CSE, the sponsor is interested in performing power calculations under several treatment effect scenarios. Focusing, for simplicity, on two scenarios (standard scenario versus optimistic scenario), the experimental treatment is expected to improve the six-minute walk distance by 40 or 50 meters compared to placebo, respectively, with the common standard deviation of 70 meters. The treatment effect assumptions used in this case study are summarized in Table 1.6. Therefore, the mean change in the placebo arm is set to $\mu = 0$ and the mean changes in the six-minute walk distance in the experimental arm are set to $\mu = 40$ (standard scenario) or $\mu = 50$ (optimistic scenario). The common standard deviation is $\sigma = 70$.

Two `Sample` objects that correspond to the two treatment arms in this trial can now be created and added to the `DataModel` object (`data.model`); see Listing 1.11. The data model specification in this case study includes two

TABLE 1.6: Treatment effect assumptions in Case study 1.1.

Scenario	Mean (SD)	
	Placebo	Treatment
Standard	0 (70)	40 (70)
Optimistic	0 (70)	50 (70)

sets of outcome parameters and three sets of sample sizes. Therefore, the resulting data model includes six assumption sets.

LISTING 1.11: Sample specification in Case study 1.1

```
# Outcome parameter set 1 (standard scenario)
outcome1.placebo = parameters(mean = 0, sd = 70)
outcome1.treatment = parameters(mean = 40, sd = 70)

# Outcome parameter set 2 (optimistic scenario)
outcome2.placebo = parameters(mean = 0, sd = 70)
outcome2.treatment = parameters(mean = 50, sd = 70)

# Sample object for Placebo and Treatment arm
data.model = data.model +
  Sample(id = "Placebo",
         outcome.par = parameters(outcome1.placebo,
                                   outcome2.placebo)) +
  Sample(id = "Treatment",
         outcome.par = parameters(outcome1.treatment,
                                   outcome2.treatment))
```

Design parameters such as the length of the enrollment and follow-up periods do not need to be specified in this data model since the trial will employ a fixed design (all patients will be followed for 16 weeks) and it will be assumed that all patients complete the trial (no dropout).

Specification of the analysis model

Just like the data model, the analysis model needs to be initialized as shown in Listing 1.4. Only one significance test is planned to be carried out in the PAH clinical trial (treatment versus placebo). The treatment effect will be assessed using the one-sided two-sample *t*-test (see Listing 1.12).

LISTING 1.12: Test specification in Case study 1.1

```
analysis.model = analysis.model +
  Test(id = "Placebo vs Treatment",
       samples = samples("Placebo", "Treatment"),
       method = "TTest")
```

According to the specifications, the two-sample t-test will be applied to Sample 1 (Placebo) and Sample 2 (Treatment). These sample IDs come from the data model defined earlier (Listing 1.11). As explained before, the sample order is determined by the expected direction of the treatment effect. In this case, an increase in the six-minute walk distance indicates a beneficial effect and a numerically larger value of the primary endpoint is expected in Sample 2 (Treatment) compared to Sample 1 (Placebo). This implies that the list of samples to be passed to the t-test should include Sample 1 followed by Sample 2.

It is recommended within the CSE approach to examine multiple alternative analysis strategies. In this clinical trial, this could include, for example, a stratified test or a more complex model-based test with an adjustment for the six-minute walk distance at baseline. Stratification factors are easily accounted for in **Mediana** by including additional samples in the data model and defining a custom test in the analysis model that accounts for the stratification factors.

To illustrate the use of the `Statistic` object, the treatment difference, i.e., the difference between the sample means in the treatment and placebo arms in the six-minute walk distance, can be computed using the `DiffMeanStat` statistic (see Listing 1.13). It is to be noted that this method calculates the difference between the mean in Sample 1 and that in Sample 2. Therefore, the `Treatment` sample is placed in the first position in `samples` followed by the `Placebo` sample.

LISTING 1.13: Analysis model specification in Case study 1.1

```
# Compute the treatment difference (difference between the
    sample means)
analysis.model = analysis.model +
  Statistic(id = "Treatment difference",
            method = "DiffMeanStat",
            samples = samples("Treatment", "Placebo"))
```

No multiplicity adjustment is specified in the analysis model since only one null hypothesis of no treatment effect is tested in this clinical trial. Therefore, the analysis model includes only one analysis strategy that will be evaluated as part of CSE.

Specification of the evaluation model

The data and analysis models specified above collectively define the clinical scenarios to be examined in the PAH clinical trial. As six assumption sets were defined in the data model and one strategy in the analysis model, there are six clinical scenarios in this case study. The performance of these scenarios is to be evaluated using success criteria or metrics that are aligned with the clinical objectives of the trial. In this trial it is most appropriate to use regular power or, more formally, *marginal power*. This criterion is specified in the evaluation model presented in Listing 1.14.

LISTING 1.14: Criterion specification (marginal power) in Case study 1.1

```
evaluation.model = evaluation.model +
  Criterion(id = "Marginal power",
            method = "MarginalPower",
            tests = tests("Placebo vs Treatment"),
            labels = c("Placebo vs Treatment"),
            par = parameters(alpha = 0.025))
```

The `tests` argument lists the IDs of the tests (previously defined in the analysis model) to which the criterion is applied (note that more than one test can be specified in the same criterion). The test IDs link the evaluation model with the corresponding analysis model. In this particular case, marginal power will be computed for the t-test that compares the mean change in the six-minute walk distance in the placebo and treatment arms (Placebo vs treatment). The resulting one-sided p-value will be compared to a significance level corresponding to the one-sided Type I error rate of 2.5% (`alpha = 0.025`).

Finally, in order to compute the average value of the statistic specified in the analysis model over the simulation runs (i.e., difference between the sample means in the treatment and placebo arms), another `Criterion` object needs to be added as shown in Listing 1.15.

LISTING 1.15: Criterion specification (mean treatment difference) in Case study 1.1

```
# Mean treatment difference (average of the treatment
    differences across the simulation runs)
evaluation.model = evaluation.model +
  Criterion(id = "Mean treatment difference",
            method = "MeanSumm",
            statistics = statistics("Treatment difference"),
            labels = c("Mean treatment difference"))
```

The `statistics` argument of this `Criterion` object lists the IDs of the statistics defined in the analysis model to which this metric is applied. In this case study, only one *Statistic* object has been defined in the analysis model which computes the difference between the sample means in the `Treatment` and `Placebo` samples.

Perform Clinical Scenario Evaluation

After the clinical scenarios (data and analysis models) and evaluation model have been defined, along with the simulation parameters (number of simulation runs, seed and processor load, see Listing 1.6), the operating characteristics of the selected clinical scenarios are evaluated by calling the `CSE` function.

As shown in Listing 1.16, the function call specifies the three CSE components in this case study as well as the simulation parameters.

LISTING 1.16: Performing Clinical Scenario Evaluation in Case study 1.1

```
# Perform clinical scenario evaluation
results = CSE(data.model,
              analysis.model,
              evaluation.model,
              sim.parameters)
```

Simulation-based results for this case study are presented in Table 1.7 (based on 100,000 simulation runs). It should be noted that the mean treatment difference is not strictly equal to the true treatment difference in the two scenarios, i.e., to 40 and 50 in the standard and optimistic scenarios, respectively, due to Monte Carlo error.

TABLE 1.7: Simulation results in Case study 1.1.

Assumption set	Sample size per arm	Marginal power	Mean treatment difference
Standard	N = 50	81.1%	40.0
	N = 60	87.6%	40.1
	N = 70	92.1%	40.2
Optimistic	N = 50	94.6%	50.2
	N = 60	97.3%	50.2
	N = 70	98.7%	50.2

1.2.4 Case study 1.2: Clinical trial with two time-to-event endpoints

This case study illustrates a more complex setting where the trial's primary and secondary objectives are formulated in terms of analyzing the time to a clinically important event (progression or death in an oncology setting). Therefore, data and analysis models can be set up based on a multivariate exponential distribution and the log-rank test. Moreover, due to the multiplicity of tests, a multiple testing procedure will be utilized to protect the Type I error rate. This case study with two endpoints helps showcase the package's ability to model complex design and analysis strategies in trials with multivariate outcomes.

Consider a Phase III trial which will be conducted to evaluate the efficacy of a new treatment for metastatic colorectal cancer (MCC). Patients will be randomized in a 2:1 ratio to an experimental treatment or placebo (in addition to best supportive care). Progression-free survival (PFS) is the primary endpoint in this clinical trial and overall survival (OS) serves as the key secondary endpoint, which provides supportive evidence of treatment efficacy. A hierarchical testing approach will be utilized in the analysis of the two endpoints. The PFS analysis will be performed first at $\alpha = 0.025$ (one-sided), followed by the OS analysis at the same level if a significant effect on PFS is established. The resulting testing procedure is known as the fixed-sequence procedure and controls the overall Type I error rate. For more information on this multiple testing procedure, see Chapter 2.

Specification of the data model

To define a data model in the MCC clinical trial, the total event count in the trial is assumed to range between 390 and 420. This trial utilizes an unbalanced design with a 2:1 randomization ratio. This ratio needs to be specified in the Event object (Listing 1.17). It is important to note that the number of events is specified for the primary endpoint only.

LISTING 1.17: Event object specification in Case study 1.2

```
data.model = data.model +
  Event(n.events = c(390, 420),
        rando.ratio = c(1,2))
```

An event-driven design with a variable patient follow-up will be used in this trial. The total trial duration will be 30 months, which includes a 12-month enrollment (accrual) period and a minimum follow-up of 18 months. Based on historical information, it is anticipated that 50% of the patients will be enrolled at the 75% point of the accrual period. A convenient way to model non-uniform enrollment is to use a beta distribution, where the distribution parameters are derived from the expected enrollment at a specific timepoint. For example, if half of the patients are expected to be enrolled by the 75% point, a beta distribution with the shape parameters $a = \log(0.5)/\log(0.75)$ and $b = 1$ can be used. Generally, if q denotes the proportion of patients enrolled at $100p\%$ of the enrollment period, patient enrollment can be modeled using a beta distribution which is derived as follows:

- If $q < p$, the beta distribution is Beta$(a, 1)$ with $a = \log(q)/\log(p)$.

- If $q > p$, the beta distribution is Beta$(1, b)$ with $b = \log(1 - q)/\log(1 - p)$.

- Otherwise the beta distribution is Beta$(1, 1)$.

The set of design parameters also includes the dropout distribution and its parameters. In this clinical trial, the dropout distribution is exponential with the rate determined from historical data. These design parameters are specified in the Design object (see Listing 1.18).

LISTING 1.18: Design object specification in Case study 1.2

```
# Enrollment parameters
enroll.par = parameters(a = log(0.5)/log(0.75),
```

```
                         b = 1)

# Dropout parameters
dropout.par = parameters(rate = 0.0115)

# Design parameters
data.model = data.model +
  Design(enroll.period = 9,
         study.duration = 21,
         enroll.dist = "BetaDist",
         enroll.dist.par = enroll.par,
         dropout.dist = "ExpoDist",
         dropout.dist.par = dropout.par)
```

Listing 1.18 defines a single set of design parameters and, based on CSE principles, it is important to examine other sets that may correspond, for example, to less aggressive patient enrollment assumptions.

The treatment effect assumptions that will be used in the Clinical Scenario Evaluation are listed in Table 1.8. The table shows the hypothesized median times along with the corresponding hazard rates for the primary and secondary endpoints.

TABLE 1.8: Treatment effect assumptions in the MCC clinical trial.

Endpoint	Placebo	Treatment
Progression-free survival		
Median time (months)	6	9
Hazard rate	0.116	0.077
Hazard ratio	0.077/0.116 = 0.67	
Overall survival		
Median time (months)	15	19
Hazard rate	0.046	0.036
Hazard ratio	0.036/0.046 = 0.79	

For simplicity, a single set of treatment effect assumptions is considered in this case study but, as above, it is recommended to explore multiple alternatives based on more optimistic assumptions as well as more pessimistic assumptions that may represent the worst-case scenario.

It follows from Table 1.8 that the median time to disease progression is assumed to be $t_0^{PFS} = 6$ months and $t_1^{PFS} = 9$ months in the placebo and treatment arms, respectively. Under an exponential distribution assumption, the median times correspond to the following hazard rates

$$\lambda_0^{PFS} = \log 2/t_0^{PFS} = 0.116, \quad \lambda_1^{PFS} = \log 2/t_1^{PFS} = 0.077,$$

and the resulting hazard ratio for PFS is $0.077/0.116 = 0.67$. Similarly, focusing on the OS assumptions, the median time to death is assumed to be 15 months and 19 months in the placebo and treatment arms, respectively, corresponding to the hazard ratio of 0.79. The table shows that the hypothesized effect size is much larger for PFS compared to OS (PFS hazard ratio is lower than OS hazard ratio).

In this clinical trial, two endpoints are evaluated for each patient (PFS and OS) and thus their joint distribution needs to be specified. A bivariate exponential distribution will be used in this example and samples from this bivariate distribution will be generated using the `MVExpoPFSOSDist` function which implements multivariate exponential distributions. The function utilizes the copula method, i.e., random variables that follow a bivariate normal distribution will be generated and then converted into exponential random variables. For simplicity, if the generated OS time is lower than the PFS time, the PFS time will be truncated at the OS time.

The next several statements specify the parameters of the bivariate exponential distribution:

- Parameters of the marginal exponential distributions, i.e., the hazard rates.

- Correlation matrix of the underlying multivariate normal distribution used in the copula method.

The hazard rates for PFS and OS in each treatment arm that serve as the key data model parameters are defined based on the information presented in Table 1.8 (`placebo.par` and `treatment.par`). The correlation matrix (`corr.matrix`) serves as a supportive parameter in the data model and is specified based on historical information. For the purpose of illustration, the correlation between the two endpoints will be set to 0.3. These parameters are combined to define the outcome parameter sets (`outcome.placebo` and `outcome.treatment`) that will be included in the sample-specific set of data model parameters (`Sample` objects).

LISTING 1.19: Sample object specification in Case study 1.2

```
# Outcome parameters: Progression-free survival
median.time.pfs.placebo = 6
rate.pfs.placebo = log(2)/median.time.pfs.placebo
outcome.pfs.placebo = parameters(rate = rate.pfs.placebo)

median.time.pfs.treatment = 9
rate.pfs.treatment = log(2)/median.time.pfs.treatment
outcome.pfs.treatment = parameters(rate = rate.pfs.
    treatment)

# Outcome parameters: Overall survival
median.time.os.placebo = 15
rate.os.placebo = log(2)/median.time.os.placebo
outcome.os.placebo = parameters(rate = rate.os.placebo)
```

```
median.time.os.treatment = 19
rate.os.treatment = log(2)/median.time.os.treatment
outcome.os.treatment = parameters(rate = rate.os.treatment)

# Parameters lists
placebo.par = parameters(parameters(rate = rate.pfs.placebo
   ),
                        parameters(rate = rate.os.placebo)
   )

treatment.par = parameters(parameters(rate = rate.pfs.
    treatment),
                        parameters(rate = rate.os.
    treatment))

# Correlation between two endpoints
corr.matrix = matrix(c(1.0, 0.3,
                       0.3, 1.0), 2, 2)

# Outcome parameters
outcome.placebo = parameters(par = placebo.par,
                             corr = corr.matrix)
outcome.treatment = parameters(par = treatment.par,
                               corr = corr.matrix)

# Data model
data.model = data.model() +
  OutcomeDist(outcome.dist = "MVExpoPFSOSDist",
             outcome.type = c("event", "event")) +
  Sample(id = list("Placebo PFS",
                   "Placebo OS"),
         outcome.par = parameters(outcome.placebo)) +
  Sample(id = list("Treatment PFS",
                   "Treatment OS"),
         outcome.par = parameters(outcome.treatment))
```

It is important to note that a separate sample ID needs to be assigned to each endpoint within the two samples (e.g., Placebo PFS, Placebo OS, Treatment PFS and Treatment OS) corresponding to the two treatment arms. This will enable the user to construct analysis models for examining the treatment effect on each endpoint.

Specification of the analysis model

The treatment comparisons for both endpoints will be carried out based on the log-rank test (method = "LogrankTest"). As indicated in Listing 1.20, the two tests included in the analysis model reflect the twofold objective of this trial. The first test focuses on a PFS comparison between the two treatment arms (`id = "PFS test"`) whereas the other test is carried out to assess the treatment effect on OS (`id = "OS test"`)

LISTING 1.20: Test object specification in Case study 1.2

```
# Log-rank tests for PFS and OS
analysis.model = analysis.model +
  Test(id = "PFS test",
       samples = samples("Placebo PFS",
                         "Treatment PFS"),
       method = "LogrankTest") +
  Test(id = "OS test",
       samples = samples("Placebo OS",
                         "Treatment OS"),
       method = "LogrankTest")
```

As alternative analysis strategies to the basic log-rank test, a stratified version of the log-rank test or a more complex test based on the Cox proportional-hazards model could be considered.

Further, as was stated earlier, the two endpoints will be tested hierarchically using a multiplicity adjustment procedure known as the fixed-sequence procedure. This procedure is applied to the null hypotheses tested in this clinical trial:

- H_1: Null hypothesis of no difference between the two arms with respect to PFS.

- H_2: Null hypothesis of no difference between the two arms with respect to OS.

Based on the fixed-sequence procedure, the null hypothesis H_1 is tested first at the full α level (one-sided $\alpha = 0.025$). If this null hypothesis is rejected, i.e., a significant treatment effect on PFS is established, the treatment effect on OS is evaluated by testing the null hypothesis H_2 at the full α level. However, if the PFS test is not significant (H_1 cannot be rejected), the OS test will not be carried out. The fixed-sequence procedure can be easily implemented using the `FixedSeqAdj` method specified in a `MultAdjProc` object.

LISTING 1.21: MultAdjProc object specification in Case study 1.2

```
# Fixed-sequence procedure
analysis.model = analysis.model +
  MultAdjProc(proc = "FixedSeqAdj")
```

It is worth mentioning that, for the purpose of simplification, if no tests are defined in the `tests` argument of the `MultAdjProc` object, all tests specified in an analysis model will be examined in the order specified in the model. In this case study, as the test for the null hypothesis of PFS was specified first in the analysis model, it will be tested first by the fixed-sequence procedure.

The fixed-sequence procedure used in the multiplicity adjustment tends to lack flexibility and alternative approaches to addressing multiplicity in this clinical trial ought to be considered; see, for example, a detailed discussion of optimal adjustment selection in Chapter 2.

Finally, since the target number of events is fixed in this case study and some patients will not reach the event of interest (and will be censored), it will be important to estimate the number of patients to be enrolled in the trial in order to achieve the required number of events. In the **Mediana** package, this can be accomplished by selecing a descriptive statistic named `PatientCountStat`, specified in a `Statistic` object, for each treatment arm (see Listing 1.22).

LISTING 1.22: Statistic object specification in Case study 1.2

```
# Number of patients
analysis.model = analysis.model +
  Statistic(id = "Number of patients (Placebo arm)",
            samples = samples("Placebo PFS"),
            method = "PatientCountStat") +
  Statistic(id = "Number of patients (Treatment arm)",
            samples = samples("Treatment PFS"),
            method = "PatientCountStat")
```

Specification of the evaluation model

The evaluation model specifies the most basic criterion for assessing the probability of success in the PFS and OS analyses (marginal power). A criterion based on *disjunctive power*, i.e., the probability of establishing a significant effect on PFS or OS, could be considered as well; however, it would not provide additional information in this particular setting. Indeed, due to the hierarchical testing approach, the probability of detecting a significant treatment effect on at least one endpoint is simply equal to the probability of establishing a significant PFS effect.

LISTING 1.23: Criterion specification (marginal power) in Case study 1.2

```
evaluation.model = evaluation.model +
  Criterion(id = "Marginal power",
            method = "MarginalPower",
            tests = tests("PFS test",
                          "OS test"),
            labels = c("PFS test",
                       "OS test"),
            par = parameters(alpha = 0.025))
```

To compute the average value of the number of enrolled patients in each sample, another `Criterion` object will be included, in addition to the one specified to obtain the marginal power. The IDs of the corresponding `Statistic` objects will be included in the `statistics` argument of the two Criterion objects.

LISTING 1.24: Criterion specification (average of number of patients) in Case study 1.2

```
# Average number of patients across the simulation runs
evaluation.model = evaluation.model +
  Criterion(id = "Average number of patients",
            method = "MeanSumm",
            statistics = statistics("Number of patients (
  Placebo arm)",
                                     "Number of patients (
  Treatment arm)"),
            labels = c("Average number of patients (Placebo
   arm)",
                       "Average number of patients (
  Treatment arm)"))
```

Perform Clinical Scenario Evaluation

As in Case study 1.1, the simulation-based clinical scenario evaluation is performed by passing the data, analysis and evaluation models defined above as well as the simulation parameters to the CSE function as shown in Listing 1.25.

LISTING 1.25: Perform the Clinical Scenario Evaluation in Case study 1.2

```
# Perform clinical scenario evaluation
results = CSE(data.model,
              analysis.model,
              evaluation.model,
              sim.parameters)

# Print the simulation results in the R console
summary(results)
```

Simulation results based on 100,000 simulation runs are summarized in Table 1.9.

TABLE 1.9: Simulation results in Case study 1.2.

Total number of events	Marginal power		Average number of patients	
	PFS test	OS test	Treatment	Placebo
390	90.9%	38.4%	386	193
420	92.7%	40.9%	416	208

1.3   Clinical trial optimization

An important application of the general Clinical Scenario Evaluation (CSE) approach introduced in Section 1.2 is the broad field of *clinical trial optimization*. Clinical trial optimization can be defined in a general sense as a class of methods aimed at quantifying the impact of design scenarios and analysis strategies on the pre-specified success criteria, which naturally leads to identifying optimal designs and analyses in a clinical trial. Numerous recent publications dealt with the general topic of clinical trial optimization, mostly with emphasis on applying decision-theoretic approaches; see, for example, Hee and Stallard (2012), Krisam and Kieser (2015), Ondra et al. (2016).

As a rigorous quantitative approach to the assessment of candidate designs and statistical analysis techniques, CSE facilitates the process of identifying the individual components and parameters in a general optimization problem and thus provides a solid foundation for developing and applying optimization methods. This book provides a survey of CSE-based approaches to identifying best-performing analysis strategies and decision rules in clinical trials. Special emphasis is placed on practical solutions and software implementation to facilitate the process of applying optimization algorithms to real-life clinical trials. This section introduces the guiding principles for development of optimization strategies. A detailed discussion of key components of broadly used clinical trial optimization methods is provided in Sections 1.4 and 1.5. Numerous examples with a thorough exploration of practical aspects of clinical trial optimization can be found in Chapters 2 and 3.

Just like the general CSE approach, clinical trial optimization relies on a structured framework that facilitates the formulation of an optimization problem as well as selection and application of appropriate optimization strategies. In broad strokes, CSE-based clinical trial optimization focuses on identifying data models or analysis models (and, occasionally, components of evaluation models) with optimal performance based on relevant criteria. While it is less common to consider optimal selection of data models, optimization methods can be applied to identify data models with an optimal randomization scheme. For example, Stucke and Kieser (2012) studied the problem of determining an optimal allocation of patients in multi-arm clinical trials with the goal of minimizing the total sample size. Along the same line, optimal selection of randomization schemes and other design-related optimization problems in the context of group-sequential trials were investigated by Schlömer and Brannath (2013). Most attention in publications on CSE-based optimization has been given to problems of identifying optimal analysis models, which includes optimal selection of statistical tests, multiplicity adjustments, decision rules in adaptive trials, etc. To give a few examples, Benda et al. (2010) described a CSE-driven exercise aimed at optimization of the sample size adaptation rule in an adaptive design. Dmitrienko, Paux and Brechenmacher (2015) considered optimal selection of complex multiplicity adjustment strategies in clinical trials with multiple objectives. Further, Dmitrienko et al. (2016) developed optimization criteria for determining the best futility stopping rule in a clinical trial with a single interim analysis.

To set up an optimization problem in a clinical trial or development program, the sponsor first needs to build a CSE framework, which involves a detailed specification of plausible data models, applicable analysis models and appropriate evaluation criteria. These criteria are expected to be aligned with the clinical objectives of a trial or program. In a sense, optimization criteria "quantify" the clinical objectives by providing an explicit definition of "success" or "win" in one or more clinical trials. When considering available options, it is important to bear in mind that multiple criteria are typically applicable to any optimization problem. The trial's sponsor needs to carefully examine these criteria to choose the most meaningful criteria for a given setting.

An optimization problem is then defined by specifying a set of candidate analysis models and selecting a general optimization strategy. With a discrete set of analysis models, e.g., in problems with a family of statistical tests that can be used to assess the treatment effect, optimization relies on performing a series of fairly straightforward head-to-head comparisons. In more complex settings, analysis models are indexed by one or more parameters, e.g., parameters of decision rules, known as *target parameters*. In this case optimization focuses on identifying optimal configurations of these parameters that maximize the selected evaluation criterion or criteria.

The following two classes of optimization strategies will be investigated in this book. *Direct optimization strategies* are broadly used in clinical trials with a single objective or multiple objectives that are related to each other and focus on identifying an analysis model that maximizes pre-specified evaluation criteria. Optimal configurations of analysis model parameters are found using univariate or multivariate grid-search algorithms. *Tradeoff-based optimization* arises in clinical trials with several competing objectives. The goal of this approach is to choose an analysis model or configurations of the target parameters that achieves a desirable balance among the competing objectives.

After an optimal set of target parameters has been identified, it is important to ensure that the conclusions are robust against deviations from the underlying assumptions, i.e., deviations from the data models assumed in the optimization algorithm. It is important to remember that optimal analysis models are only *locally optimal*, which is conceptually similar to locally optimal designs in the theory of optimal design (see, for example, Atkinson and Donev, 1992). Optimal analysis models are likely to depend on the hypothesized treatment effects or design parameters. Therefore it is important to run a series of *sensitivity assessments* to determine the impact of possible deviations from the assumed data model on the performance of the optimal analysis model.

The three components of clinical trial optimization defined above, namely, selection of an optimization strategy, identification of optimal or nearly optimal values of the target parameters, and sensitivity assessments, are discussed in Sections 1.3.1, 1.3.2 and 1.3.3. As noted above, Sections 1.4 and 1.5 will provide an in-depth look at commonly used optimization strategies, namely, direct and tradeoff-based strategies. Case studies based on real clinical trials will be used in the two sections to illustrate the key steps in setting up and applying optimization algorithms that utilize these strategies. For the sake of concreteness, it will be assumed throughout the rest of the chapter that clinical trial optimization is applied to build an optimal analysis model in a single clinical trial. The general approaches defined below and illustrated in Sections 1.4 and 1.5 are easily extended to other optimization problems such as optimal selection of data and analysis models in development programs that include several trials.

1.3.1   Optimization strategies

As emphasized above, the key to successful implementation of clinical trial optimization lies in a careful review of relevant information to define an optimization problem and select the most sensible optimization strategy. This section provides an overview of popular approaches to defining optimization algorithms in clinical trials, including direct optimization and tradeoff-based optimization strategies.

Direct optimization

Direct optimization methods are commonly considered in settings when optimization is performed to pursue a single goal or several closely related goals. When it is relevant to explore multiple related goals in a clinical trial, the goals of interest are typically combined into a single goal. In this case, a single optimization criterion is set up and an optimal analysis model is identified via direct optimization. However, if the goals conflict with each other, the problem can be solved by finding an optimal compromise among the goals. Tradeoff-based optimization strategies can be applied in the latter case.

To define a formal framework, consider a set of CSE models introduced in Section 1.2, i.e., data, analysis and evaluation models, in a given clinical trial. Suppose that the data model is indexed by θ and the analysis model is indexed by λ (in general, both θ and λ are multivariate parameters). The vector θ may include both key and supportive data model parameters. The optimization algorithm focuses on finding an optimal analysis model and λ serves as the target parameter in this optimization problem. The evaluation criterion based on the selected evaluation model is denoted by $\psi(\lambda|\theta)$. A higher value of this criterion is associated with improved performance of the analysis model. Within the direct optimization framework, an optimal value of the target parameter λ is found by maximizing this criterion given the data model parameter $\boldsymbol{\theta}$. Examples of direct optimization algorithms are provided in Section 1.4 as well as Chapters 2 and 3.

The straightforward direct optimization strategy is easily extended to define *constrained optimization algorithms*. Constrained optimization is defined as a strategy aimed at selecting an optimal analysis model that maximizes an appropriate criterion, e.g., $\psi_1(\boldsymbol{\lambda}|\boldsymbol{\theta})$, subject to a set of constraints, e.g.,

$$\psi_2(\boldsymbol{\lambda}|\boldsymbol{\theta}) \in C,$$

where C is a pre-defined univariate or multivariate region. Most of the time, constraints are defined in terms of simple inequalities, e.g., a constrained optimization strategy may be applied to maximize power (ψ_1) in such a way that the Type I error rate (ψ_2) is protected. Constrained optimization algorithms are illustrated in Chapter 3.

It was mentioned above that in optimization problems with several related goals, it is often convenient to aggregate the goals into a single goal. This can be accomplished using the general approaches developed in the literature on optimal designs. Specifically, a *compound criterion*, e.g., minimum criterion or average criterion, can be defined by combining the goal-specific criterion functions. If $\psi_i(\boldsymbol{\lambda})$ denotes the evaluation criterion corresponding to the ith goal, $i = 1, \ldots, m$, the minimum criterion is defined as

$$\psi_M(\boldsymbol{\lambda}) = \min_{i=1,\ldots,m} \psi_i(\boldsymbol{\lambda}).$$

The minimum criterion takes a minimax-type approach to the optimization problem in the presence of several goals. For each value of the target parameter $\boldsymbol{\lambda}$, the worst-case scenario is identified by computing the minimum across the goal-specific criterion functions. Further, the average criterion is computed by averaging the criterion functions across the m goals, i.e.,

$$\psi_A(\boldsymbol{\lambda}) = \sum_{i=1}^{m} w_i \psi_i(\boldsymbol{\lambda}).$$

The average criterion is based on ideas that are conceptually similar to those used in Bayesian model averaging and can incorporate prior information on how important each goal is within a given clinical trial. Specifically, w_i is a positive value that quantifies the available prior information on the ith goal and $w_1 + \ldots + w_m = 1$.

Tradeoff-based optimization

The second class of optimization strategies considered in this book is the class of tradeoff-based optimization strategies. Optimization algorithms of this kind are encountered in clinical trials with multiple competing objectives and are aimed at identifying an analysis model that provides a balance among these objectives. It is instructive to draw an analogy with tradeoff-based designs considered in the theory of optimal design for regression models. Multiple criteria aimed at achieving balance between two goals have been studied in the optimal design literature. For example, DT-optimal designs are constructed as designs that balance the goals of model discrimination and parameter estimation in a class of regression models. The underlying criterion is defined as a convex combination of the criteria used in the problems of optimal model discrimination and parameter estimation (Atkinson, 2008).

To define tradeoff-based optimization strategies, consider the problem of finding an optimal analysis model in a clinical trial. As before, this model is indexed by a multivariate parameter $\boldsymbol{\lambda}$ which serves as the target parameter in this optimization problem. Suppose that there are two ways to evaluate the performance of the analysis model that conflict with each other and thus define two competing goals. Let $\psi_1(\boldsymbol{\lambda}|\boldsymbol{\theta})$ and $\psi_2(\boldsymbol{\lambda}|\boldsymbol{\theta})$ define the functions that quantify the performance of the model with respect to these goals. These functions are known as *performance functions* and it is assumed that a higher value of each function is associated with better performance.

To illustrate a "tag of war" between the two goals, suppose that $\psi_1(\boldsymbol{\lambda}|\boldsymbol{\theta})$ is a monotonically increasing function of the target parameter and $\psi_2(\boldsymbol{\lambda}|\boldsymbol{\theta})$ is a monotonically decreasing function of the same parameter. The first performance function is then maximized by selecting a larger value of $\boldsymbol{\lambda}$ but, to maximize the second performance function, $\boldsymbol{\lambda}$ needs to be set to a smaller value. As in the optimal design literature, a convex combination of the two functions can be computed to define an overall criterion. This criterion serves as an example of additive tradeoff-based criteria:

$$\psi_{AT}(\boldsymbol{\lambda}|\boldsymbol{\theta}) = w_1\psi_1(\boldsymbol{\lambda}|\boldsymbol{\theta}) + w_2\psi_2(\boldsymbol{\lambda}|\boldsymbol{\theta}),$$

where w_1 and w_2 are positive values that determine the relative importance of the two goals (the values add up to 1). This criterion supports the identification of target parameters that achieve a desirable compromise between the two competing goals. When formulating optimization problems in clinical trials with competing goals, it is critical to ensure that the resulting tradeoff-based criterion is a concave function of the target parameter $\boldsymbol{\lambda}$. This assumption may be violated if the selected performance functions are linearly related to each other, which leads to a collinearity problem. The consequences of collinearity in trials with conflicting goals are illustrated in Chapter 3 (see Case study 3.2).

An important underlying assumption used in additive tradeoff-based criteria is that the selected performance functions are measured on the same scale, i.e., each function represents the probability of success for the corresponding goal. If different scales are used, it is recommended to consider a bivariate tradeoff-based criterion, which is defined as

$$\psi_{BT}(\boldsymbol{\lambda}|\boldsymbol{\theta}) = g(\psi_1(\boldsymbol{\lambda}|\boldsymbol{\theta}), \psi_2(\boldsymbol{\lambda}|\boldsymbol{\theta})),$$

where $g(x, y)$ is a monotonically increasing function of both x and y. An optimal value of the target parameter $\boldsymbol{\lambda}$ is found by maximizing the bivariate criterion to achieve an optimal balance between the two goals. Utility of additive and bivariate tradeoff-based criteria is assessed in Section 1.5.

1.3.2 Optimization algorithm

After an optimization problem has been formulated and appropriate strategy, e.g., direct optimization or tradeoff-based optimization, has been selected, an optimal analysis model or a set of nearly optimal models are found using grid search. To describe the details of this algorithm, the notation introduced in Section 1.3.1 will be utilized. Consider an optimization problem with a data model indexed by $\boldsymbol{\theta}$ and an analysis model indexed by $\boldsymbol{\lambda}$. Assume that $\boldsymbol{\lambda}$ is the target parameter in this problem. Let Λ denote the set of possible values of $\boldsymbol{\lambda}$ and, lastly, let $\psi(\boldsymbol{\lambda} \,|\, \boldsymbol{\theta})$ denote the main criterion in this optimization problem. As above, higher values of this criterion are desirable. An optimal value of the target parameter, denoted by $\boldsymbol{\lambda}^*$, is found by maximizing this criterion, i.e.,

$$\boldsymbol{\lambda}^* = \arg\max_{\boldsymbol{\lambda} \in \Lambda} \psi(\boldsymbol{\lambda} \,|\, \boldsymbol{\theta}).$$

The optimal value depends on the data model parameter ($\boldsymbol{\theta}$) but, to simplify notation, this dependence will be suppressed.

In most clinical trial applications, the optimization criterion needs to be evaluated using a simulation-based approach and a univariate or multivariate grid search is employed based on Monte Carlo approximations to the criterion function. It is therefore important to account for uncertainty around the true optimal value of the target parameter due to simulation or other approximation errors. With relatively flat criterion functions, the value of $\boldsymbol{\lambda}$ that maximizes the criterion is very likely to be variable. It is recommended to report the "point estimate" of the optimal parameter, i.e., $\boldsymbol{\lambda}^*$, as well as a "confidence interval" or "confidence region," known as the *optimal interval* or *optimal region*, that defines a set of plausible values of λ^* that may be thought of as nearly optimal values. Examining analysis models with nearly optimal parameter values helps inform the overall decision-making process even if the criterion function is not flat around its maximum.

In a general multivariate optimization problem, a "confidence region" for the optimal target parameter is defined as the set of values for which the criterion function is sufficiently close to its maximum value. Optimal regions are conceptually similar to support or likelihood intervals for parameters of interest (Edwards, 1992). Within a general likelihood-based inferential framework, the most appropriate estimate of a parameter is found by maximizing the likelihood function. A support or likelihood confidence interval is then defined by identifying the parameter values for which the likelihood function is close to its maximum.

This notion of an optimal region is formalized as follows. A $100\eta\%$ optimal region for $\boldsymbol{\lambda}^*$ is denoted by $I_\eta(\boldsymbol{\theta})$ and is defined as the set of target parameters

for which
$$I_\eta(\boldsymbol{\theta}) = \{\boldsymbol{\lambda} \in \Lambda : \ \psi(\boldsymbol{\lambda}\,|\,\boldsymbol{\theta}) \geq \eta\psi(\boldsymbol{\lambda}^*\,|\,\boldsymbol{\theta})\},$$
where η is a pre-defined level ($0 < \eta < 1$). As an example, in a univariate optimization problem, a 99% optimal interval is defined as the set of λ's such that the criterion is no more than 1% lower than its maximum value. From a practical perspective, these nearly optimal values of the target parameters are almost as informative as the optimal value.

Optimal regions play a central role in assessing consistency of alternative data models and defining a robust optimal analysis model when there is considerable uncertainty around the data model parameters in a clinical trial. Based on key CSE principles, sponsors are encouraged to examine several sets of data model parameters, e.g., $\boldsymbol{\theta}_1, \ldots, \boldsymbol{\theta}_m$. In this case sets of nearly optimal values of the target parameter based on appropriate optimal regions can be identified for the selected data models and simple consistency checks can be performed. In particular, let $I_\eta(\boldsymbol{\theta}_i)$ denote the $100\eta\%$ optimal region based on $\boldsymbol{\theta}_i$, $i = 1, \ldots, m$. The *joint optimal region* is defined as the intersection of the resulting optimal regions, i.e.,

$$I_\eta = \bigcap_{i=1}^{m} I_\eta(\boldsymbol{\theta}_i).$$

If the joint optimal region is not empty, it is fair to conclude that the data models chosen by the trial's sponsor are reasonably consistent or compatible. Additionally, the joint optimal region guides the selection of an analysis model that provides optimal or nearly optimal performance across the selected data models.

1.3.3   Sensitivity assessments

An important feature of the optimization algorithm described in Section 1.3.2 is that optimal values of the target parameters may depend heavily on the underlying data model. In this sense, optimal analysis models are locally optimal and are generally unlikely to be globally optimal. Returning to the analogy with optimal designs for regression models used in Section 1.3.1, a locally optimal analysis model is a direct analogy of a locally optimal design which is derived based on a particular set of regression parameters. It is critical to perform a comprehensive sensitivity assessment of optimal or nearly optimal analysis models to help identify models that perform optimally under a broad range of assumptions.

This section provides an overview of easy-to-implement sensitivity assessments that are incorporated into the general clinical trial optimization framework. There are two commonly used approaches to performing sensitivity analyses, termed *qualitative* and *quantitative* sensitivity analyses. Qualitative assessments may be thought of as *pivoting-based* assessments in the sense that the most likely set of assumptions, known as the *main data model*, is selected and this data model is "pivoted" in a number of directions to set up qualitatively different alternative data models with improved or reduced treatment effects. By contrast, the quantitative approach examines the "robustness profile" of an optimal analysis model using a large set of data models that are only quantitatively different from the main model. These models are obtained using random perturbations of the main model and, for this reason, quantitative sensitivity assessments can be viewed as *perturbation-based* assessments. Both types of sensitivity assessments will be illustrated later in this chapter (see Sections 1.4 and 1.5) and throughout this book.

Qualitative sensitivity assessments

As explained above, robustness of optimal data models in clinical trial optimization problems is assessed by carrying out a series of "stress tests" that include qualitative sensitivity assessments. Sensitivity assessments in general and qualitative assessments in particular are justified by the well-known fact that statistical assumptions used in power calculations, e.g., sets of assumed treatment effects in a data model, tend to be quite unreliable and are often subject to "optimism bias." It is strongly recommended to perform a thorough and critical review of the treatment effect scenarios and understand how the optimal analysis model performs across these scenarios. At first glance, it may be desirable to explore a very broad class of data models based on alternative treatment effect scenarios; however, this is likely to be a daunting task. A discrete set of data models or, equivalently, sets of data model parameters is likely to be a good approximation and much more attractive from a practical perspective as long as the data models are *qualitatively* different and correspond to clinically distinct scenarios. For example, it is often sufficient to consider around five models that cover a range of optimistic and pessimistic assumptions.

Using the notation introduced at the end of Section 1.3.2, consider a set of m data models corresponding to the vector parameters $\boldsymbol{\theta}_1, \ldots, \boldsymbol{\theta}_m$. The first data model is treated as the main model and the others represent alternative models included in the qualitative sensitivity assessment. Optimal values of the target parameter $\boldsymbol{\lambda}$ are computed under each data model, i.e., $\boldsymbol{\lambda}_i^*$ is found by maximizing $\psi(\boldsymbol{\lambda} \mid \boldsymbol{\theta}_i)$, $i = 1, \ldots, m$. An initial sensitivity assessment is performed by studying the clustering of the optimal values or identifying important trends across the chosen data models.

A more formal consistency check can be carried out by employing joint optimal regions introduced in Section 1.3.2. Using appropriate optimal regions computed under the individual models, i.e., $I_\eta(\boldsymbol{\theta}_i)$, $i = 1, \ldots, m$, the joint optimal region, denoted by I_η, is obtained as the intersection of the data model-specific regions. It is helpful to evaluate the size of I_η relative to the size of the target parameter space. Even if the optimal values of the target parameter under the alternative data models may not be numerically close to the optimal value derived from the main model, there may be a considerable overlap among the optimal regions. This indicates that the data model-specific optimal values are, in fact, reasonably consistent and the optimization algorithm is robust against qualitative deviations from the main data model.

Consistency analyses based on joint optimal regions can be augmented using compound criteria, i.e., minimum and average criteria, introduced in Section 1.3.1. In this case the criteria computed from the individual data models are treated as if they correspond to different goals within the same trial. Let $\psi(\boldsymbol{\lambda}|\boldsymbol{\theta}_i)$ denote the evaluation criterion of interest computed from the ith data model, $i = 1, \ldots, m$. The minimum criterion can then be defined as

$$\psi_M(\boldsymbol{\lambda}) = \min_{i=1,\ldots,m} \psi(\boldsymbol{\lambda}|\boldsymbol{\theta}_i).$$

This compound criterion supports an investigation of optimal analysis models under the worst-case scenario. Similarly, the average criterion is given by

$$\psi_A(\boldsymbol{\lambda}) = \sum_{i=1}^{m} w_i \psi(\boldsymbol{\lambda}|\boldsymbol{\theta}_i),$$

where $w_1, \ldots, w_m$ determine the relative importance of the individual data models. The weight of the main data model is typically greater than that of the alternative models but, in the absence of reliable prior information, the data models can be treated as being equally likely, i.e., $w_i = 1/m$, $i = 1, \ldots, m$.

Using either compound criterion, optimal parameters of the analysis model of interest are found in a standard way. Analysis models based on the resulting values of the target parameter can be referred to as robust optimal analysis models.

Quantitative sensitivity assessments

While sensitivity analyses within the qualitative framework consider a relatively small family of pre-specified alternative data models, the quantitative approach examines the robustness of an optimal analysis model using a large set of data models. The overall goal of quantitative sensitivity assessments in optimization problems is to carry out a comprehensive characterization of the performance of an optimal analysis model under *quantitative* deviations from the main data model. Alternative data models used in this analysis are randomly generated from the main data model. These models, known as *bootstrap data models*, are constructed by assigning certain distributions to the individual parameters of the main data model and applying a perturbation-based approach that relies on the parametric bootstrap. These distributions may be specified by the trial's sponsor or may represent posterior distributions of the data model parameters computed from earlier trials (see Chapter 4 for more information). Multiple sets of data model parameters are computed by sampling from the selected distributions. Bootstrap data models are defined based on each set of model parameters and, lastly, the optimal analysis model is evaluated under each bootstrap data model.

When considering bootstrap-based perturbations, it is helpful to discuss the relationship between parametric bootstrap algorithms and a general Bayesian framework. The connections between the parametric bootstrap and Bayesian methods were studied in multiple papers, including Efron (2012). In simple terms, the implementation of the parametric bootstrap in the context of quantitative sensitivity assessments amounts to assigning a prior-type distribution to selected parameters of the data model and generating multiple samples that are used for building alternative data models.

To introduce a general algorithm for performing quantitative sensitivity assessments, consider an optimization problem with the data and analysis models denoted by $D(\boldsymbol{\theta})$ and $A(\boldsymbol{\lambda})$. Using a criterion based on a selected evaluation model, denoted by $\psi(\boldsymbol{\lambda} \,|\, \boldsymbol{\theta})$, an optimal value of the target parameter $\boldsymbol{\lambda}$ is found by maximizing the criterion. As before, the optimal value is denoted by $\boldsymbol{\lambda}^*$. To study the robustness of the optimal analysis model based on $\boldsymbol{\lambda}^*$, a distribution is assigned to selected data model parameters and k sets of bootstrap model parameters are generated. Some of the data model parameters, including supportive parameters, can be "frozen" in the sense that their values will be kept constant across the bootstrap samples. The vectors of bootstrap data model parameters are denoted by $\boldsymbol{\theta}_i'$, $i = 1, \ldots, k$. The distributions are indexed by a parameter, known as the *uncertainty parameter*, that determines the magnitude of random deviations from the assumed data model.

Using each vector of bootstrap parameters, bootstrap data models, denoted by $D(\boldsymbol{\theta}_1'), \ldots, D(\boldsymbol{\theta}_k')$, are set up and the optimization criterion is evaluated for the optimal analysis model and each of the bootstrap data models. The resulting criterion values under bootstrap sampling are given by

$$\psi_i = \psi(\boldsymbol{\lambda}^* \,|\, \boldsymbol{\theta}_i'), \; i = 1, \ldots, k.$$

An empirical distribution is easily constructed based on $\psi_1, \ldots, \psi_k$ and sheds light on the sensitivity of the optimal target parameter to deviations from the original data model. It is recommended to study the effect of the uncertainty parameter on the shape of this empirical distribution, which can be done by computing standard descriptive statistics. In addition, relevant quantities such as the probability of performance loss due to data model uncertainty can be derived. This probability is estimated based on the number of bootstrap samples that satisfy the following condition:

$$\psi(\lambda^*|\boldsymbol{\theta}_i') \leq (1 - r)\psi(\lambda^*|\boldsymbol{\theta}), \; i = 1, \ldots, k.$$

where r is a positive value. For example, with $r = 0.1$, this analysis yields the probability of observing more than a 10% reduction (on a relative scale) in the evaluation criterion due to a given level of uncertainty around the assumed data model.

1.4   Direct optimization

The goal of this section is to provide a high-level overview of key considerations related to direct optimization strategies and discuss their implementation using a Phase III clinical trial with two patient populations of interest. The key concepts introduced in Section 1.3 will be illustrated in this section. This includes detailed examples of qualitative and quantitative sensitivity assessments and characterization of optimal values of a target parameter using optimal intervals under several sets of treatment effect scenarios.

The direct optimization approach will also be used in several case studies in Chapters 2 and 3. For example, Case study 2.1 in Chapter 2 will apply and extend this approach to perform a head-to-head comparison of two multiplicity adjustment procedures. Case study 3.1 in Chapter 3 will present a more comprehensive review of optimization algorithms and sensitivity assessments aimed at selecting the best-performing multiplicity adjustment procedure in a similar setting of a multi-population clinical trial.

1.4.1   Case study 1.3: Clinical trial with two patient populations

The clinical trial example used in this section is based on a Phase III clinical trial for prevention of venous thromboembolism (VTE) described in Cohen et al. (2013, 2014). A CSE framework for this clinical trial will be defined below; however, the main focus will be on defining the components of the optimization algorithm in this trial and many important CSE techniques such as a review of alternative data and analysis models will be omitted. For a detailed review of CSE-based clinical trial optimization; see Chapters 2, 3 and 4.

Data, analysis and evaluation models

As stated in Section 1.2, the data model in a clinical trial includes the specification of key elements of the trial design and outcome distribution. The patient population to be studied in the trial is the population of acute medically ill patients who remain at risk for VTE. A simple two-arm design will be utilized with patients randomly allocated in a 1:1 ratio to receive a novel treatment or control (short course of prophylaxis with enoxaparin followed by placebo). The primary endpoint in the VTE trial is a composite binary endpoint based on deep-vein thrombosis, nonfatal pulmonary embolism or VTE-related death at Day 35. The experimental treatment is expected to reduce the event rate based on this composite endpoint compared to the control.

An important element of the trial design is a pre-defined marker, namely, the baseline D-dimer level, which is believed to be a moderator of treatment response. In general, D-dimer concentration is often used as a prognostic marker that helps diagnose thrombosis. In this particular trial, patients with elevated D-dimer levels at baseline are expected to experience greater therapeutic benefit compared to those with lower D-dimer levels. A binary classifier is defined based on a clinically meaningful threshold and a multi-population design will be employed in this clinical trial. The two populations of interest are defined as follows

- General population of patients (commonly known as the *all-comers* population).

- Population of *marker-positive* patients with elevated D-dimer levels at baseline (above the pre-specified threshold).

Note that the general population also includes *marker-negative* patients with reduced D-dimer levels but the efficacy profile of the new treatment is not planned to be evaluated in this population. The multi-population design will be used to maximize clinical benefit and optimize patient selection for treatment. For more information on the use of prognostic and predictive markers in multi-population trials; see Chapter 3.

The data model is denoted by $D(\boldsymbol{\theta})$, where

$$\boldsymbol{\theta} = (\theta_1, \ldots, \theta_5)$$

is the vector of key and supportive parameters. The list of key data model parameters consists of the event rates in the four samples included in the model, i.e.,

- Sample 1 consists of marker-negative patients in the control arm.

- Sample 2 consists of marker-positive patients in the control arm.

- Sample 3 consists of marker-negative patients in the treatment arm.

- Sample 4 consists of marker-positive patients in the treatment arm.

The event rates in the four samples are denoted by θ_1 through θ_4. The supportive parameter in this data model, denoted by θ_5, is the prevalence of marker-positive patients in the general patient populations. This prevalence rate was set to 40%.

The event rate assumptions to be used in this clinical trial were derived from historical data and available information on the pre-defined marker. The event rate in the control arm was assumed to be 7.5%. The marker status (positive versus negative) was not expected to have any impact on the event rate in this arm; in other words, the event rate was set to 7.5% in Sample 1 as well as Sample 2. As noted above, the experimental treatment was expected to result in a reduction in the event rate with much greater benefit in patients with a marker-positive status. The assumed values of the key data model parameters are listed in Table 1.10.

TABLE 1.10: Event rates under four scenarios in the VTE trial in Case study 1.3.

Sample	Scenario 1	Scenario 2	Scenario 3	Scenario 4
Sample 1	$\theta_1 = 0.075$	$\theta_1 = 0.075$	$\theta_1 = 0.075$	$\theta_1 = 0.075$
Sample 2	$\theta_2 = 0.075$	$\theta_2 = 0.075$	$\theta_2 = 0.075$	$\theta_2 = 0.075$
Sample 3	$\theta_3 = 0.06$	$\theta_3 = 0.06$	$\theta_3 = 0.06$	$\theta_3 = 0.06$
Sample 4	$\theta_4 = 0.04125$	$\theta_4 = 0.045$	$\theta_4 = 0.04875$	$\theta_4 = 0.0525$

This table summarizes the event rates under four scenarios. Scenario 1 defined the most likely set of event rates in the trial and the data model based on this scenario will be referred to as the *main data model*. Under Scenario 1, the relative risk reduction in the marker-positive subset was equal to 45%. By contrast, the relative risk reduction in the complementary subset of marker-positive patients was only 20%. In other words, this scenario is based on the assumption that the selected marker is a strong predictor of treatment response and helps identify a patient subgroup with enhanced treatment effect. Even though this particular scenario appears most likely based on the results of clinical trials conducted prior to the current trial, it is important to examine alternative sets of event rates that may be less optimistic. Scenarios 2, 3 and 4 presented in Table 1.10 defined alternative sets of event rates in the four samples. These scenarios corresponded to the cases where the marker exhibits gradually decreasing predictive strength. It follows from this table that the relative risk reduction in the subset of marker-positive patients under Scenarios 2, 3 and 4 was assumed to be 40%, 35% and 30%, respectively. From a practical perspective, the marker was close to being non-informative in Scenario 4 in the sense that, under this set of assumptions, the treatment effect was assumed to be virtually homogeneous across the trial population.

The analysis model in this clinical trial example includes several components such as the test for evaluating the significance of the treatment effect and a multiplicity adjustment. The significance will be assessed using the Cochran-Mantel-Haenszel (CMH) method with an adjustment for pre-defined stratification factors. A fairly quick sample size calculation was performed under the s data model to support the clinical trial optimization exercise. The sample size was selected to achieve a sufficiently high probability of detecting a statistically significant treatment effect (marginal power) in the general trial population as well as marker-positive subpopulation. The calculation was run based on the CMH test with a two-sided $\alpha = 0.05$ and no multiplicity adjustment was applied in this initial calculation. With the total sample size (treatment and control arms) set to 3800 patients, marginal power was equal to 81.3% and 81.1% in the general population and subpopulation of marker-positive patients, respectively. When the alternative sets of statistical assumptions were considered (Scenarios 2, 3 and 4), the total sample size in the general population was adjusted upward to keep the overall probability of

TABLE 1.11: Sample sizes in the general population and marker-positive subpopulation under four scenarios in Case study 1.3.

Population	Scenario 1	Scenario 2	Scenario 3	Scenario 4
General population	3800	4400	5000	5600
Subpopulation	1520	1760	2000	2240

success in the trial at a sufficiently high level. The resulting sample sizes are presented in Table 1.11.

The treatment effect test will be viewed as a fixed component of the analysis model and the model will be optimized with respect to multiplicity adjustment. Given the multi-population design employed in the trial, two null hypotheses of no effect will be tested:

- Null hypothesis of no effect in the general population (H_0).

- Null hypothesis of no effect in the subpopulation of marker-positive patients (H_1).

A multiplicity adjustment is required in this trial to protect the overall Type I error rate at the nominal level (two-sided $\alpha = 0.05$) due to multiple opportunities to claim treatment effectiveness (in the general population and marker-positive subpopulation). A multiplicity adjustment will be performed based on the Holm procedure. This procedure was selected mostly because it utilizes a simple set of decision rules and alternative approaches to multiplicity adjustment that could have been used in this setting, including the Hochberg procedure, will be described in Chapter 3 (see Case study 3.1).

To define the multiplicity adjustment rules used in the Holm procedure, let p_0 and p_1 denote the two-sided treatment effect p-values computed from the CMH test. The two goals pursued in this trial, i.e., the goals of establishing a significant treatment effect in the general population and marker-positive subpopulation, are not equally important. From the sponsor's perspective, it will be more desirable to demonstrate a beneficial effect in the general population. The Holm procedure supports an option to account for the differential importance of the two null hypotheses. The degree of differential importance is controlled by a parameter denoted by λ, where $0 \leq \lambda \leq 1$.

The Holm procedure relies on a data-driven testing sequence and testing begins with the null hypothesis corresponding to the smaller p-value. The following two cases will need to be considered:

- Case 1: $p_0 < p_1$. The Holm procedure will reject the null hypothesis of no effect in the general population (H_0) if $p_0 \leq \alpha(1 - \lambda)$. If H_0 is rejected, the null hypothesis of no effect in the pre-defined subpopulation (H_1) will be tested next. This null hypothesis will be rejected if $p_1 \leq \alpha$. Otherwise, if H_0 is not rejected, the null hypothesis H_1 will be accepted and no beneficial effect can be claimed in the subpopulation.

- Case 2: $p_1 < p_0$. Testing will begin with H_1 and this null hypothesis will be rejected if $p_1 \leq \alpha\lambda$. The null hypothesis H_0 will be tested next provided H_1 is rejected, namely, H_0 will be rejected if $p_0 \leq \alpha$. However, as in Case 1, if H_1 is not rejected, the null hypothesis H_0 will be automatically accepted without testing.

It is worth noting that λ may be viewed as the weight of the subpopulation test in this multiplicity adjustment procedure. However, this interpretation of λ is likely to be misleading since it follows from the testing algorithm defined above that a significant treatment effect can be established in the marker-positive subpopulation even if λ is set to 0. Indeed, the null hypothesis H_1 will be rejected by the Holm procedure with $\lambda = 0$ in Case 1 provided $p_0 \leq \alpha$ and $p_1 \leq \alpha$. For this reason, it is advisable to treat λ as the general parameter of the Holm procedure that impacts power of the tests in the general population and pre-defined subpopulation.

The resulting analysis model based on the Holm procedure with a pre-defined λ is denoted by $A(\lambda)$. Given the importance of the λ parameter, it is natural to consider a problem of identifying an optimal value of λ in this clinical trial. In this optimization problem, λ will serve as the target parameter and a direct optimization strategy based on an appropriate evaluation criterion can be applied. Multiple criteria can be considered in this setting. For the sake of illustration, the criterion derived from disjunctive power, i.e., the probability of at least one significant outcome in this trial, will be used as the main criterion in this evaluation model:

$$\psi(\lambda \,|\, \boldsymbol{\theta}) = P(\text{Reject } H_0 \text{ or Reject } H_1 \,|\, D(\boldsymbol{\theta}), A(\lambda)).$$

This probability is evaluated for the selected analysis model $A(\lambda)$ and the underlying data model $D(\boldsymbol{\theta})$. An optimal value of λ will be found by maximizing this disjunctive criterion for a given data model $D(\boldsymbol{\theta})$.

As a quick comment, evaluation criteria based on disjunctive power have a number of limitations and alternative approaches to defining evaluation criteria for this and similar optimization problems will be introduced in Chapters 2 and 3; see, for example, Case studies 2.1 and 3.1. In addition, it is good practice to investigate several relevant criteria in a particular problem. Evaluation criteria may not be uniquely defined in trials with several clinical objectives and application of multiple criteria enables the trial's sponsor to better "quantify" the plurality of objectives.

The problem of selecting an optimal multiplicity adjustment in this clinical trial will be considered in the next three sections. Sections 1.4.2 and 1.4.3 will provide a summary of pivoting-based and perturbation-based sensitivity assessments of the Holm procedure to determine its performance under systematic (qualitative) and random (quantitative) deviations from an assumed data model. A direct optimization approach will be utilized in Section 1.4.4 to identify an optimal value of the target parameter λ that defines the weighting scheme in the Holm procedure as well as ranges of nearly optimal values. Optimization will be performed based on the disjunctive criterion defined above.

1.4.2   Qualitative sensitivity assessment

As stressed in Section 1.3.3, a key component of any optimization exercise is a set of sensitivity assessments, including qualitative and quantitative sensitivity analyses. Most commonly, these assessments are performed after an optimization algorithm has been applied to identify the best-performing analysis model in a clinical trial. However, as will be shown below, sensitivity assessments can be conducted independently of optimization algorithms. For example, when the performance of multiplicity adjustments is evaluated, sensitivity assessments can be conducted to compare and contrast the "robustness profile" of a given multiplicity adjustment method to that of a basic analysis method that employs no multiplicity adjustment.

Qualitative or pivoting-based assessments focus on studying the impact of model uncertainty using a small number of qualitatively different treatment effect scenarios. In this particular case, pivoting-based sensitivity assessments will focus on the overall performance of the Holm procedure across the four scenarios defined in Table 1.10. It was explained in Section 1.4.1 that the three alternative scenarios address potential "optimism bias" in the main model by considering weaker differential effects between the marker-positive and marker-negative subpopulations. For example, an impressive relative risk reduction of 45% within the marker-positive subpopulation assumed in Scenario 1 shrinks to a 30% reduction within the same subpopulation in Scenario 4.

To establish a reference point for qualitative sensitivity assessments for the Holm procedure, Figure 1.2 provides a summary of the key metrics in the VTE clinical trial, i.e., the operating characteristics of the treatment effect tests in the general population and marker-positive subpopulation, using the basic unadjusted method. This method utilized no multiplicity adjustment and each test was simply carried out at a two-sided $\alpha = 0.05$. The characteristics included the marginal probabilities of a significant outcome for each test as well as the disjunctive probability, i.e., the probability of establishing a significant treatment effect in either population. It can be seen that the probability of achieving success in the general population was approximately the same across the scenarios due to the fact that the sample size was appropriately adjusted when reduced treatment effects were assumed in the subpopulation in Scenarios 2, 3 and 4 (see Table 1.11). However, the sample size adjustments were clearly not sufficient to prevent the probability of success in the subpopulation of marker-positive patients from dropping quite rapidly across the scenarios (from 81.1% in Scenario 1 to from 59.0% in Scenario 4). Disjunctive power was driven mostly by the probability of success in the general population and decreased at a relatively slow rate with the shrinking treatment effect in the subpopulation.

It is of interest to compare the characteristics of the unadjusted method presented in Figure 1.2 to those of the Holm procedure under the same four sets of treatment effect assumptions. In this preliminary assessment, it was

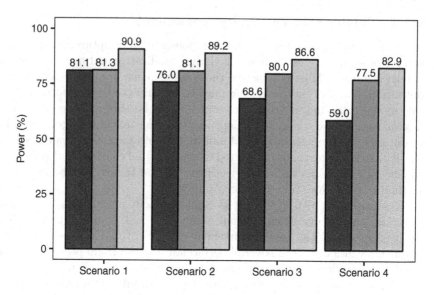

FIGURE 1.2: Probability of establishing a significant treatment effect in the marker-positive subpopulation (black bars), general trial population (dark gray bars) and disjunctive probability (light gray bars) under the four scenarios without a multiplicity adjustment in Case study 1.3.

assumed that the main parameter of this procedure was set to $\lambda = 0.5$, i.e., the smaller p-value was to be tested at a 0.025 level and, if it was significant, the larger p-value would be tested at a 0.05 level. Figure 1.3 provides a summary of the same characteristics as in Figure 1.2 and presents a virtually identical overall pattern of marginal and disjunctive probabilities. The marginal and disjunctive probabilities were lower in Figure 1.3 compared to Figure 1.2 due to a multiplicity adjustment but it is clear that the two analysis methods were very similar to each other in terms of general sensitivity to the statistical assumptions in this clinical trial.

1.4.3 Quantitative sensitivity assessment

In this particular clinical trial example, a small set of alternative data models was considered and the pivoting-based sensitivity analysis included a rather basic set of assessments. However, quantitative or perturbation-based stress tests defined in Section 1.3.3 can be quite informative even in this setting. Unlike qualitative assessments, perturbation-based sensitivity assessments focus on one of the pre-defined data models, e.g., the main data model, and examine a large number of closely related data models.

Using the general framework for performing quantitative sensitivity as-

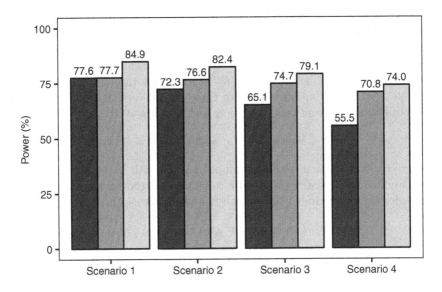

FIGURE 1.3: Probability of establishing a significant treatment effect in the marker-positive subpopulation (black bars), general trial population (dark gray bars) and disjunctive probability (light gray bars) under the four scenarios with the Holm-based multiplicity adjustment in Case study 1.3.

sessments, the overall goal of quantitative assessments in this clinical trial example is to study the performance of the Holm-adjusted and unadjusted analysis models under alternative data models (bootstrap data models) that are only quantitatively different from the main model. By sampling from pre-defined distributions assigned to selected data model parameters, bootstrap data models will be defined. Characteristics of the Holm procedure as well as the analysis strategy without a multiplicity adjustment will be computed from each bootstrap data model.

This parametric bootstrap algorithm was run to perform perturbation-based sensitivity assessments based on the main data model that corresponds to Scenario 1 in Table 1.10. Let $\boldsymbol{\theta} = (\theta_1, \ldots, \theta_5)$ denote the vector of the data model parameters in this scenario, i.e.,

$$\boldsymbol{\theta} = (0.075, 0.075, 0.06, 0.04125, 0.4).$$

It was shown in Section 1.3.3 that the first step of the algorithm involves assigning suitable distributions to selected parameters of the data model. If data from earlier trials with the same treatment and patient population are available, it is sensible to compute the posterior distributions of these data model parameters based on relevant prior distributions. In this case it is recommended to identify several sets of prior distributions that represent different levels of confidence about the assumed parameter values (this approach is considered in Chapter 4). In general, a more straightforward way of performing quantitative sensitivity assessments relies on a direct specification of the distributions for the parameters of interest.

In this case study, since the key data model parameters, i.e., the first four parameters in $\boldsymbol{\theta}$, define the event rates in Samples 1 through 4, it is natural to assign a beta distribution to each of these parameters. Specifically, multiple sets of bootstrap event rates are generated as follows:

$$\theta'_{ij} \sim \text{Beta}(\alpha_j, \beta_j), \ j = 1, \ldots, 4, \ i = 1, \ldots, k,$$

where θ'_{ij} is the event rate for Sample j in the ith bootstrap set and k is the number of bootstrap sets. For compactness, the parameter vector that includes the event rates from the ith bootstrap set can be defined:

$$\boldsymbol{\theta}'_i = (\theta'_{i1}, \theta'_{i2}, \theta'_{i3}, \theta'_{i4}), \ i = 1, \ldots, k.$$

The shape parameters of the beta distributions for the key data model parameters are chosen to ensure that the mean of the event rates in a bootstrap set is equal to the event rate in the same sample assumed under Scenario 1. In other words,

$$\frac{\alpha_j}{\alpha_j + \beta_j} = \theta_j, \ j = 1, \ldots, 4.$$

In addition, a free parameter that will be referred to as the *uncertainty parameter* and denoted by c ($c > 0$) is introduced to quantify the amount of variability around the specified mean values. This parameter can be defined as a common coefficient of variation for the four bootstrap distributions. Given this coefficient of variation and using well-known properties of beta distributions, the shape parameters of the bootstrap distributions are computed from the following two equations

$$\alpha_j = \frac{1 - \theta_j}{c^2} - \theta_j, \ \beta_j = \frac{\alpha_j(1 - \theta_j)}{\theta_j}, \ j = 1, \ldots, 4.$$

It is easy to see that, with a larger value of the uncertainty parameter, greater deviations from the assumed data model parameters should be expected in the bootstrap sets.

Finally, the fifth element of $\boldsymbol{\theta}$ is the supportive parameter that defines the prevalence of marker-positive patients in the general population. Again, a beta distribution could be assigned to this parameter or, for the sake of simplicity, this parameter can be set to a fixed value, i.e., $\theta'_{i5} = 0.4, \ i = 1, \ldots, k$.

A large number of bootstrap data models is typically generated and a simulation-based approach is applied to compute appropriate characteristics of the selected procedures from each bootstrap data model. Using disjunctive power for the Holm procedure as an example, bootstrap-based disjunctive power is computed from the bootstrap data models as follows

$$\psi_i = \psi(\lambda \,|\, \boldsymbol{\theta}'_i), \ i = 1, \ldots, k.$$

TABLE 1.12: Key parameters in three bootstrap data models and associated disjunctive power for the Holm procedure in Case study 1.3.

Bootstrap set	Bootstrap event rates	Disjunctive power
Bootstrap set 1	$\theta'_1 = (0.0654, 0.0649, 0.0607, 0.0303)$	0.858
Bootstrap set 2	$\theta'_2 = (0.0799, 0.0745, 0.0576, 0.0371)$	0.953
Bootstrap set 3	$\theta'_3 = (0.0767, 0.0665, 0.0678, 0.0467)$	0.403

Bootstrap-based probabilities of significant treatment effects in the general population and marker-positive subpopulations can be computed in a similar way.

The following quick example illustrates the process of generating bootstrap data models and computing evaluation criteria from these data models in this clinical trial. Table 1.12 lists three sets of key data model parameters. The key data model parameters were generated using the algorithm described above with the uncertainty parameter set to $c = 0.1$ and the supportive data model parameter set to 0.4 in all three bootstrap sets. Multiple evaluation criteria can be computed in this setting and, for the sake of illustration, disjunctive power, i.e., the probability of detecting a significant treatment effect in the general population or pre-defined subpopulation, was computed for each bootstrap data model. The probability was evaluated via additional simulations based on each bootstrap data model with the Holm-based multiplicity adjustment (λ was set to 0.5 in the Holm procedure).

Beginning with Bootstrap set 1 in Table 1.12, the event rates in this bootstrap sample were generally consistent with the rates assumed under Scenario 1 with a lower rate among marker-positive patients assigned to the treatment arm ($\theta'_{14} = 0.0303$). Disjunctive power for the Holm procedure computed from the bootstrap data model based on these parameters (85.8%) was fairly close to disjunctive power obtained under Scenario 1 (see Figure 1.3).

The same algorithm was applied to compute disjunctive power for the other two bootstrap sets. The control event rate in the subset of marker-negative patients ($\theta'_{21} = 0.0799$) was higher than expected and, at the same time, the treatment event rate in the subset of marker-positive patients ($\theta'_{24} = 0.0371$) was lower than expected in Bootstrap set 2. This resulted in improved disjunctive power (95.3%). By contrast, the event rate in the treatment arm within the marker-positive subset turned out to be quite high in Bootstrap set 3 ($\theta'_{34} = 0.0467$) and this drove disjunctive power to a very low level (40.3%).

By examining the empirical distribution of bootstrap-based characteristics of the Holm procedure and unadjusted strategy, e.g., disjunctive power, the trial's sponsor can determine the impact of random deviations from the assumed data model on the two analysis strategies and see if the Holm procedure is as sensitive or perhaps more sensitive to uncertainty around the true values of the data model parameters. As part of this assessment, it is advisable to study the shape of the empirical distribution as a function of the uncertainty parameter c. In addition, descriptive statistics such as the mean and median disjunctive power can be computed for the Holm procedure and unadjusted analysis strategy and compared to the values of disjunctive power derived from the original model.

The uncertainty parameter c defines the variance of bootstrap distributions assigned to data model parameters and thus it plays a central role in perturbation-based sensitivity assessments. It is helpful to discuss rules for selecting appropriate values of this parameter. Given the similarities between approaches based on the parametric bootstrap and Bayesian inferences, it appears natural to review general guidelines for choosing prior distributions discussed in the Bayesian literature. For example, Herson (1979) introduced a set of straightforward rules to facilitate the process of specifying conjugate prior distributions (beta distributions) for binary endpoints. Based on these rules, a beta prior distribution with the coefficient of variation of 0.1 can be thought of as a rather "aggressive" or high-confidence prior and increasing values of this parameter correspond to decreasing levels of confidence. For example, the case where the coefficient of variation is close to 0.5 defines a low-confidence prior.

If this general approach is extended to bootstrap-based sensitivity analyses, the uncertainty parameter $c = 0.1$ will correspond to a "high-confidence" or "low-uncertainty" setting where the trial's sponsor is quite confident about the treatment effect assumptions. With greater values of c, the level of confidence will decrease but, in most practical scenarios, uncertainty parameters above 0.5 define an unusually high level of variability around the original set of assumptions. Of course, the trial's sponsor needs to be careful with a blind application of similar general guidelines. They can certainly serve as a starting point but need to be fine-tuned on a case by case basis.

Figure 1.4 provides a quick illustration of the rules for selecting the uncertainty parameter in perturbation-based sensitivity assessments. This figure plots the beta distributions for the event rates in the four samples corresponding to three values of the uncertainty parameter ($c = 0.05$, $c = 0.1$ and $c = 0.15$)[1]. Examining the shapes of the bootstrap distributions with $c = 0.05$, it is easy to see that there is a minimal overlap between the adjacent distributions. Therefore, it is fair to say that this uncertainty parameter defines a low-uncertainty setting where the trial's sponsor anticipates some variability but is reasonably confident about the selected values of the event rates in the individual samples. Further, with the uncertainty parameter set to 0.1, the degree of overlap is considerably increased. As a result, the probability of reversal in the marker-negative subpopulation, e.g., the probability that

---

[1]Note that there should have been four beta distributions assigned to the four key parameters in the data model. In this particular case, the same event rate was assumed within the subpopulations of marker-positive and marker-negative patients in the placebo arm, i.e., $\theta_1 = \theta_2$, and the same beta distribution was assigned to θ_1 and θ_2.

the control event rate is greater than the treatment event rate in a bootstrap sample, is non-trivial in this case. It would be most appropriate to refer to this setting as a medium-uncertainty setting. Finally, the amount of overlap grows dramatically if the uncertainty parameter increases to 0.15 and the distributions assigned to the event rates become almost indistinguishable. For this reason, the case with $c = 0.15$ may be thought of as a high-uncertainty setting.

The considerations presented above led to a decision to focus on perturbation-based sensitivity assessments with the uncertainty parameter set to 0.05 and 0.1 in this clinical trial example. Sensitivity assessments based on the beta distributions for the key parameters of the main data model were run with $k = 1,000$ bootstrap sets. The key characteristics of the unadjusted and Holm procedures, e.g., the marginal probabilities of a significant effect in the two patient populations as well as the disjunctive probability, were computed from the data models based on these bootstrap sets.

As the very first step in examining the bootstrap-based characteristics of the two analysis methods, it is helpful to plot the empirical distributions of each characteristic. For example, Figure 1.5 displays the empirical probability density functions of the probabilities of success in the general population and marker-positive subpopulation for the two selected values of uncertainty parameter ($c = 0.05$ and $c = 0.1$). The empirical distributions were compared to the corresponding marginal probabilities of success based on the original data model, i.e., 81.3% in the general population and 81.1% in the subpopulation. It can be seen from the figure that, in a low-uncertainty setting with $c = 0.05$, the bootstrap-based marginal probabilities were clustered reasonably closely around their expected values represented by the vertical lines. The distributions were not symmetric around the vertical lines and were slightly skewed to the left, which means that the probabilities were low in a large number of the bootstrap samples. The empirical distributions were much more skewed and exhibited a long left tail when the medium-uncertainty setting ($c = 0.1$) was considered in the sensitivity assessment. The number of bootstrap samples that resulted in low probabilities of success increased and, in a handful of bootstrap samples, the probabilities dropped to or below 25%. At the same time, the mode of each distribution shifted to the right. This suggested that, on average, the marginal probabilities of success in the two patient populations computed from the bootstrap data models were nearly the same as the values obtained from the main model. For example, the medians of the empirical distributions appeared to be fairly close to the vertical lines.

The distribution plots presented in Figure 1.5 help visualize the impact of perturbations and, as the next step, it is natural to perform a quantitative comparison of the bootstrap-based characteristics of the unadjusted and Holm procedures. Multiple descriptive statistics can be computed from the empirical distributions, including the mean and median. Since the mean is likely to be unduly affected by the outliers, i.e., bootstrap models that result in very low probabilities of relevant outcomes, it is more sensible to focus on the

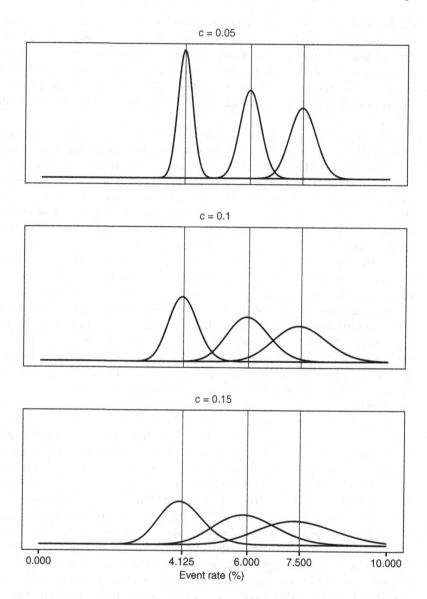

FIGURE 1.4: Assumed distributions of the event rates used in the permutation-based sensitivity assessments under the main data model with three values of the uncertainty parameter (c) in Case study 1.3. The vertical lines are drawn at the event rates assumed under the main data model.

median probabilities. It is also helpful to compute the proportion of bootstrap models where the probability of interest falls below the reference probability

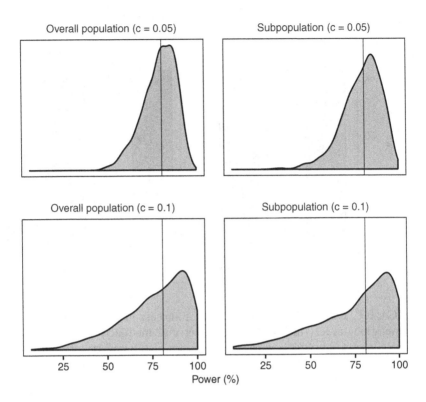

FIGURE 1.5: Distribution of the bootstrap-based marginal probabilities of significant treatment effects in the general population and marker-positive subpopulation for two values of the uncertainty parameter (c) in Case study 1.3. The probabilities are computed without an adjustment for multiplicity. The vertical lines identify the corresponding probabilities evaluated under the main data model.

computed from the main data model. This quantity helps the trial's sponsor estimate how frequently the selected analysis methods will underperform with increasing uncertainty about the treatment effects in this clinical trial. Along the same line, a specific threshold can be introduced to find the likelihood of *relevant loss*. For example, the proportion of bootstrap models with a reduction of more than 10% on an absolute scale in the probability of interest can be computed to determine how often the analysis methods will exhibit a tangible drop in performance if the original assumptions are not deemed reliable.

Figure 1.6 sheds more light on the effect of increasing uncertainty on the performance of the unadjusted analysis method and Holm procedure. This figure directly compares the marginal probabilities of a significant treatment

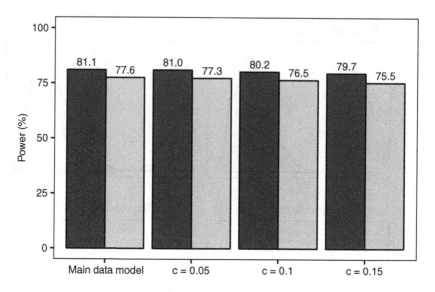

FIGURE 1.6: Marginal probability of success in the marker-positive subpopulation under the main data model and median probability of success under bootstrap models with several values of the uncertainty parameter (c) in Case study 1.3. The probabilities are computed based on the unadjusted analysis method (black bars) and Holm procedure (gray bars).

effect in the marker-positive subpopulation to their bootstrap-based counterparts. The median was used as a measure of central tendency and the median of the bootstrap-based probabilities were computed for the three values of the uncertainty parameter ($c = 0.05$, $c = 0.1$ and $c = 0.15$) that were examined in Figure 1.4. Figure 1.6 supports the hypothesis formulated above and shows that, despite increasing variability associated with larger values of the uncertainty parameter, the median probabilities were virtually unaffected. For example, as the uncertainty parameter increased from the low-uncertainty level to the high-uncertainty level, the unadjusted probability of success in the subpopulation decreased by less than 3 percentage points (from 81.1% to 79.7%). A similar slight downward trend was observed for the Holm procedure. This set of sensitivity analyses demonstrates that, as in Section 1.4.2, the "robustness profiles" of the analysis model with the Holm-based adjustment was nearly identical to that of the unadjusted analysis model. In general, a more detailed description of empirical distributions is recommended and the reader will find a good example of using violin plots in quantitative sensitivity assessments in Chapter 2 (see Case study 2.1).

A permutation-based approach to performing sensitivity assessments is a useful tool but it may be difficult to interpret the results if a meaningful range for the uncertainty parameter has not been established. Figure 1.5 shows that variability in any characteristic of an analysis method will keep increasing with the increasing uncertainty parameter unless there is a cap on the uncertainty parameter. As pointed out earlier in this section and will be stressed again in Chapters 2 and 3, the definition of low and high uncertainty is application-specific and the value of c needs to be calibrated in each setting. In addition, it was demonstrated above that it is very useful to identify a reference analysis model and perform a comparative analysis of the "robustness profiles" of the analysis model of interest and reference model. This approach can be utilized in any optimization problem focusing on optimal selection of multiplicity adjustments. The reference analysis model can be defined based on another multiplicity adjustment strategy or basic analysis strategy that employs no multiplicity adjustment.

1.4.4 Optimal selection of the target parameter

This section will focus on the problem of identifying an optimal multiplicity adjustment method in a family of the Holm-based adjustments indexed by λ. Optimal values of the target parameter λ will be found using the direct optimization algorithm, i.e., using a univariate grid search, under the main data model and three alternative models defined in Table 1.10.

An optimal value of λ will be defined as the value that maximizes the disjunctive criterion, i.e., results in the highest value of the probability of a significant treatment effect in the general trial population or subpopulation of patients with a marker-positive status at baseline after the Holm-based multiplicity adjustment. Formally, optimization will focus on maximizing

$$\psi(\lambda \,|\, \boldsymbol{\theta}_i) = P(\text{Reject } H_0 \text{ or Reject } H_1 \,|\, D(\boldsymbol{\theta}_i), A(\lambda)), \ i = 1, 2, 3, 4,$$

where $A(\lambda)$ defines the analysis model with the Holm procedure that sets the initial weight of the subpopulation test to λ ($0 \leq \lambda \leq 1$) and the data model $D(\boldsymbol{\theta}_i)$ is constructed using the vector of data model parameters corresponding to Scenario i.

Figure 1.7 plots the disjunctive criterion as a function of the target parameter under the four pre-defined scenarios. The general conclusion that can be drawn from Figure 1.7 is that the criterion was either maximized or quite high when the target parameter was small. The optimal values of λ are listed in Table 1.13 (optimal intervals listed in this table will be discussed below). It is clear from this table that the treatment effect test in the subpopulation of marker-positive patients should not be given much initial weight in the Holm procedure if optimization is aimed at improving the probability of a significant treatment effect in either patient population.

Once again, the target parameter determines the initial weight of the subpopulation test in this multiplicity problem. This weight is updated during testing and the final weight of this test is driven by the ordering of the hypothesis p-values. For example, considering the optimization problem under

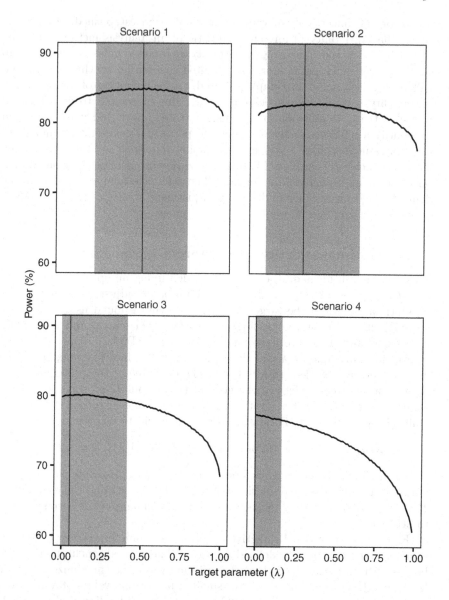

FIGURE 1.7: Disjunctive criterion as a function of the target parameter (λ) under the four scenarios with the Holm-based multiplicity adjustment in Case study 1.3.

Scenario 2, it follows from Table 1.13 that the optimal value of the target parameter was 0.29. This means that, if $p_0 < p_1$, the null hypothesis of no effect in the general population will be tested at 0.71α. If it is rejected, the

TABLE 1.13: Optimal value and optimal intervals for the target parameter (λ) based on the disjunctive criterion under the four treatment effect scenarios with the Holm-based multiplicity adjustment in Case study 1.3.

Scenario	Optimal value	99% optimal interval
Scenario 1	0.50	$(0.20, 0.78)$
Scenario 2	0.29	$(0.06, 0.64)$
Scenario 3	0.05	$(0.00, 0.41)$
Scenario 4	0.00	$(0.00, 0.16)$

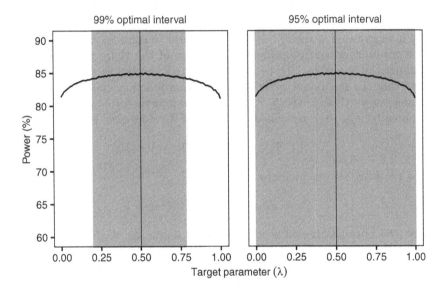

FIGURE 1.8: Optimal value and optimal intervals for the target parameter (λ) based on the disjunctive criterion under the main data model (Scenario 1) with the Holm-based multiplicity adjustment in Case study 1.3. The vertical line represents the optimal value of λ and the gray rectangles define the 99% optimal interval (left-hand panel) and 95% optimal interval (right-hand panel).

full α level will be utilized in the subpopulation test. On the other hand, if $p_1 < p_0$, the null hypothesis of no effect in the subpopulation will be tested first at 0.29α and, after that, the null hypothesis of no effect in the general population will be tested at α provided the first hypothesis in the testing sequence is rejected.

It was pointed out in Section 1.3.2 that it may be misleading to report only the single value of the target parameter at which the criterion function is maximized if this function is fairly flat around its maximum. Indeed, it can be seen from Figure 1.7 that the range of the disjunctive criterion is quite narrow under the more optimistic sets of treatment effect assumptions (Scenario 1 and 2). In this case the focus needs to shift from the "point estimate" of the optimal target parameter to a "confidence interval" which is obtained by considering all values of the target parameter for which the criterion function is close to its maximum.

To illustrate the derivation of a "confidence interval" for the optimal value of λ, consider the optimization problem under the main data model (Scenario 1). The disjunctive criterion under this data model is plotted in the two panels of Figure 1.8. This figure shows that the disjunctive criterion was maximized at $\lambda = 0.5$. This value, denoted by λ^*, is represented by the vertical line in both panels. In addition to the point estimate associated with the highest value of the criterion, it is natural to consider ranges of λ values that resulted in nearly optimal performance of the Holm procedure in this optimization problem. To define these ranges, known as optimal intervals, note that the maximum value of the criterion function under the main data model was $\psi(\lambda^* \mid \boldsymbol{\theta}_1) = 0.85$. A 99% optimal interval for λ^* under Scenario 1, denoted by $I_{0.99}(\boldsymbol{\theta}_1)$, is defined as the set of λ values such that

$$\psi(\lambda \mid \boldsymbol{\theta}_1) \geq 0.99\psi(\lambda^* \mid \boldsymbol{\theta}_1) = 0.8415.$$

The resulting set was given by

$$I_{0.99}(\boldsymbol{\theta}_1) = (0.2, 0.78).$$

The 99% optimal interval is represented by a gray rectangle in the left-hand panel of Figure 1.8. The interval was fairly wide, which reflects the fact that the criterion function was quite flat around λ^*. From a practical perspective, a single-point reduction on a relative scale, i.e., reduction from 85% to 84.2%, in the probability of success is virtually trivial. It is fair to treat the λ values within the 99% optimal interval as if they were optimal values of the target parameter.

Similarly, a 95% optimal interval for the target parameter, denoted by $I_{0.95}(\boldsymbol{\theta}_1)$, is computed from

$$\psi(\lambda \mid \boldsymbol{\theta}_1) \geq 0.95\psi(\lambda^* \mid \boldsymbol{\theta}_1) = 0.8075.$$

The 95% optimal interval, shown in the right-hand panel of Figure 1.8, was extremely wide. This interval actually extended over the entire range of λ, i.e.,

$$I_{0.95}(\boldsymbol{\theta}_1) = (0, 1).$$

There were clearly limited opportunities for optimization under this particular set of assumptions. This optimal interval demonstrates that, if a 5% drop in disjunctive power on a relative scale was acceptable to the trial's sponsor, the target parameter could be set to any value between 0 and 1 in Scenario 1.

Using the same algorithm, 99% optimal intervals were computed under the other three treatment effect scenarios. When Scenarios 2, 3 and 4 were examined, the optimal intervals for λ^* were tighter and consequently more informative than that derived under Scenario 1. The resulting sets of nearly optimal values of the target parameter are listed in Table 1.13. The optimal intervals presented in this table back up the conclusion based on the point estimates of λ^*. With the exception of the main data model that relied on the assumption of a strong predictive biomarker, the optimal sets of λ values were shifted toward 0 and supported the decision to "upweight" the general population test in this clinical trial.

A review of the point estimates of the optimal target parameter in Table 1.13 suggests that the results are quite inconsistent across the four treatment effect scenarios. An important application of optimal intervals in optimization problems is that they facilitate consistency assessments across multiple scenarios. This can be accomplished by computing a joint optimal interval which is defined as the intersection of the scenario-specific intervals. For example, a joint 99% optimal interval for λ^* is given by

$$I_{0.99} = \bigcap_{i=1}^{4} I_{0.99}(\boldsymbol{\theta}_i).$$

It is easy to verify that the 99% optimal interval in this clinical trial is empty, which provides support to the hypothesis of lack of consistency across the chosen scenarios. The four scenarios are qualitatively different and a single Holm-based multiplicity adjustment that exhibits optimal or nearly optimal performance under all of these scenarios cannot be constructed.

An alternative method for combining criterion functions across several sets of treatment effect assumptions can be developed based on the compound criteria introduced in Section 1.3.1. The compound criteria, i.e., minimum and average criteria, approach the problem of pooling the disjunctive power functions from a different perspective. The two criteria, denoted by $\psi_M(\lambda)$ and $\psi_A(\lambda)$, respectively, are defined in the context of this optimization problem as follows:

$$\psi_M(\lambda) = \min_{i=1,\dots,4} \psi(\lambda \mid \boldsymbol{\theta}_i),$$

$$\psi_A(\lambda) = \sum_{i=1}^{4} w_i \psi(\lambda \mid \boldsymbol{\theta}_i).$$

The weights in the average criterion reflect the likelihood of each scenario and, for simplicity, it will be assumed that the four scenarios were equally likely, i.e., $w_1 = \dots = w_4 = 1/4$.

The resulting criterion functions are plotted in Figure 1.9. Recall that the four treatment effect scenarios were introduced to capture a progressively shrinking treatment effect in the subpopulation of interest and, consequently,

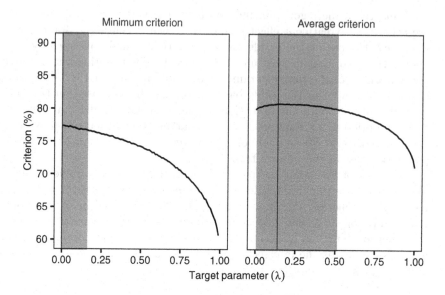

FIGURE 1.9: Minimum and average criteria as functions of the target parameter (λ) with the Holm-based multiplicity adjustment in Case study 1.3. The vertical lines represent the optimal value of the target parameter based on the two criteria and the gray rectangles define the 99% optimal intervals.

in the general trial population. Therefore, it is not surprising that the minimum criterion in the left-hand panel of Figure 1.9 is virtually identical to the criterion evaluated under the scenario with the lowest relative risk reduction in the marker-positive subpopulation (Scenario 4). The criterion in the right-hand panel of this figure is defined as the mean of the four disjunctive criterion functions and its shape resembles that of the disjunctive criterion under Scenario 3.

An optimal value of the target parameter λ can be found based on each of the two criterion functions in a straightforward manner. Using a simple grid search, the minimum criterion was maximized at $\lambda^* = 0$ whereas the optimal value derived under the average criterion was $\lambda^* = 0.14$. This means that, if the trial's sponsor was interested in applying a minimax approach based on the minimum criterion, an optimal Holm procedure would correspond to the lowest possible value of the target parameter. The optimal value of λ under the average criterion was not that extreme but was still quite small.

The last step involves a general characterization of nearly optimal values of λ based on optimal intervals. The 99% optimal intervals for λ^* are shown in Table 1.14. As expected from Figure 1.9, the 99% optimal interval was very tight for the minimum criterion and a wider optimal interval was established based on the average criterion. To summarize the findings presented

TABLE 1.14: Optimal value and 99% optimal interval for the target parameter (λ) based on the minimum and average criteria with the Holm-based multiplicity adjustment in Case study 1.3.

Criterion	Optimal value	99% optimal interval
Minimum criterion	0.00	$(0.00, 0.16)$
Average criterion	0.14	$(0.01, 0.51)$

in Table 1.14, the compound criteria suggest that the initial weight of the subpopulation test should be set to a small value in the Holm procedure.

1.5 Tradeoff-based optimization

This section will focus on optimization problems that utilize tradeoff-based strategies, i.e., deal with determining an optimal balance between competing goals. As in Section 1.4, key components of optimization algorithms defined in Section 1.3 will be illustrated. This includes a careful review of available optimization criteria, optimal selection of a single target parameter under multiple treatment effect scenarios and identification of nearly optimal sets of parameters using optimal intervals. Sensitivity assessments were discussed in detail in Section 1.5 and will not be emphasized in this section.

The general concepts and examples presented in this section will be utilized and expanded in the subsequent chapters. Specifically, tradeoff-based optimization algorithms will be applied to select an optimal multiplicity adjustment in Case study 2.3 and to identify an optimal decision-making approach in multi-population clinical trials in Case study 3.3.

1.5.1 Case study 1.4: Clinical trial with an adaptive design

Tradeoff-based optimization methods will be illustrated using a clinical trial with a simple adaptive design. The case study used in this section is based on a Phase II clinical trial in patients with severe sepsis (Lewis et al., 2013) and also follows a clinical trial example introduced in Dmitrienko et al. (2016). As before, CSE models will be set up for this trial and then the problem of optimal selection of data-driven decision rules in this adaptive trial will be introduced.

Data, analysis and evaluation models

The case study considered in this section is built around an exploratory Phase II trial in the population of patients with severe sepsis. The main goal of this trial is to efficiently characterize the dose-response relationship and support dose selection decisions for the subsequent confirmatory Phase III trial. This clinical trial will be conducted to evaluate the efficacy and safety of three doses of a novel treatment for septic shock versus placebo. Patients in all trial arms will receive the current standard of care for severe sepsis. The three doses will be labelled

- Dose L (low dose).

- Dose M (medium dose).

- Dose H (high dose).

A randomization scheme with an equal allocation of patients to the four trial arms ($n = 100$ patients per arm) will be utilized in this trial.

The primary endpoint in this Phase II trial is the change from baseline to 48 hours in the Sequential Organ Failure Assessment (SOFA) score. This endpoint is approximately normally distributed. This endpoint serves as a surrogate for 28-day all-cause mortality that will be used as the primary endpoint in the subsequent Phase III trial. An adaptive design with a single interim analysis will be utilized in the trial. An early evaluation of the efficacy profile of each dose (treatment effect on the SOFA score) will be performed at the interim look to select the best doses and terminate patient enrollment in underperforming dosing arms.

Based on this information, the data model will include four samples, i.e.,

- Sample 1 includes patients allocated to placebo.

- Sample 2 includes patients allocated to Dose L.

- Sample 3 includes patients allocated to Dose M.

- Sample 4 includes patients allocated to Dose H.

The data model is indexed by a vector of effect sizes in the three treatment arms. The vector of data model parameters is denoted by

$$\boldsymbol{\theta} = (\theta_1, \theta_2, \theta_3),$$

where θ_1 is the assumed effect size at Dose L, i.e., the mean treatment difference between Dose L and placebo divided by the common standard deviation. The effect sizes θ_2 and θ_3 are defined in the same way based on the comparisons between Dose M and placebo, and Dose H and placebo, respectively. No supportive data model parameters will be considered in this setting. The resulting data model is denoted by $D(\boldsymbol{\theta})$.

Using historical information, the trial's sponsor is interested in examining three qualitatively different sets of effect sizes. The assumed sets of effect sizes in the three treatment arms, labeled Scenarios 1, 2 and 3, are defined in Table 1.15. The corresponding vectors of effect sizes will be denoted by

TABLE 1.15: Effect sizes under three scenarios in Case study 1.4.

Comparison	Scenario 1	Scenario 2	Scenario 3
Dose L vs. placebo	$\theta_1 = 0.30$	$\theta_1 = 0$	$\theta_1 = 0$
Dose M vs. placebo	$\theta_2 = 0.35$	$\theta_2 = 0.35$	$\theta_2 = 0$
Dose H vs. placebo	$\theta_3 = 0.40$	$\theta_3 = 0.40$	$\theta_3 = 0.40$

θ_1, θ_2 and θ_3, respectively. In Scenario 1, all three doses of the experimental treatment were assumed to be effective and the treatment effects followed a linear dose-response relationship. The other two scenarios were introduced to study the key characteristics of the adaptive design, namely, its ability to detect the doses with reduced treatment effects at the interim analysis. For example, in Scenario 2 the same pattern of effect sizes at the two higher doses was considered but Dose L was assumed ineffective. The final scenario assumed that only one dose (Dose H) was effective in this trial. The data model based on Scenario 1 will be referred to as the main data model in this clinical trial example.

Continuing to the analysis model in this clinical trial, the first component of the model is the treatment effect test. The tests for the three dose-placebo comparisons will be carried out based on the analysis of covariance with an adjustment for the baseline value of the SOFA score and a continuous score that predicts 28-day mortality based on a set of demographic and clinical characteristics observed at baseline. For the purpose of this optimization exercise, the basic two-sample t-test will be used in the analysis model. No multiplicity adjustment will be employed in this exploratory trial and each dose-placebo test will be carried out at a one-sided $\alpha = 0.025$. Using the total sample size of 400 patients, the probability of establishing a significant treatment effect at one or more doses (disjunctive power) was slightly greater than 90% under the main data model.

The second and more important component of the analysis model is the data-driven decision rule to be applied in this trial. As stated above, a two-stage adaptive design with an interim analysis will be utilized. The interim look will be taken after 200 patients have been enrolled in the trial. Patients in the first stage, i.e., patients with a 48-hour SOFA assessment prior to the interim analysis, will be randomly allocated to all four trial arms. The magnitude of the treatment effect in each dosing arm (Dose L, Dose M and Dose H) compared to placebo will be examined at the interim decision point. A *futility rule* will be applied to ensure that only the most promising doses are retained. Patient enrollment in a dosing arm will discontinue if the observed treatment effect is too small. Note that the trial will be terminated at this decision point if all three doses are dropped due to futility. If at least one dosing arm is retained, patients in the second stage, i.e., patients enrolled after the interim analysis, will be randomly allocated to the remaining dosing arms and placebo.

The futility rule will be defined based on the concept of *predicted probability of success*. Formally, a dosing arm will be dropped at the interim analysis if the appropriately defined predicted probability of success at the final analysis is below a pre-specified threshold. Predicted probability of success can be defined using a frequentist or Bayesian approach and, in this clinical trial example, conditional power (Lan, Simon and Halperin, 1982) will be utilized to define the predicted probability of success. Conditional power will be computed for each dose-placebo comparison and will be defined as the conditional probability of a significant treatment difference between the individual dose and placebo at the final analysis given the interim analysis data. Let n_1 denote the common sample size per trial arm in the first stage and n_2 denote the common sample size per arm in the second stage of the trial. Further, let Z_{i0} and Z_{i1} denote the test statistics for assessing the treatment difference between the ith dose and placebo at the interim and final analyses, respectively (Doses L, M and H are referred to as the first, second and third doses). Conditional power in the ith dosing arm is computed as follows

$$\begin{aligned} \mathrm{CP}_i(\theta) &= P_\delta(Z_{i1} \geq z_{1-\alpha} \mid Z_{i0}) \\ &= \Phi\left(\sqrt{\frac{n_1}{n_2}}Z_{i0} + \sqrt{\frac{n_2}{2}}\theta - \sqrt{\frac{n_1+n_2}{n_2}}z_{1-\alpha}\right), \ i = 1, 2, 3. \end{aligned}$$

Here $z_{1-\alpha}$ is the $(1-\alpha)$-quantile of the standard normal distribution, i.e., $z_{1-\alpha} = 1.96$, and $\Phi(x)$ is the cumulative probability function of the standard normal distribution. The probability is evaluated under the assumption that the true effect size in the selected dosing arm after the interim analysis is equal to θ. Most commonly, θ is set to the sample estimate of the effect size at the interim analysis, i.e., $\hat{\theta}_i$. Using this approach, the futility rule will be met in the ith dosing arm if $\mathrm{CP}_i(\hat{\theta}_i)$ is below a pre-specified threshold denoted by λ $(0 < \lambda < 1)$. In this case, the predicted probability of success will be considered unacceptably low and the ith dosing arm will be dropped.

The parameter of the futility rule (λ) plays a central role in the adaptive design. If a low value of this parameter is chosen, the data-driven decision rule will be overly liberal in the sense that patient enrollment will be discontinued in a dosing arm only if the predicted probability of success is close to 0. With this futility rule, all three doses will be retained most of the time at the interim analysis which will be inconsistent with the goals of the trial. The other extreme is the case where λ is large, which leads to a very conservative futility rule and frequent decisions to terminate the trial. The analysis model with the futility rule based on the threshold set to λ will be denoted by $A(\lambda)$. The trial's sponsor is likely to be interested in finding an optimal value of λ in this analysis model and an optimization problem can be set up with λ serving the role of the target parameter.

A tradeoff-based approach will be applied to set up the criterion for this optimization problem. To motivate this criterion, recall that adaptive designs tend to provide an advantage over traditional designs with a fixed sample size. In particular, adaptive designs may result in improved power if the average sample size (i.e., the expected number of patients enrolled in the trial) is set to the same value as the sample size in the traditional design. On the other hand, an adaptive approach to trial design may require a smaller average sample size to achieve the same level of power as in traditional designs. The goals of maximizing power and minimizing the average sample size are, in fact, competing goals in virtually all adaptive design settings, including the simple adaptive design introduced above. An optimal value of the target parameter λ can be selected by applying a tradeoff-based strategy which is formulated in terms of these two goals.

The following notation will be used to define the optimization criterion in this adaptive trial. Let $\psi_1(\lambda \mid \boldsymbol{\theta})$ and $\psi_2(\lambda \mid \boldsymbol{\theta})$ denote the performance functions associated with the two goals of maximizing power and minimizing the average sample size, respectively. The performance functions depend on the target parameter through the analysis model $A(\lambda)$ and they also depend on the underlying data model $D(\boldsymbol{\theta})$.

The first performance function is defined as

$$\psi_1(\lambda \mid \boldsymbol{\theta}) = 1 - \psi_A(\lambda \mid \boldsymbol{\theta}),$$

where $\psi_A(\lambda \mid \boldsymbol{\theta})$ is an appropriately defined overall probability of success at the final analysis in the adaptive trial. Since multiple dose-placebo contrasts are examined in this trial, it is most sensible to define $\psi_A(\lambda \mid \boldsymbol{\theta})$ as disjunctive power. Therefore, $1 - \psi_A(\lambda \mid \boldsymbol{\theta})$ is equal to the Type II error rate associated with the adaptive design. It can be shown that disjunctive power decreases and the Type II error rate increases with the increasing futility threshold. As a consequence, this performance function is a monotonically increasing function of the target parameter.

The second performance function is defined based on the average number of patients enrolled in the adaptive trial, denoted by $N(\lambda \mid \boldsymbol{\theta})$. In other words,

$$\psi_2(\lambda \mid \boldsymbol{\theta}) = N(\lambda \mid \boldsymbol{\theta}).$$

The average sample size, as was explained above, decreases with λ and thus the second performance function is a monotonically decreasing function of the target parameter. Specifically, with $\lambda = 0$, no futility rule is applied at the interim analysis and the adaptive design simplifies to the traditional design with 100 patients per trial arm. However, if the futility threshold is set to 1, all trial arms will be terminated at the interim look and the average number of enrolled patients per arm will be close to 50 (this number will be greater than 50 due to the patients who have been enrolled in the trial but not included in the interim analysis database).

Figure 1.10 depicts the performance functions $\psi_1(\lambda \mid \boldsymbol{\theta}_1)$ and $\psi_2(\lambda \mid \boldsymbol{\theta}_1)$ over the $[0, 1]$ interval. Note that the vector $\boldsymbol{\theta}_1$ corresponds to Scenario 1 and thus the two functions were evaluated under the main data model. It follows from the figure that the performance functions are, in fact, increasing and decreasing functions of the target parameter λ, respectively. To identify the

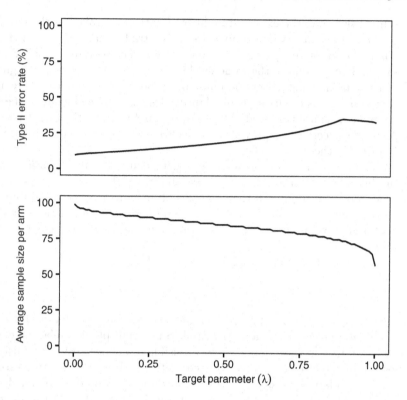

FIGURE 1.10: Performance functions based on the Type II error rate (top panel) and average sample size (bottom panel) in the adaptive design evaluated under the main data model (Scenario 1) in Case study 1.4.

value of λ that strikes a meaningful balance between the increasing Type II error rate and decreasing average number of patients enrolled in the trial, a tradeoff-based optimization criterion needs to be set up.

It was shown in Section 1.3.1 that there are several ways to define a tradeoff-based criterion in a given optimization problem, including additive and bivariate criteria. A additive criterion can be considered as the first candidate for a tradeoff-based criterion in this clinical trial. This criterion focuses on a simple weighted sum of the two performance functions:

$$\psi_{AT}(\lambda \mid \boldsymbol{\theta}) = w\psi_1(\lambda \mid \boldsymbol{\theta}) + (1 - w)\psi_2(\lambda \mid \boldsymbol{\theta}),$$

where w $(0 < w < 1)$ is a pre-defined quantity that determines the importance of the goal of improving power relative to the goal of reducing the average sample size in the adaptive design. If w is set to a smaller value, the additive tradeoff-based criterion will be dominated by the goal of maximizing the average sample size and, if w is close to 1, the goal of maximizing power will play a dominating role. An optimal value of the target parameter λ can be found by maximizing this criterion function over the $[0, 1]$ interval.

While the additive approach to defining a tradeoff-based optimization criterion may seem reasonable at first glance, there are two important considerations that limit its practical applications. The additive criterion implicitly relies on a linear approximation in the sense that it treats power as a linear function of the sample size. A linear approximation may be justified only if a narrow range of sample sizes is considered; however, in general, this approximation is unlikely to be accurate. Further, the additive tradeoff-based criterion is based on two performance functions that are defined on different scales. The first function is related to the probability of success whereas the second function measures the average sample size. With two different scales employed in the criterion, it is difficult to select a relevant value for w and this parameter may be difficult to interpret.

As an alternative to the basic additive tradeoff-based criterion, a bivariate criterion can be considered. This criterion utilizes the following bivariate function:

$$g(x, y) = 1 - x - \psi_T(y),$$

where $\psi_T(y)$ is the overall probability of success at the final analysis, e.g., disjunctive power, in the traditional design with the common sample size per arm set to y. This power function of the traditional design with a fixed sample size serves as a reference function for the adaptive design. The two arguments (x and y) are based on the two performance functions introduced above, i.e.,

$$x = \psi_1(\lambda \mid \boldsymbol{\theta}) \text{ and } y = \psi_2(\lambda \mid \boldsymbol{\theta}).$$

The problem of identifying an optimal value of the target parameter λ is then reduced to the problem of maximizing the bivariate tradeoff-based criterion which is given by

$$\psi_{BT}(\lambda \mid \boldsymbol{\theta}) = g(\psi_1(\lambda \mid \boldsymbol{\theta}), \psi_2(\lambda \mid \boldsymbol{\theta})) = \psi_A(\lambda \mid \boldsymbol{\theta}) - \psi_T(N(\lambda \mid \boldsymbol{\theta})).$$

It immediately follows from this formula that, in this setting, the bivariate tradeoff-based criterion quantifies the power advantage of the adaptive design over the traditional design when the sample size in the traditional design is equal to the expected sample size of the adaptive design. This means that the bivariate criterion admits a simple interpretation and, in addition, this approach to defining optimization criteria does not require a pre-specification of parameters similar to the w parameter in the additive tradeoff-based criterion.

A key consideration related to the choice of an optimization criterion in this setting is related to a multiplicity-based calibration. As stated earlier in this section, no multiplicity adjustment will be applied when the retained doses are compared to placebo at the final analysis. However, when a direct comparison of the power functions of the adaptive and traditional designs is conducted, it is critical to account for the fact that the adaptive design is likely to underperform due to the potentially lower number of doses analyzed at the end of the trial. The number of doses retained at the interim analysis within the adaptive design framework becomes a confounding factor. Indeed, as increasingly more aggressive futility stopping rules with a higher threshold λ are applied, the expected number of doses retained at the interim analysis will decrease. If no multiplicity-based calibration is applied, more dose-placebo tests will be carried out in the traditional design compared to the adaptive design and, since each test is carried out at a one-sided $\alpha = 0.025$, this will result in a higher overall probability of success for the traditional design. More formally, for any vector of effect sizes $\boldsymbol{\theta}$, $\psi_A(\lambda \mid \boldsymbol{\theta})$ will decrease at a much faster rate than $\psi_T(N(\lambda \mid \boldsymbol{\theta}))$ at larger values of λ. As a result, the criterion function $\psi_{BT}(\lambda \mid \boldsymbol{\theta})$ may not be a reliable measure of the power advantage of the adaptive design over the traditional design. A multiplicity-based calibration helps ensure that the two power functions are directly comparable to each other. With a proper multiplicity adjustment, the more dose-placebo tests are carried out at the final analysis, the lower the adjusted significance level used in each dose-placebo test. When this sliding scale is applied, the adaptive design will no longer be penalized for dropping ineffective doses at the interim analysis.

To perform a multiplicity-based calibration, the Dunnett procedure, which is commonly used in clinical trials with several dose-control comparisons, will be utilized. To compute Dunnett-adjusted significance levels, let t_1, t_2 and t_3 denote the test statistics for the comparisons between placebo and Doses L, M and H, respectively, at the final analysis. Since the primary endpoint is normally distributed, under the global null hypothesis of no effect, the test statistics follow a central trivariate t distribution with known pairwise correlations (pairwise correlation are equal to 0.5 in this balanced design). The marginal distribution of each test statistic is the t distribution with $\nu = 2(n-1)$ degrees of freedom, where $n = 100$ is the common sample size in the four trial arms. Without a multiplicity adjustment, each dose is declared statistically significant if the corresponding test statistic exceeds the critical value of this t distribution, e.g., $t_{1-\alpha}(\nu) = 1.97$, where $t_{1-\alpha}(\nu)$ is the $(1-\alpha)$-quantile of the central t distribution with ν degrees of freedom. With a calibration based on the Dunnett procedure, the common critical value is adjusted upward or, in other words, the significance level is adjusted downward. For example, if all three doses are retained at the interim analysis, the adjusted critical value for each test statistic, denoted by $c_{1-\alpha}$, is computed from

$$P(t_1 \geq c_{1-\alpha} \text{ or } t_2 \geq c_{1-\alpha} \text{ or } t_3 \geq c_{1-\alpha}) = \alpha.$$

This adjusted critical value is equal to 2.35 and the corresponding adjusted significance level is 0.0094 (one-sided). Similarly, if two doses are retained at the interim analysis, the adjusted critical value is found using the joint distribution of two test statistics under the global null hypothesis. This results in the adjusted critical value of 2.21 and one-sided significance level of 0.0135. Finally, with a single dose retained at the interim analysis, the one-sided significance level is simply set to 0.025. Depending on the decision made at the interim analysis, the correct significance level for the dose-placebo tests is computed at the final analysis and incorporated into the power function of the adaptive design, i.e., $\psi_A(\lambda \mid \boldsymbol{\theta})$, which is then included in the bivariate tradeoff-based criterion.

1.5.2 Optimal selection of the target parameter

With the optimization criterion defined, an optimal value of the target parameter λ that represents the threshold for the predicted probability of success in the futility rule is easily determined via a univariate grid search. Figure 1.11 plots the bivariate tradeoff-based criterion as a function of the target parameter λ under the pre-defined effect size scenarios. Scenario-specific optimal values of λ were determined by maximizing the corresponding criterion functions (these values are listed in Table 1.16). Figure 1.11 shows that, as ineffective doses were introduced in the data model, the optimal futility thresholds shifted toward 0. However, they were fairly consistent across the three qualitatively different sets of assumptions.

An important pattern is observed in Figure 1.11. Consider first the scenario that corresponds to a linear-dose relationship with no ineffective doses (Scenario 1). In this scenario, the criterion function had a concave shape with the highest value achieved around $\lambda = 0.4$. With the maximum value of the criterion function close to 6%, the optimal adaptive design resulted in a 6% improvement in multiplicity-adjusted disjunctive power compared to the traditional design. This power gain was relatively modest which illustrates a well-known fact that adaptive designs with futility stopping rules are unlikely to provide much improvement over designs with a fixed sample size when the treatment is effective at all dose levels. However, when the scenarios with one or more ineffective doses were examined (Scenarios 2 and 3), there was a considerable increase in the highest value of the criterion function. Figure 1.11 shows that the optimal adaptive design under Scenario 2 provided an 11.3% power gain over the comparable traditional design and, under Scenario 3, this power gain went up to 19.8%. This trend should not be surprising since, with a larger number of ineffective doses in a trial, a futility stopping rule serves as an increasingly efficient filter for underperforming dosing arms. This results in improved performance over traditional designs that do not incorporate an option to select the most promising doses at an interim look.

When reviewing the shapes of the criterion functions in Figure 1.11, it is clear that the curves are far from being smooth. The lack of smoothness is caused by rounding (note that the average sample size in the adaptive design had to be rounded off to support a direct comparison to the traditional design) and, in the presence of rounding, the error margin associated with "point estimates" of the optimal values of λ increases. In this context, it is sensible to put more emphasis on the values of the target parameter that are very likely to be declared optimal. The 99% optimal intervals for the optimal value of λ were first computed in this optimization problem but they turned

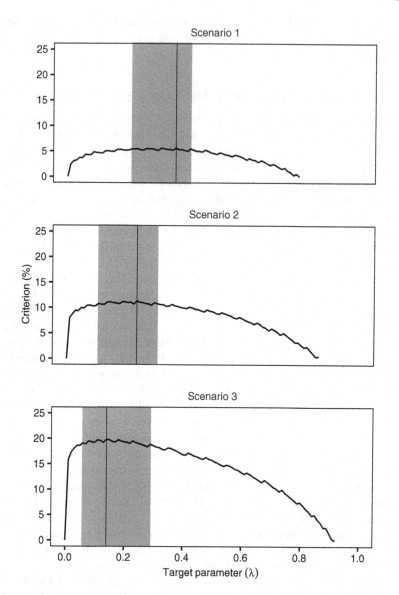

FIGURE 1.11: Bivariate criterion as a function of the target parameter λ under the three scenarios in Case study 1.4. The vertical lines represent the optimal values of the target parameter for each scenario and the gray rectangles define the 95% optimal intervals.

out to be very tight and virtually non-informative. For this reason, Table 1.16 presents the 95% optimal intervals for λ^* based on the three sets of effect sizes.

TABLE 1.16: Optimal value and optimal intervals for the target parameter (λ) based on the bivariate tradeoff-based criterion under the three pre-defined scenarios in Case study 1.4.

Scenario	Optimal value	95% optimal interval
Scenario 1	0.37	$(0.22, 0.42)$
Scenario 2	0.24	$(0.11, 0.31)$
Scenario 3	0.14	$(0.06, 0.29)$

As shown in Table 1.16, the 95% optimal intervals for the optimal futility threshold were also fairly narrow. Given the uncertainty around the true values of the treatment effects at the three doses examined in this trial, it will be ideal from the sponsor's perspective to identify a futility rule which is optimal or nearly optimal under the three scenarios of interest. To accomplish this, a joint optimal interval was derived by taking the intersection of the optimal values presented in Table 1.16. The 95% joint optimal interval was equal to

$$I_{0.95} = (0.22, 0.29).$$

If a futility rule is defined based on a threshold selected from this interval, the resulting adaptive design will be close to optimal across the three effect size scenarios. For the sake of example, the mid-point of the joint interval, i.e., $\lambda = 0.25$, serves as a robust choice for the target parameter in this optimization problem.

This section has focused mostly on the derivation and application of tradeoff-based criteria in optimization problems with competing goals. It is helpful to mention other important components of the optimization exercise that need to be considered by the trial's sponsor. The sponsor can explore, for example, compound criteria similar to those discussed in Section 1.4 to find robust solutions to the optimization problem considered in this clinical trial. Further, it has been emphasized multiple times throughout this chapter that sensitivity assessments are an integral part of any optimization exercise. Note that a qualitative assessment based on three realistic sets of treatment effects has been incorporated into the optimization algorithm. In addition, it will be informative to perform a series of perturbation-based quantitative assessments under one of the data models, e.g., the main data model. These assessments will support a comprehensive evaluation of the robustness of the adaptive design based on the optimal value of the futility threshold identified above.

2

Clinical Trials with Multiple Objectives

Alex Dmitrienko

Mediana Inc.

Gautier Paux

Institut de Recherches Internationales Servier

2.1 Introduction

It is very common to evaluate multiple clinical objectives in clinical trials, especially in confirmatory Phase III trials. In a confirmatory setting, trial sponsors are often interested in pursuing a number of regulatory claims for experimental treatments that reflect their effects on several clinical endpoints or in multiple patient populations. In a traditional setting, the individual clinical objectives may represent the same source of multiplicity, e.g., in a clinical trial with a single primary endpoint multiplicity may be induced by the analysis of several dose-placebo comparisons. More challenging multiplicity problems arise in clinical trials where combinations of two or more sources of multiplicity are examined, e.g., the efficacy profile of an experimental treatment may be evaluated at several different dose levels with respect to the primary and a few secondary endpoints. An assessment of "multivariate" objectives of this kind enables sponsors to better differentiate novel treatments from available treatments and enrich the product labels.

The main regulatory requirement in trials with complex clinical objectives is strict control of the overall Type I error rate across all key objectives, including objectives based on secondary endpoints or secondary tests that may be included in the product label. The importance of pre-defining statistical methods for addressing potential Type I error rate inflation in confirmatory trials is emphasized in regulatory documents, including the guidance on multiplicity issues in clinical trials published by the European Medicines Agency (EMA, 2002; EMA, 2017) and draft guidance on multiple endpoints in clinical trials released by the U.S. Food and Drug Administration (FDA, 2017). The recently published FDA and EMA guidance documents discussed the issues of error rate control in traditional settings as well as more advanced settings where a confirmatory trial is designed to pursue multiple hierarchically ordered clinical objectives.

Methodological advances in the field of multiple comparisons have led to the development of powerful multiplicity adjustment strategies aimed at protecting the overall Type I error rate in traditional settings with a single source of multiplicity and more advanced settings with several multiplicity dimensions. A detailed review of the underlying theory and commonly used multiplicity adjustments can be found in Dmitrienko, Tamhane and Bretz (2009) as well as recently published review papers on multiplicity issues in clinical drug development, including Dmitrienko, D'Agostino and Huque (2013), Dmitrienko and D'Agostino (2013), Alosh, Bretz and Huque (2014) and Wang et al. (2015). Statistical methods utilized in advanced multiplicity problems, known as gatekeeping procedures, have been discussed in Dmitrienko and Tamhane, (2011, 2013) and Dmitrienko, Kordzakhia and Brechenmacher (2016).

From the sponsor's perspective, it is important to identify efficient multiplicity adjustments with the ultimate goal of maximizing the probability of success in a single trial or development program. It is therefore critical to carefully evaluate the applicable multiplicity adjustment strategies and perform a comprehensive assessment of their operating characteristics under trial-specific assumptions. These assessments can be facilitated using the general Clinical Scenario Evaluation (CSE) techniques presented in this book. A broader application of CSE-based review of available options will help extend the current standards for addressing multiplicity issues in confirmatory trials. For instance, it is still very common to apply basic corrections for multiplicity such as Bonferroni-based corrections that may result in reduced probability of success.

CSE-based approaches to systematic and quantitative evaluation of candidate multiplicity adjustment strategies in traditional and advanced settings will be investigated in this chapter. The CSE framework introduced in Chapter 1 will be employed to develop easy-to-implement clinical trial optimization strategies. These strategies focus on selection of optimal methods for addressing multiplicity that are robust against possible deviations from the statistical assumptions made in a trial.

The general CSE framework in the context of trials with multiple clinical objectives will be defined in Section 2.2. The overview of key CSE considerations will be followed by three case studies that focus on optimization problems arising in trials with several dose-placebo comparisons and clinical endpoints; see Sections 2.3, 2.4 and 2.5. R code based on the **Mediana** package will be included at the end of each case study to provide software implementation of CSE-based assessments in each case study. See Chapter 1 for more information on this R package.

2.2   Clinical Scenario Evaluation framework

The CSE principles defined in Chapter 1 will be utilized in this chapter to support a quantitative approach to selecting the most efficient and robust multiplicity adjustments in clinical trials with complex objectives. To apply the key principles, the following three components will need to be explicitly defined:

- Data models define the mechanism for generating patient data in a clinical trial or across several trials within a development program. The key and supportive parameters of the data model such as the expected treatment effects or correlations among the test statistics corresponding to the multiple objectives need to be specified.

- Analysis models define the statistical tests for assessing the treatment effect in the trial as well as multiplicity adjustment procedures.

- Evaluation models define the criteria to be applied to the selected analysis models. The criteria represent different definitions of "success" based on the analysis of individual objectives in a clinical trial. When selecting the evaluation criteria, it is critical to ensure that they are fully aligned with the clinical objectives of the trial.

A detailed review of the individual components of this general framework in the context of clinical trials with multiple objectives will be provided in Sections 2.2.1, 2.2.2 and 2.2.3.

The CSE framework supports a broad range of practical approaches to clinical trial optimization. Commonly used optimization strategies will be illustrated in this chapter. This includes the more straightforward direct optimization algorithms based on a univariate or multivariate grid search as well as more advanced tradeoff-based optimization algorithms aimed at determining an optimal balance between two conflicting goals in a clinical trial (see Chapter 1 for more information on optimization strategies). Optimization algorithms will be applied to choose the most efficient adjustment from the set of candidate adjustments and optimal parameters of the selected multiplicity adjustment will be identified.

An additional important consideration that will be emphasized throughout this chapter deals with robustness of the resulting optimal multiplicity adjustments. For example, Case study 2.1 will focus on the problem of identifying the most efficient multiplicity adjustment in a clinical trial with several dose-placebo comparisons that is also robust with respect to possible deviations from the hypothesized data model. Robustness will be assessed by carrying out a series of "stress tests" that rely on qualitative and quantitative sensitivity assessments (common approaches to performing sensitivity assessments were discussed in Chapter 1).

2.2.1   Data models

A variety of different data models arise in clinical trials with several clinical objectives to define data generation mechanisms for the individual sources of multiplicity. The models are characterized by the structure of samples, i.e., independent groups of patients, and distributions of the outcome variables, i.e., clinical endpoints.

Beginning with clinical trials with one primary endpoint, a single sample is defined for each trial arm and a univariate outcome distribution is specified. As an example, consider the data model in Case study 2.1 which is set up for a clinical trial with three trial arms (placebo and two doses of an experimental treatment) and a single endpoint. In this case, three samples included in this data model directly correspond to the three arms.

This approach is easily extended to settings with several endpoints that are measured on the same patient. Case studies 2.2 and 2.3 provide an example of a clinical trial with three trial arms (placebo and two doses of a novel treatment) and two clinical endpoints (primary endpoint and key secondary endpoint). Again, three samples based on the three trial arms need to be defined and a bivariate distribution needs to be specified for each patient's outcome.

2.2.2   Analysis models

Analysis models used in this setting are similar to those utilized in other clinical trial settings in that they include a specification of statistical methods for evaluating the treatment effect. A unique feature of analysis models arising in trials with multiple objectives is that several candidate procedures for performing multiplicity adjustments are often incorporated into the model and an optimal analysis model is built by identifying the most efficient multiplicity adjustment method. This section provides a high-level survey of commonly used multiple testing procedures for traditional and advanced multiplicity problems.

Multiplicity problems

To set the stage for a discussion of multiplicity adjustments, it is helpful to begin with a classification of multiplicity problems encountered in clinical trials and define key concepts such as the concept of strong Type I error rate control.

Consider a problem of testing m null hypotheses in a trial with a simple set of clinical objectives. The hypotheses, denoted by $H_1, \ldots, H_m$, correspond to several assessments of an experimental treatment compared to control. The assessments may be based on multiple endpoints or multiple dose-control contrasts. The hypothesis H_i is defined using a treatment parameter denoted by θ_i with a larger value of θ_i corresponding to a beneficial treatment effect, i.e.,

$$H_i : \ \theta_i \leq \delta_i, \ i = 1, \ldots, m.$$

Here δ_i is a pre-specified constant that defines a clinically relevant threshold. It is worth noting that this formulation of a hypothesis testing problem covers both superiority and non-inferiority testing strategies (non-inferiority tests correspond to negative values of $\delta_1, \ldots, \delta_m$). The null hypotheses are tested versus the one-sided alternatives given by

$$K_i : \ \theta_i > \delta_i, \ i = 1, \ldots, m.$$

As an example, the null hypotheses of no effect are defined in Case study 2.1 in terms of two dose-placebo comparisons. The treatment parameters are the mean treatment differences and the thresholds are set to 0, i.e., $\delta_1 = \delta_2 = 0$.

The marginal p-values for testing the null hypotheses are denoted by $p_1, \ldots, p_m$. In addition, let $p_{(1)} < \ldots < p_{(m)}$ denote the ordered p-values, i.e., $p_{(1)}$ denotes the most significant p-value in the family and $p_{(m)}$ denotes the least significant p-value. The corresponding ordered hypotheses will be denoted by $H_{(1)}, \ldots, H_{(m)}$.

It is well known that the probability of one or more incorrect conclusions is inflated when multiple null hypotheses are tested in a clinical trial. Control of the appropriately defined error rate is mandated in confirmatory Phase III trials and it is the sponsor's responsibility to identify a correction for multiplicity to protect the overall Type I error rate at a nominal level, e.g., at a one-sided $\alpha = 0.025$. The Type I error rate or, more formally, *familywise error rate*, is to be controlled in the strong sense, which means that the probability of erroneously rejecting any true null hypothesis in the family of hypotheses must be less than or equal to the pre-defined α level regardless of the actual subset of the true null hypotheses. Strong familywise error rate control streamlines the formulation of regulatory claims since the probability of incorrectly making a regulatory claim is preserved for any set of clinical objectives.

The problem defined above is often referred to as a traditional multiplicity problem with a *single source of multiplicity* since there is no underlying hierarchical structure in this problem and the hypotheses can be thought of as belonging to the same family. As pointed out in the introduction, hierarchically ordered objectives play an increasingly more important role in confirmatory clinical trials. The objectives are associated with the evaluation of multiple aspects of the treatment's effect, e.g., assessments based on primary and secondary endpoints that are performed simultaneously with assessments in multiple patient populations. In the presence of ordered clinical objectives, multiple families of null hypotheses are defined to account for the underlying hierarchical structure of the objectives. For example, the first family may contain null hypotheses of no effect based on the primary endpoint and other families may be set up based on supportive endpoints such as secondary and tertiary endpoints. The resulting multiplicity problems are characterized by having *several sources of multiplicity* and will be referred to as advanced multiplicity problems throughout this chapter.

TABLE 2.1: Classification of commonly used multiple testing procedures in traditional multiplicity problems.

Distributional information	Logical restrictions	
	Data-driven testing sequence	Pre-specified testing sequence
Nonparametric procedures	Holm	Fixed-sequence
	Nonparametric chain procedures	
Semiparametric procedures	Hochberg Hommel	No procedures
Parametric procedures	Dunnett	
	Parametric chain procedures	

Multiplicity adjustments in advanced problems will be discussed in Case studies 2.2 and 2.3 using a clinical trial with two ordered clinical endpoints (primary endpoint and key secondary endpoint). The analysis of these endpoints defines the first source of multiplicity and the other source of multiplicity is induced by two dose-placebo tests that are carried out for each endpoint.

When advanced multiplicity problems with several families of null hypotheses are considered, the definition of strong familywise error rate control is naturally extended to cover all families of hypotheses and can be thought of as global familywise error rate control which needs to be contrasted with error rate control within each individual family.

Classification of multiple testing procedures

Numerous multiple testing procedures have been developed in the literature to correct for multiplicity in traditional and advanced settings. This section provides a summary of key features of multiple testing procedures that help define a useful classification scheme. The classification scheme will be formulated for multiplicity adjustments used in a traditional setting with a single source of multiplicity and can be extended to procedures designed for advanced settings with several sources of multiplicity, known as *gatekeeping procedures*. A detailed review of the commonly used multiple testing procedures will be provided below.

The classification scheme is presented in Table 2.1. When considering available options for multiplicity corrections in a given problem, it is critical to assess the amount of available clinical information, i.e., information on logical restrictions among the hypotheses of interest, and statistical information, i.e., information on the joint distribution of the hypothesis test statistics.

Beginning with the discussion of logical restrictions, it is important to differentiate between the cases where the hypotheses are ordered based on clinical or regulatory considerations and cases where the hypotheses are interchangeable. In the former case, multiple testing procedures that examine the null hypotheses according to the pre-defined ordering need to be considered. If the latter case holds, procedures that support a data-driven hypothesis ordering are to be chosen. With a data-driven ordering, hypotheses are tested in the order determined by the significance of the test statistics. Table 2.1 gives examples of multiple testing procedures that utilize a pre-defined or data-driven testing sequence. Note that two classes of multiple testing procedures span over the two columns in the table (nonparametric and parametric chain procedures). This is due to the fact that most procedures in these classes can be constructed using algorithms with a data-dependent testing sequence as well as a pre-specified testing sequence.

Using the multiplicity problem with two dose-placebo comparisons from Case study 2.1 as an example, if limited information on the dose-response relationship is available, it may not be clear how to arrange the comparisons and associated null hypotheses in a logical way. In this case, it will be difficult to justify the use of the fixed-sequence or similar procedures that rely on a pre-specified testing sequence, i.e., the treatment effect at the high dose is tested first followed by the test of the treatment effect at the low dose. The most sensible strategy will be to set up a multiplicity adjustment based on a procedure with a data-driven testing sequence, e.g., the Holm procedure that first examines the null hypothesis associated with the most significant treatment effect p-value.

Distributional information also plays an important role in the selection of most appropriate multiplicity adjustments in a given problem. Three classes of multiple testing procedures that make different assumptions about the joint distribution of the hypothesis test statistics are shown in Table 2.1. Nonparametric procedures are basic p-value-based procedures that impose no distributional assumptions, which results in power loss. Despite their limitations, nonparametric multiple testing procedures are surprisingly popular in clinical trials. Examples of simplistic multiplicity adjustments based on nonparametric methods are given in Chapter 1, including the enzalutamide trial in metastatic prostate cancer (Beer et al., 2014). By contrast, semiparametric procedures are also set up using marginal p-values but gain efficiency by making additional assumptions on the joint distribution. Finally, parametric procedures protect the familywise error rate only under specific distributional assumptions.

In what follows, key ideas behind nonparametric, semiparametric and parametric procedures arising in traditional multiplicity problems as well as gatekeeping procedures used in advanced multiplicity problems will be introduced. For a detailed description of the underlying testing algorithms; see Dmitrienko, D'Agostino and Huque (2013) and Dmitrienko and D'Agostino (2013).

Nonparametric multiple testing procedures

When considering nonparametric multiple testing procedures, it is useful to focus on a class of nonparametric *chain* procedures. This class includes a large number of popular methods for multiplicity adjustment, including the fixed-sequence and Holm procedures, that are ultimately derived from the Bonferroni procedure. Most chain procedures utilize flexible decision rules that are formalized as α-*allocation* and α-*propagation* rules. The first rule defines the process of distributing the overall Type I error rate among the null hypotheses of interest and the second rule governs the process of updating the hypothesis weights during the testing process. An α-propagation rule hinges upon the "use it or lose it" principle (Dmitrienko, Wiens and Tamhane, 2008) which states that, after a hypothesis is rejected, the fraction of the overall error rate assigned to this hypothesis can be "recycled" by splitting it among the remaining non-rejected hypotheses.

To illustrate the concepts of α-allocation and α-propagation, consider a problem of testing three null hypotheses denoted by H_1, H_2 and H_3. These hypotheses may represent the null hypotheses of no effect in a clinical trial with three doses of a novel treatment compared to placebo. Some of the hypotheses may be more important than the others and the relative importance of the individual hypotheses can be taken into account by assigning hypothesis weights denoted by w_1, w_2 and w_3. The weights are non-negative and sum to 1. The hypothesis weights are defined by the α-allocation rule specified by the trial's sponsor.

The α-propagation rule describes the process of re-distributing the available error rate among the non-rejected hypotheses after each rejection. This rule specifies the *transition parameters* that are denoted by g_{ij}, $i, j = 1, 2, 3$. The parameter g_{ij} defines the fraction of the error rate which is carried over from the hypothesis H_i to the hypothesis H_j after H_i is rejected. It is not meaningful to apply any fraction of the error rate back to the hypothesis that has been rejected and thus $g_{ii} = 0$, $i = 1, 2, 3$. The transition parameters are typically organized in a matrix format. In this multiplicity problem, a 3×3 transition matrix is defined as follows

$$T = \begin{bmatrix} 0 & g_{12} & g_{13} \\ g_{21} & 0 & g_{23} \\ g_{31} & g_{32} & 0 \end{bmatrix}.$$

The transition parameters are non-negative and the sum of the parameters in each row does not exceed 1, i.e.,

$$g_{i1} + g_{i2} + g_{i3} \leq 1, \ i = 1, 2, 3.$$

If the row sums in a transition matrix are all equal to 1, the chain procedure is known as an α-*exhaustive procedure* because all of the error rate "released" after a rejection is transferred to the non-rejected hypotheses. Note that the transition parameters are also updated after each rejection.

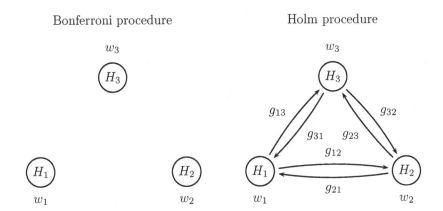

FIGURE 2.1: Decision rules used in the Bonferroni and Holm procedures.

Figure 2.1 presents two diagrams that visualize the α-allocation and α-propagation rules for two popular multiple testing procedures (Bonferroni and Holm procedures). Each hypothesis is represented by a circle and the value next to each circle defines the initial weight assigned to this hypothesis according to the α-allocation rule. The connections between the hypotheses are governed by the α-propagation strategy and visualize the process of re-distributing the error rate after each rejection.

As shown in the figure, the two multiple testing procedures utilize the same α-allocation strategy, i.e., a general set of potentially unequal hypothesis weights is considered and the procedure-specific vectors of initial weights are denoted by

$$W_B = [w_1 \; w_2 \; w_3], \; W_H = [w_1 \; w_2 \; w_3].$$

A trivial α-propagation rule is used in the Bonferroni procedure. With the Bonferroni-based multiplicity adjustment, each hypothesis is tested independently of the other hypotheses using the weight vector W_B. This means that the hypothesis H_i is rejected if $p_i \leq \alpha w_i$, $i = 1, 2, 3$. No α propagation is applied in the sense that $g_{ij} = 0$, $i, j = 1, 2, 3$, in the transition matrix T_B and this is why the hypotheses in the left-hand panel of Figure 2.1 are not connected to each other.

Lack of α propagation leads to an overly conservative multiplicity adjustment and, by contrast, the Holm procedure shown in the right-hand panel of Figure 2.1 serves as an example of a procedure that efficiently utilizes α propagation. Suppose that the transition matrix used in this procedure is given by

$$T_H = \begin{bmatrix} 0 & 0.5 & 0.5 \\ 0.5 & 0 & 0.5 \\ 0.5 & 0.5 & 0 \end{bmatrix}.$$

It is easy to verify that all row sums in the matrix are equal to 1 and thus this Holm procedure is an α-exhaustive procedure.

It is informative to quickly compare the rejection rules employed by the two procedures defined in Figure 2.1. Consider a testing algorithm that begins with the hypothesis H_1. As stated above, this hypothesis is rejected by the Bonferroni if $p_1 \leq \alpha w_1$. The same rejection rule is used by the Holm; however, unlike the Bonferroni, this procedure supports α-propagation. Specifically, after H_1 is rejected, the significance level utilized in this test, i.e., αw_1, is distributed between the other two hypotheses according to the transition matrix T_H. Since $g_{12} = 0.5$ and $g_{13} = 0.5$, the updated weights of H_2 and H_3 are equal to

$$w_2 + 0.5w_1 \text{ and } w_3 + 0.5w_1,$$

respectively. If H_2 is the next hypothesis in the testing sequence, it will be rejected if $p_2 \leq \alpha(w_2 + 0.5w_1)$. With this and any other efficient chain procedure, the hypotheses are re-weighted after each rejection and, in fact, the weight of H_3 will be updated again if the test of H_2 is significant.

Figure 2.1 gives examples of fairly basic nonparametric chain procedures. Chain procedures with more complex α-propagation rules will be introduced in Case study 2.2. Also, as pointed out in Table 2.1, chain procedures can be constructed using testing algorithms with a pre-specified or data-driven testing sequence.

Three procedures from the class of nonparametric multiple testing procedures will be examined in detail later in this chapter as well as in Chapter 3, namely, the Bonferroni, fixed-sequence and Holm procedures. Therefore, it is helpful to explicitly define the testing algorithms used in these procedures. Consider, as before, a multiplicity problem with m null hypotheses and let $w_1, \ldots, w_m$ denote the hypothesis-specific weights. As shown above, the Bonferroni procedure utilizes a very basic set of rejection rules, i.e.,

$$\text{Reject } H_i \text{ if } p_i \leq \alpha w_i, \ i = 1, \ldots, m.$$

The fixed-sequence procedure relies on a *sequentially rejective algorithm* with a pre-specified hypothesis ordering. The hypotheses H_1 through H_m are tested sequentially beginning with H_1 and a hypothesis is rejected if its test and the tests for the hypotheses placed earlier in the sequence are all significant at the α level. In other words, the following stepwise algorithm is utilized in the fixed-sequence procedure:

- Step 1. Reject H_1 if $p_1 \leq \alpha$. If H_1 is rejected, continue to the next step. Otherwise, accept all hypotheses.

- Step 2. Reject H_2 if $p_2 \leq \alpha$. If H_2 is rejected, continue to the next step. Otherwise, accept the hypotheses H_2 through H_m.

- Step i ($i = 3, \ldots, m-1$). Reject H_i if $p_i \leq \alpha$. If H_i is rejected, continue to the next step. Otherwise, accept the hypotheses H_i through H_m.

- Step m. Reject H_m if $p_m \leq \alpha$.

The Holm procedure utilizes a *step-down algorithm*, which is a sequentially rejective algorithm with a data-driven testing sequence that begins with the hypothesis corresponding to the most significant p-value. To define the algorithm, assume that the hypothesis weights are all positive and consider the ordered p-values ($p_{(1)} < \ldots < p_{(m)}$), ordered hypotheses ($H_{(1)}, \ldots, H_{(m)}$) and ordered hypothesis weights ($w_{(1)}, \ldots, w_{(m)}$). Also, let

$$v_i = w_{(i)} + \ldots + w_{(m)}, \ i = 1, \ldots, m.$$

The Holm procedure uses the following stepwise algorithm:

- Step 1. Reject $H_{(1)}$ if $p_{(1)} \leq \alpha w_{(1)}/v_1 = \alpha w_{(1)}$. If $H_{(1)}$ is rejected, continue to the next step. Otherwise, accept all hypotheses.

- Step 2. Reject $H_{(2)}$ if $p_{(2)} \leq \alpha w_{(2)}/v_2$. If $H_{(2)}$ is rejected, continue to the next step. Otherwise, accept the hypotheses $H_{(2)}$ through $H_{(m)}$.

- Step i ($i = 3, \ldots, m-1$). Reject $H_{(i)}$ if $p_{(i)} \leq \alpha w_{(i)}/v_i$. If $H_{(i)}$ is rejected, continue to the next step. Otherwise, accept the hypotheses $H_{(i)}$ through $H_{(m)}$.

- Step m. Reject $H_{(m)}$ if $p_{(m)} \leq \alpha w_{(m)}/v_m = \alpha$.

This testing algorithm is easily extended to the case where some of the hypothesis weights are set to 0.

Semiparametric multiple testing procedures

An important feature of the class of chain procedures introduced above is that they represent extensions of the Bonferroni procedure, which implies that, just like the basic Bonferroni procedure, they cannot utilize available information on the distribution of the hypothesis test statistics in a multiplicity problem. More efficient multiplicity adjustments can be set up by incorporating distributional information. Multiple testing procedures derived from the Simes test serve as examples of more powerful procedures that impose fairly flexible distributional assumptions on the hypothesis test statistics. For this reason, they are known as semiparametric procedures.

The class of semiparametric procedures contains several procedures, the most well known of which are the Hochberg and Hommel procedures. Consider again a multiplicity problem with m hypotheses that may be unequally important and assume that all hypothesis weights are positive. The Hochberg procedure uses a *step-up algorithm* that examines the ordered p-values beginning with the least significant p-value, i.e.,

- Step 1. Reject all hypotheses if $p_{(m)} \leq \alpha w_{(m)}/v_m = \alpha$. If this condition is not satisfied, accept the hypothesis $H_{(m)}$ and continue to the next step.

- Step 2. Reject the hypotheses $H_{(1)}$ through $H_{(m-1)}$ if $p_{(m-1)} \leq \alpha w_{(m-1)}/v_{m-1}$. If this condition is not satisfied, accept the hypothesis $H_{(m-1)}$ and continue to the next step.

- Step i ($i = 3, \ldots, m-1$). Reject the hypotheses $H_{(1)}$ through $H_{(m-i+1)}$ if $p_{(m-i+1)} \leq \alpha w_{(m-i+1)}/v_{m-i+1}$. If this condition is not satisfied, accept the hypothesis $H_{(m-i+1)}$ and continue to the next step.

- Step m. $H_{(1)}$ is rejected if $p_{(1)} \leq \alpha w_{(1)}/v_1 = \alpha w_{(1)}$.

As before, the stepwise testing algorithm utilized by the Hochberg procedure can be extended to the case where some of the hypothesis weights are set to 0. The Hommel procedure relies on a conceptually similar step-up testing algorithm.

Multiplicity adjustments based on semiparametric procedures are known to be uniformly more powerful than those based on nonparametric procedures. For example, the Hochberg procedure is uniformly more powerful than the Holm procedure. This means that, for any hypothesis in a multiplicity problem, the probability of rejection by the Hochberg is no less and may be strictly greater than the probability of rejection by the Holm. Further, the Hommel procedure is uniformly more powerful than the Hochberg procedure and the two procedures are identical to each other in multiplicity problems with two null hypotheses.

Since semiparametric procedures are derived from the Simes test, they may not always protect the familywise error rate. The issue of potential error rate inflation for Simes-based procedures, including the Hochberg and Hommel procedures, has been studied in Sarkar and Chang (1997), Sarkar (1998) and Sarkar (2008). It has been shown that these procedures do, in fact, provide error rate control if the hypothesis test statistics follow a multivariate normal distribution with non-negative pairwise correlation coefficients. This assumption is quite flexible and is met in a large number of clinical trial settings. Examples include multiplicity problems in trials with several dose-placebo comparisons considered in Case studies 2.1 and 2.2 as well as trials with one or more pre-defined patient subgroups considered in Case study 3.1.

Parametric multiple testing procedures

Multiple testing procedures in this class, which includes the Dunnett and related procedures, can be utilized in multiplicity problems with a known joint distribution of the hypothesis test statistics. Parametric procedures are more powerful than their nonparametric or semiparametric counterparts and, for this reason, have found numerous applications in clinical trials.

To define a general multiplicity adjustment framework based on a parametric approach, consider a problem of testing the null hypotheses $H_1, \ldots, H_m$ and let $t_1, \ldots, t_m$ denote the hypothesis test statistics. Suppose that the joint distribution of these statistics is known in advance, e.g., they follow a multivariate t or normal distribution as in trials with several doses of an experimental treatment compared to a common control. Multiplicity adjustments can be derived directly from this joint distribution under the global null hypothesis, i.e., under the assumption that all m hypotheses are simultaneously true. The basic Dunnett procedure, for example, is defined by computing a common adjusted significance value for the test statistics. This value, denoted by c, is computed from

$$P(t_1 \geq c \text{ or } \ldots \text{ or } t_m \geq c) = \alpha,$$

where, as stated above, the probability is evaluated under the global null hypothesis. The Dunnett procedure rejects the hypothesis H_i if $t_i \geq c$, $i = 1, \ldots, m$. The resulting parametric procedure is uniformly more powerful than the Bonferroni procedure.

This simple parametric approach to setting up a multiplicity adjustment has been generalized in a number of directions. First of all, hypothesis weights are easily incorporated into the decision rules of parametric procedures. Further, just as the basic Dunnett procedure can be viewed as a parametric extension of the Bonferroni, Dunnett-type multiplicity adjustments have been defined based on step-down and step-up testing algorithms. These parametric procedures can be thought of as extensions of the Holm and Hochberg procedures, respectively. A parametric approach can also be applied to extend the class of Bonferroni-based chain procedures to set up parametric chain procedures for multiplicity problems where the joint distribution of the hypothesis test statistics is known at the trial's design stage.

Comparison of multiple testing procedures

From a practitioner's point of view, it is helpful to formulate guidelines for selecting most appropriate multiplicity adjustments for a given trial with several clinical objectives. General guidelines of this kind were presented, for example, in Dmitrienko and D'Agostino (2013). To provide a concise summary of the recommendations, nonparametric multiple testing procedures can be applied in any multiplicity problem but tend to be rather conservative, which leads to power loss. Parametric procedures, on the other hand, offer the most powerful approach to multiplicity adjustment but impose restrictive assumptions on the joint distribution of the hypothesis test statistics. Semiparametric procedures strike a balance between the two extremes in the sense that they are quite efficient and, at the same time, they are not overly sensitive to distributional assumptions.

As an illustration, consider a clinical trial conducted to evaluate the efficacy of several doses of a novel treatment versus a common control. The key advantage of parametric multiple testing procedures is that they lead to more powerful inferences compared to nonparametric and semiparametric procedures if the joint distribution of the test statistics in a multiplicity problem is specified, e.g., the test statistics follow a multivariate normal distribution with known pairwise correlations. This assumption is justified in this clinical trial, e.g., if the trial design is balanced and every patient completes the trial, the pairwise correlation coefficients are all equal to 0.5. However, if there are missing observations with a complex missingness pattern, it may be challenging or even impossible to compute the exact values of the pairwise correlations. In this case, adjusted significance levels of a parametric procedure cannot be computed and the trial's sponsor will need to consider a multiplicity adjustment based on a nonparametric or semiparametric procedure. With a semiparametric approach, familywise error rate control is guaranteed in a multivariate normal setting as long as the pairwise correlations are non-negative. It can be shown that in trials with several dose-control comparisons these correlation coefficients are indeed non-negative regardless of the missingness pattern. Semiparametric multiple testing procedures such as the Hommel procedure can then be considered as "robust" alternatives to powerful but potentially inflexible parametric procedures.

Gatekeeping procedures

The three classes of multiple testing procedures (nonparametric, semiparametric and fully parametric) described above were originally developed for a traditional setting with a single source of multiplicity or, more formally, with a single family of null hypotheses of no effect. Most of these procedures can be extended to define more sophisticated adjustments for advanced multiplicity problems where the hypotheses of interest are grouped into two or more families. These complex problems arise in clinical trials with ordered multiple objectives, e.g., clinical trials with primary and key secondary endpoints evaluated in several patient populations. The resulting procedures are commonly referred to as gatekeeping procedures.

A key requirement for gatekeeping procedures is that they should protect the familywise error rate not only within each family of hypotheses but also across the families. In addition, gatekeeping procedures are expected to efficiently incorporate the hierarchical structure of the families, i.e., account for the fact that some families are more important than the others and a family can serve as a gatekeeper for other families. Several classes of gatekeeping procedures have been developed in the literature to accommodate different types of gatekeepers. This includes procedures that support *serial gatekeepers*, *parallel gatekeepers* and *general gatekeepers*. Within the general gatekeeping framework, arbitrary logical relationships among the families can be taken into account when setting up a procedure.

A flexible method for constructing gatekeeping procedures that support general logical relationships, known as the *mixture method*, has found multiple applications in clinical trials with ordered objectives. This includes an important class of trials that are conducted to assess the effect of several doses of an experimental treatment on a single primary endpoint and several key secondary endpoints. A clinically relevant restriction imposed in these trials prevents the sponsor from claiming a significant treatment effect on an endpoint if the effect at the same dose on a higher-ranked endpoint is not significant. This means that, if the null hypothesis related to one endpoint cannot be rejected, the hypotheses associated with the less important endpoints are accepted without testing. Mixture-based gatekeeping procedures enable the trial's sponsor to build multiplicity adjustments in this and similar settings using *component procedures* such as Hochberg or Hommel procedures that are more powerful than basic Bonferroni-based procedures. For example, efficient Hochberg- and Hommel-based gatekeeping procedures were successfully used to handle several sources of multiplicity in Phase III lurasidone trials for the treatment of schizophrenia (Meltzer et al., 2011; Nasrallah et al., 2013). Another important advantage of mixture-based gatekeeping procedures is that they may be implemented using stepwise testing algorithms similar to those utilized in chain procedures. An example of a mixture-based gatekeeping procedure with a stepwise testing algorithm is provided in Case study 2.3.

2.2.3 Evaluation models

To define a general framework for constructing evaluation criteria for settings with several clinical objectives, consider a trial with m objectives. Let $D(\theta)$ denote the data model in this trial, where θ is a vector of key and supportive data model parameters. The null hypotheses associated with the objectives of interest are denoted by $H_1, \ldots, H_m$ and may be placed in a single family or several hierarchically arranged families. The analysis model in the trial incorporates a multiplicity adjustment, which is indexed by a parameter vector λ, e.g., λ may define the set of hypothesis-specific weights. This parameter vector serves as the target parameter in the optimization problem. The evaluation criterion, as a function of λ, will be denoted by $\psi(\lambda)$. Note that the criterion also depends on θ but this dependence will be suppressed.

It is instructive to consider first a clinical trial with a single objective, e.g., a two-arm clinical trial with a single primary endpoint and no pre-specified secondary endpoints. In this setting power is defined simply as the probability of a statistically significant treatment effect. With several pre-defined null hypotheses and corresponding sets of possible trial outcomes, multiple definitions of power or multiple evaluation criteria can be considered. Most commonly, these criteria belong to the class of *exceedence criteria* (e.g., disjunctive and conjunctive power) or *expectation criteria* (e.g., weighted power). In addition, evaluation criteria can be defined based on the concept of *multiplicity penalties.*

The evaluation criteria defined in this section are more relevant in traditional multiplicity problems with a single family of null hypotheses. More options for defining criteria are available when more complex multiplicity problems with multiple families of hypotheses are considered. For example, that evaluation criteria in multi-family problems can account for the hierarchical relationships among the families, including the relative importance of each family, in addition to incorporating hypothesis weights within each family. Examples of evaluation criteria designed for settings with several sources of multiplicity that define several families of hypotheses are given in Case studies 2.2 and 2.3.

As the final comment, the evaluation criteria defined in this section can be applied with different optimization approaches, including the direct and tradeoff-based optimization strategies defined in Chapter 1. For example, a direction optimization algorithm based on disjunctive and weighted criteria will be used to select optimal multiplicity adjustments in Case study 2.2. Case study 2.3 will illustrate the process of applying a tradeoff-based optimization approach with the same evaluation criteria in a similar optimization problem.

Disjunctive power and related criteria

Evaluation criteria in the class of exceedence criteria are broadly used in clinical trials. These criteria are defined in terms of the probability of exceeding a pre-specified number of rejections in a family of null hypotheses. The most popular member of this class is the criterion based on *disjunctive power*. The criterion, denoted by ψ_D, is defined based on the probability of the disjunctive event, i.e., the probability of rejecting at least one null hypothesis in the family:

$$\psi_D(\boldsymbol{\lambda}) = P\left(\sum_{i=1}^m r_i \geq 1\right),$$

where r_i denotes an indicator variable with $r_i = 1$ if the null hypothesis H_i is rejected and 0 otherwise, $i = 1, \ldots, m$. The probability is evaluated under a specific set of alternative hypotheses using an analysis model (multiple testing procedure) corresponding to the target parameter $\boldsymbol{\lambda}$.

The evaluation criterion based on disjunctive power can be generalized in a variety of ways. For example, in a setting with multiple families of hypotheses that arises in advanced problems with several sources of multiplicity, an extended disjunctive criterion, known as the *subset disjunctive criterion*, can be defined as the probability of rejecting one or more hypotheses within every family. To illustrate, consider a multiplicity problem with two families of hypotheses and let M denote the index set of all hypotheses, i.e., $M = \{1, \ldots, m\}$. Suppose that the first m_1 hypotheses are included in the first family and the remaining m_2 hypotheses are included in the second family ($m_1 + m_2 = m$). The corresponding index sets are denoted by M_1 and M_2. The subset disjunctive criterion, denoted by ψ_{SD}, is equal to the probability of at least one rejection in the first family and at least one rejection in the second family, i.e.,

$$\psi_{SD}(\boldsymbol{\lambda}) = P \left(\sum_{i \in M_1} r_i \geq 1 \text{ and } \sum_{j \in M_2} r_j \geq 1 \right).$$

Another popular evaluation criterion in the class of exceedence criteria is the *conjunctive criterion*, denoted by ψ_C, which is defined based on the probability to reject all null hypotheses in the family:

$$\psi_C(\boldsymbol{\lambda}) = P \left(\sum_{i=1}^{m} r_i = m \right).$$

Criteria based on disjunctive power typically provide a preliminary assessment of the probability of success in a clinical trial with multiple objectives and other approaches to defining evaluation criteria, e.g., criteria based on weighted power, are preferable to the exceedence criteria. Potential limitations of the disjunctive and related criteria were discussed in several publications (see, for example, Millen and Dmitrienko, 2011). These limitations are related to the fact that these criteria are symmetric with respect to the pre-defined null hypotheses. In addition, the criteria do not provide any information on the number of rejected hypotheses and do not support an option to assign hypothesis-specific weights to account for the relative importance of the individual hypotheses. Detailed comparisons of criteria based on disjunctive and weighted power are provided in Case studies 2.1 through 2.3.

Weighted power criteria

Expectation evaluation criteria are defined based on the expected number of clinically relevant events, e.g., the expected number of rejected null hypotheses. A simple example of expectation evaluation criteria is the *simple weighted criterion*, which is defined as a weighed sum of the marginal power functions:

$$\psi_{SW}(\boldsymbol{\lambda}) = \sum_{i=1}^{m} v_i \psi_i(\boldsymbol{\lambda}),$$

where $\psi_i(\boldsymbol{\lambda})$ denotes the marginal power function for the test of H_i, i.e., the probability to reject this null hypothesis as a function of $\boldsymbol{\lambda}$. Note that

$$E(r_i) = P(\text{Reject } H_i) = \psi_i(\boldsymbol{\lambda}), \ i = 1, \ldots, m.$$

Also, $v_1, \ldots, v_m$ are the pre-specified importance parameters that determine the relative importance or "value" of the clinical objectives associated with the null hypotheses. The importance parameters are assumed to be non-negative and are often standardized to ensure that they add up to 1.

It is helpful to note that, if the importance parameters are equal to each other, i.e.,

$$v_1 = \ldots = v_m = \frac{1}{m},$$

weighted power is closely related to the expected number of rejected null hypotheses. Indeed, it is easy to check that

$$m\psi_{SW}(\boldsymbol{\lambda}) = \sum_{i=1}^{m} \psi_i(\boldsymbol{\lambda}) = \sum_{i=1}^{m} P(\text{Reject } H_i) = E\left(\sum_{i=1}^{m} r_i\right).$$

Further, the trial's sponsor may introduce unequal parameters if one or more clinical objectives are viewed as being more important than the others. For example, consider a multiplicity problem with three null hypotheses H_1, H_2 and H_3. Suppose that rejection of the first hypothesis is as important as simultaneous rejection of the other two null hypotheses. This implies that the importance parameters are set to

$$v_1 = \frac{1}{2}, \ v_2 = \frac{1}{4}, \ v_3 = \frac{1}{4},$$

and

$$4\psi_{SW}(\boldsymbol{\lambda}) = E(2r_1 + r_2 + r_3).$$

This expression shows that the hypothesis H_1 is "counted twice" when the expected number of rejections is computed.

A natural extension of the simple weighted criterion is a family of *partition-based weighted criteria*. These criteria offer a more nuanced approach to assigning the importance values to the original null hypotheses and their combinations. This general approach to defining evaluation criteria is closely related to decision-theoretic approaches in the sense that it relies on assigning "gains" to the outcomes of interest. The family of partition-based weighted criteria includes as special cases the disjunctive and simple weighted criteria introduced above.

To illustrate the key ideas behind partition-based weighted criteria, consider the problem of testing null hypotheses based on two dose-placebo contrasts in a clinical trial, it is helpful to explicitly formulate the outcomes of interest corresponding to specific regulatory claims that can be formulated at the end of the trial. The available claims include the claims of treatment effectiveness at each dose (with the other dose being ineffective) and the claim of treatment effectiveness at both doses. Switching to the corresponding null hypotheses of no effect at the two doses (H_1 and H_2), this is equivalent to partitioning the disjunctive event that defines the successful outcome in the trial, i.e.,

$$\{\text{Reject } H_1 \text{ or Reject } H_2\} = \{r_1 + r_2 \geq 1\},$$

into three mutually exclusive events:

$$\{\text{Reject } H_1 \text{ only}\} = \{r_1 = 1, r_2 = 0\},$$
$$\{\text{Reject } H_2 \text{ only}\} = \{r_1 = 0, r_2 = 1\},$$
$$\{\text{Reject } H_1 \text{ and } H_2\} = \{r_1 = 1, r_2 = 1\}.$$

Using the event-specific parameters, denoted by v_1, v_2 and v_{12}, the partition-based weighted criterion is defined as:

$$\begin{aligned} \psi_{PW}(\boldsymbol{\lambda}) \quad = \quad & v_1 P(r_1 = 1, r_2 = 0) + v_2 P(r_1 = 0, r_2 = 1) \\ + \quad & v_{12} P(r_1 = 1, r_2 = 1). \end{aligned}$$

The three pre-defined importance parameters quantify the desirability of demonstrating a beneficial effect at each dose and simultaneously at both doses (these parameters are non-negative and, as above, it is often helpful to standardize them to ensure that they add up to 1). The simple example considered above is easily extended to a general setting with an arbitrary number of hypotheses by considering a partition of the corresponding disjunctive event.

Criteria based on multiplicity penalties

A common feature of the exceedence and expectation evaluation criteria defined earlier in this section is that they support an indirect comparison of candidate multiple testing procedures. For example, when comparing two procedures in terms of their disjunctive power, one cannot determine how often one procedure rejects more null hypotheses than the other. Multiplicity penalties are introduced to evaluate the key characteristics of a multiple testing procedure at a more granular level. Multiplicity penalties provide a direct evaluation of a procedure's performance relative to a reference procedure. The most natural choice for a reference procedure is the basic procedure without a multiplicity adjustment (unadjusted procedure). However, another multiple testing procedure can serve as a reference procedure and multiplicity penalties can be computed to perform a "head-to-head" comparison of two candidate procedures. Multiplicity penalties, often organized into matrices, provide useful insights into the decision rules used by multiple testing procedures and help identify specific settings where rejections made by the reference procedure are lost after a particular multiple testing procedure is applied.

The following notation will be used to define multiplicity penalties. As before, consider a general problem of testing m null hypotheses and let M denote the set of hypothesis indices, i.e., $M = \{1, \ldots, m\}$. Further, let I denote an arbitrary subset of the index set M, which includes an empty set. The total number of all subsets of M is 2^m. The two multiple testing procedures of interest will be denoted by Procedure A and Procedure B. Procedure A will serve as the reference procedure and a set of multiplicity penalties will be computed for Procedure B relative to Procedure A. Let $R_A(I)$ denote the following event:

$$\{\text{Procedure A rejects all hypotheses } H_i, \ i \in I\}$$

and define $R_B(I)$ in a similar way. The multiplicity penalty for a pair of index sets $I_1 \subseteq M$ and $I_2 \subseteq M$ is defined as the probability of the simultaneous occurrence of $R_A(I_1)$ and $R_B(I_2)$, i.e.,

$$P(I_1, I_2) = P(R_A(I_1), R_B(I_2)).$$

The set of multiplicity penalties can be used to provide a thorough assessment of the performance of Procedure B relative to that of Procedure A for all possible sets of rejected null hypotheses. Consider, for example, the following sum of multiplicity penalties

$$\sum_{I \subseteq M} P(I, I).$$

Since the first index set is equal to the second index set, this quantity defines the probability that the two procedures lead to the rejection of the same hypotheses or, in other words, the probability of equivalence. If the sum is computed over all index sets I_1 and I_2 such that I_1 is a proper subset of I_2, i.e.,

$$\sum_{I_1 \subset I_2} P(I_1, I_2),$$

the result is the probability that Procedure B rejects more hypotheses than Procedure A. This probability can be viewed as the probability of superiority for Procedure B and serves as a useful evaluation criterion for performing head-to-head comparisons of multiple testing procedures.

Lastly, if the unadjusted procedure is selected as the reference procedure, any multiple testing procedure will be, by definition, inferior to the reference procedure (Procedure A). In particular, the probability of superiority for Procedure B will be equal to 0. It will be of more interest to compute the probability of inferiority for Procedure B, i.e.,

$$\sum_{I_2 \subset I_1} P(I_1, I_2).$$

This probability can be thought of as the overall multiplicity penalty associated with Procedure B. A high value of this probability for a given multiple testing procedure relative to the unadjusted procedure indicates that the chosen procedure is not an efficient multiplicity adjustment. The overall multiplicity penalty can serve as an evaluation criterion in clinical trial optimization problems.

In general, the set of the multiplicity penalties for all possible pairs of index sets $I_1 \subseteq M$ and $I_2 \subseteq M$ can be organized in a matrix-like arrangement with 2^m rows and 2^m columns. Since this matrix is constructed based on a complete enumeration of all possible outcomes (sets of rejected hypotheses), its size grows extremely fast and it is not practical to consider multiplicity penalty matrices of this kind in problems with, say, five or more hypotheses.

As an alternative, a simplified approach to defining multiplicity penalty matrices that focuses on the total number of rejected hypotheses can be applied. For any $k = 0, \ldots, m$, consider the event

$$R_A(k) = \{\text{Procedure A rejects all hypotheses } H_i, \ i \in I, \text{ with } |I| = k\}$$

and let the event $R_B(k)$ be defined in a similar way. The associated multiplicity penalty for an arbitrary pair of k and l, denoted by $P(k, l)$, is equal to the probability of the simultaneous occurrence of the events $R_A(k)$ and $R_B(l)$, i.e.,

$$P(k, l) = P(R_A(k), R_B(l)), \ k, l = 0, \ldots, m.$$

It is easy to see that $P(k, l)$ is the probability that Procedure A rejects exactly k hypotheses and Procedure B rejects exactly l hypotheses.

The resulting multiplicity penalties are easy to present using an $(m+1) \times (m+1)$ matrix with the (i, j) entry equal to $P(i-1, j-1)$, $i, j = 1, \ldots, m+1$. The sum of the entries above the main diagonal in the multiplicity penalty matrix, i.e.,

$$\sum_{i<j} P(i, j),$$

is the probability of superiority for Procedure B, i.e., the probability of rejecting more hypotheses compared to Procedure A. Similarly, the sum of the below-diagonal entries is the probability of inferiority for Procedure B and defines the overall multiplicity penalty if Procedure A represents an unadjusted strategy. Note that in this case Procedure B cannot reject more hypotheses than Procedure A and thus $P(i, j) = 0$ if $i < j$.

2.3   Case study 2.1: Optimal selection of a multiplicity adjustment

The first case study in this chapter deals with a fairly straightforward clinical trial optimization problem. Using a Phase III clinical trial with two null hypotheses of no effect, an optimal analysis model will be identified, i.e., the model corresponding to the multiplicity adjustment that outperforms the other adjustments in the pre-defined family of adjustments. The case study provides a thorough exploration of the general concepts and approaches discussed in Chapter 1. A key element of Clinical Scenario Evaluation, namely, sensitivity assessments, will be utilized to study the performance of the candidate multiplicity adjustments under a data model that represents the most likely set of statistical assumptions as well as alternative models. The comprehensive assessments will support the selection of the most powerful and robust analysis model for the Phase III trial. Even though the example used in this case study is built around a simple setting with two null hypotheses, the general methodology presented below can be extended to clinical trials with any number of null hypotheses.

For the sake of simplicity, the family of multiplicity adjustments will include only two adjustment methods and a direct optimization approach will be utilized in this case study. Also, it will be assumed that procedure parameters, e.g., weights assigned to the individual hypotheses, are fixed. Optimal parameter selection can be incorporated as part of an extended optimization problem and will be considered in Case studies 2.2 and 2.3.

2.3.1   Clinical trial

The clinical trial example used in this case study is based on the Phase III clinical trial presented in Keystone et al. (2004). The trial was conducted to evaluate the efficacy and safety of a novel treatment in the population of patients with rheumatoid arthritis who had an inadequate response to methotrexate. The primary analysis was based on the American College of Rheumatology (ACR) definition of improvement and patients were classified as responders if they experienced an improvement of at least 20% in the core criteria at Week 24 (the resulting primary endpoint is known as ACR20). Two doses of the experimental treatment were tested in the trial against a placebo.

Data model

A balanced clinical trial design with $n = 100$ patients per arm will be assumed in this clinical trial example. A data model is defined in a very straightforward way with each sample (independent group of patients) corresponding to a trial arm:

- Sample 1: Placebo arm.

- Sample 2: Low dose arm (Dose L).

- Sample 3: High dose arm (Dose H).

It will be assumed, for simplicity, that all patients complete the trial. The Clinical Scenario Evaluation framework presented in this case study is easily extended to a more realistic setting with non-trivial early discontinuation rates.

Three data models based on different sets of outcome distribution parameters (i.e., proportions of patients who meet the ACR20 response criterion at Week 24) will be considered in this case study. Let π_1, π_2 and π_3 denote the ACR20 response rates in the placebo, low dose and high dose arms, respectively. The response rates under three scenarios are listed in Table 2.2.

TABLE 2.2: Three scenarios (data models) in Case study 2.1.

Scenario	ACR20 response rate		
	Placebo	Dose L	Dose H
Scenario 1	$\pi_1 = 0.30$	$\pi_2 = 0.50$	$\pi_3 = 0.50$
Scenario 2	$\pi_1 = 0.30$	$\pi_2 = 0.40$	$\pi_3 = 0.50$
Scenario 3	$\pi_1 = 0.30$	$\pi_2 = 0.50$	$\pi_3 = 0.45$

Scenario 1 defines the main data model which is based on the most likely set of ACR20 response rates, namely, the response rates at Doses L and H are assumed to be equal. The data models corresponding to Scenarios 2 and 3 represent alternative sets of statistical assumptions. Under Scenario 2, a linear dose-response relationship is assumed in the trial and, under Scenario 3, another deviation of the assumption of an equal treatment effect in the two treatment arms is considered, namely, the response rate at Dose H is slightly reduced due to potential safety issues.

The response rates defined in Table 2.2 serve as the key data model parameters and no supportive parameters are defined in this case study.

The alternative data models based on Scenarios 2 and 3 are qualitatively different from the model based on Scenario 1 and will be utilized in qualitative sensitivity assessment summarized in Section 2.3.2. Section 2.3.3 will present a quantitative approach to sensitivity assessment that relies on alternative data models obtained by perturbing the main data model.

Analysis model

The analysis model in this case study is formulated based on the evaluation of the efficacy profile of the experimental treatment. The primary efficacy analysis is built around the null hypotheses of no effect associated with the two dose-placebo contrasts:

- Null hypothesis H_1 of no treatment difference between Dose H and placebo.

- Null hypothesis H_2 of no treatment difference between Dose L and placebo.

The individual hypotheses will be tested using the Cochran-Mantel-Haenszel test stratified by important prognostic factors such as disease severity at baseline. Let p_1 and p_2 denote the one-sided p-values for H_1 and H_2 produced by this test. Also, as in Section 2.2.2, the ordered p-values are denoted by $p_{(1)} < p_{(2)}$ and associated hypotheses are denoted by $H_{(1)}$ and $H_{(2)}$.

The overall outcome in this trial will be declared successful if the treatment is shown to provide a statistically significant improvement over placebo in one or more dosing arms, i.e., if at least one of the two null hypotheses is rejected. The analysis induces multiplicity and, consequently, the key component of the analysis model is a multiplicity adjustment applied to control the overall Type I error rate at the nominal level (one-sided $\alpha = 0.025$).

When considering applicable multiplicity adjustments, it is important to first identify a set of efficient candidate adjustments. For example, even though the trial's sponsor could select the Bonferroni or Holm procedures to handle multiplicity in this setting, this would be a poor choice since these procedures are known to be dominated in terms of power by semiparametric procedures. Indeed, as shown in Section 2.2.2, the Hochberg procedure is uniformly more powerful than the Bonferroni or Holm. The only reasonable alternative to the Hochberg in the class of nonparametric procedures is the fixed-sequence procedure. The relationship between the Hochberg and fixed-sequence procedures is rather complex, e.g., depending on the underlying set of p-values, one procedure can be superior to the other and vice versa. Therefore it is not clear a priori which procedure will be more efficient in this case study. To give a quick numeric example, if $p_1 = 0.02$ and $p_2 = 0.04$, the Hochberg cannot reject either hypothesis whereas the fixed-sequence procedure rejects H_1 if testing begins with this hypothesis. On the other hand, if $p_1 = 0.03$ and $p_2 = 0.01$, the Hochberg rejects H_2 but the fixed-sequence procedure fails to reject any hypothesis since the first test in the sequence is not significant.

For the reasons presented above, the fixed-sequence and Hochberg procedures will be included in the set of candidate multiplicity adjustments in this case study. The candidate multiplicity adjustments are defined as follows:

- Procedure F is the fixed-sequence procedure which assumes that the dose-placebo tests are carried out in a pre-specified sequence starting with Dose H. The hypothesis H_1 is rejected if $p_1 \leq \alpha$. Further, if H_1 is rejected, H_2 is tested. This hypothesis is rejected if $p_2 \leq \alpha$.

- Procedure H is the Hochberg procedure which relies on a data-driven testing sequence. Testing begins with the hypothesis corresponding to the larger p-value, i.e., $H_{(2)}$. This hypothesis is rejected if $p_{(2)} \leq \alpha$. If the procedure rejects $H_{(2)}$, the other hypothesis is automatically rejected. Otherwise, $H_{(1)}$ is tested at a lower significance level. Specifically, this hypothesis is rejected if $p_{(1)} \leq \alpha/2$. Note that this procedure treats the two null hypotheses as equally important, in other words, the hypothesis weights are set to $w_1 = w_2 = 0.5$.

It is helpful to mention that a parametric multiple testing procedure from the Dunnett family (see Section 2.2.2) could have been considered in this clinical trial as well. However, parametric procedures are valid only under the assumption that the joint distribution of the statistics for testing the null hypotheses H_1 and H_2 is fully specified, which means, for example, that the correlation between the test statistics is known at the design stage. The assumption of a fixed correlation is easily justified when all patients complete a trial but missing observations are inevitable in real clinical trials. For example, it is reported in Keystone et al. (2004) that discontinuation rates could be as high as 30% in placebo-treated patients in rheumatoid arthritis trials. Various imputation methods are applied in the presence of missing data and only one of them (last observation carried forward) guarantees that the correlation between the test statistics is preserved. This imputation method is known to be suboptimal and it is generally unclear if parametric procedures protect the overall Type I error rate when more efficient imputation methods are applied. By contrast, the Hochberg procedure is a semiparametric procedure that protects the overall Type I error rate in this example provided the correlation between the test statistics is non-negative, which is clearly the case regardless of the imputation method applied. Similarly, the fixed-sequence procedure is a nonparametric procedure that makes no assumptions about the distribution of the test statistics and it is safe to use it with any imputation method.

Evaluation model

The goal of clinical trial optimization in this case study is to perform a comprehensive comparison of two candidate analysis models based on the fixed-sequence and Hochberg procedures and select the most efficient and robust approach to multiplicity adjustment. Given that the relevant procedure parameters (e.g., hypothesis weights in the Hochberg procedure) are fixed, optimization will focus on a head-to-head comparison of the two selected procedures. The comparisons will be performed based on a broad set of evaluation models that utilize the criteria introduced in Section 2.2.3. The choice of most relevant evaluation criteria in this clinical trial example will be discussed below in Sections 2.3.2 and 2.3.3.

Beginning with exceedence-based evaluation criteria, disjunctive power is defined as the probability of rejecting either H_1 or H_2 in this clinical trial, i.e.,

$$\psi_D = P(\text{Reject } H_1 \text{ or } H_2).$$

Disjunctive power serves as a starting point in a Clinical Scenario Evaluation exercise but cannot provide a solid foundation for clinical trial optimization since it lacks several useful features. When the disjunctive event, i.e.,

$$\text{Reject } H_1 \text{ or } H_2,$$

is considered, the number of rejected hypotheses or the total importance of rejected hypotheses cannot be taken into account. Additionally, an important limitation of disjunctive power in this particular setting is that Procedure F relies on a testing algorithm that always begins with the null hypothesis H_1. Thus disjunctive power for this procedure is simply equal to the probability of rejecting H_1 and does not depend on the true treatment difference between Dose L and placebo.

The evaluation criterion based on disjunctive power will be accompanied by the basic weighted and partition-based weighted criteria that enable the trial's sponsor to fine-tune the formulation of success criteria. It is shown below that the weighted criteria support an option to assign test-specific weights to take into account the "gains" associated with specific efficacy claims.

The first criterion is defined using the weighted sum of the marginal probabilities of rejecting each hypothesis and it enables the trial's sponsor to explicitly account for the perceived importance of establishing a statistically significant effect in each dosing arm. The basic weighted power criterion is defined as

$$\psi_W = v_1 P(\text{Reject } H_1) + v_2 P(\text{Reject } H_2),$$

where v_1 and v_2 are non-negative values that determine how much importance is assigned to establishing significant treatment effects at Dose H and Dose L, respectively. These importance parameters are commonly standardized to ensure that $v_1 + v_2 = 1$. As indicated in Section 2.2.3, weighted power is closely related to evaluation criteria that account for the number of rejected hypotheses. If equal importance parameters are selected, i.e., $v_1 = v_2 = 1$, ψ_W is equal to the expected number of hypotheses rejected in this multiplicity problem.

Evaluation criteria derived from partition-based weighted power define a family of criteria that includes basic weighted power as well as disjunctive power as special cases. Using the example given in Section 2.2.3, the overall outcome of interest in the rheumatoid arthritis trial (establishing a significant effect at either dose or, in other words, rejecting H_1 or H_2) is partitioned into three mutually exclusive events:

- Reject H_1 only.

- Reject H_2 only.

- Simultaneously reject H_1 and H_2.

Based on this partitioning scheme, weighted power is defined as:

$$\begin{aligned}\psi_{PW} &= v_1 P(\text{Reject } H_1 \text{ only}) + v_2 P(\text{Reject } H_2 \text{ only}) \\ &+ v_{12} P(\text{Reject } H_1 \text{ and } H_2).\end{aligned}$$

The associated parameters (v_1, v_2 and v_{12}) are conceptually very similar to the importance parameters defined above. Specifically, v_1 and v_2 reflect the importance of demonstrating a significant effect of the corresponding dose. These parameters determine the gain associated with making a single efficacy claim in this Phase III trial. The third parameter describes the importance of establishing a simultaneous beneficial effect at Doses L and H. This parameter will generally be greater than v_1 and v_2 and, as above, the three importance values can be standardized by setting their sum to 1.

It is useful to explore the specific evaluation criteria included in the family of partition-based weighted criteria defined above. Disjunctive power is a special case that corresponds to the criterion with $v_1 = v_2 = v_{12} = 1$. Indeed,

$$\begin{aligned}\psi_{PW} &= P(\text{Reject } H_1 \text{ only}) + P(\text{Reject } H_1 \text{ and } H_2) \\ &+ P(\text{Reject } H_2 \text{ only}) \\ &= P(\text{Reject } H_1 \text{ or } H_2) \\ &= \psi_D.\end{aligned}$$

Secondly, consider an additive weighting scheme, i.e., assume that $v_1 + v_2 = v_{12}$. In this case it is easy to verify that the partition-based weighted criterion simplifies to the simple weighted criterion, i.e.,

$$
\begin{aligned}
\psi_{PW} &= v_1[P(\text{Reject } H_1 \text{ only}) + P(\text{Reject } H_1 \text{ and } H_2)] \\
&+ v_2[P(\text{Reject } H_2 \text{ only}) + P(\text{Reject } H_1 \text{ and } H_2)] \\
&= v_1 P(\text{Reject } H_1) + v_2 P(\text{Reject } H_2) \\
&= \psi_W.
\end{aligned}
$$

This equality shows that a partition-based criterion is generally justified in clinical trial optimization problems if a synergistic effect of the two doses can be assumed, i.e., the importance of establishing a significant treatment effect at both doses (v_{12}) is greater than the sum of the importance values associated with a significant effect at each individual dose ($v_1 + v_2$).

The exceedence and expectation criteria defined above can be used to support indirect comparisons among candidate multiple testing procedures. As explained in Section 2.2.3, it is also of interest to perform direct comparisons of each multiple testing procedure to the unadjusted procedure (i.e., naive analysis strategy that employs no multiplicity adjustment) or a head-to-head comparison between Procedure F and Procedure H. These comparisons help explicitly quantify the advantage of one analysis strategy over another strategy and are presented using the concept of a multiplicity penalty.

Using the definition given in Section 2.2.3, a multiplicity penalty for a multiple testing procedure quantifies the amount of power loss due to this multiplicity adjustment for a particular set of rejected null hypotheses. A multiplicity penalty matrix can be constructed based on a complete set of all possible combinations of rejected hypotheses. In this case study, this amounts to computing penalties for the settings with no rejected hypotheses, rejection of H_1 only, rejection of H_2 only and simultaneous rejection of H_1 and H_2. Alternatively, a simplified approach that focuses on the total number of rejected hypotheses can be applied.

Assuming the simplified approach, let u denote the total number of hypotheses of no effect rejected by the unadjusted analysis strategy and, similarly, let f denote the total number of rejections for Procedure F. The multiplicity penalty matrix for Procedure F, denoted by P_F, is a 3×3 matrix with the (i, j) entry set to the probability of the following outcome:

$$
O_F(i - 1, j - 1) = \{u = i - 1 \text{ and } f = j - 1\}, \ i, j = 1, 2, 3.
$$

In other words, the (i, j) entry of the multiplicity penalty matrix P_F is given by

$$
P_F(i - 1, j - 1) = P(O_F(i - 1, j - 1)), \ i, j = 1, 2, 3.
$$

As an example, the outcome $O_F(1, 0)$ corresponds to the case where the unadjusted procedure rejects exactly one hypothesis but no hypothesis can be rejected after Procedure F is applied. Note that, with the simplified approach to defining multiplicity penalties, hypothesis-specific decisions are lumped together. As a consequence, $O_F(1,1)$ covers the case where the unadjusted procedure and Procedure F reject the same null hypothesis as well as the case in which the first procedure rejects one hypothesis and the second procedure rejects the other hypothesis in this multiplicity problem. Further, a multiplicity penalty matrix for Procedure H, denoted by P_H, is defined in a similar way.

When examining the multiplicity penalty matrix of any multiple testing procedure, it is important to bear in mind that the number of rejected hypotheses after this procedure is applied cannot exceed the number of rejections before the adjustment. Consequently, all entries above the main diagonal are equal to 0. The entries below the main diagonal provide useful information on the performance of the selected procedure or, to be more precise, performance loss compared to the unadjusted analysis strategy. The performance loss is expressed in terms of probabilities of specific outcomes. Using the multiplicity penalty matrix for Procedure F as an example, the three below-diagonal entries are equal to the probabilities of the following outcomes:

$$O_F(1,0), O_F(2,0) \text{ and } O_F(2,1).$$

Considering these outcomes, it is natural to define the overall multiplicity penalty for Procedure F as a composite measure based on their probabilities. The most straightforward approach to computing the overall multiplicity penalty relies on the sum of the below-diagonal entries in the matrix, i.e.,

$$\psi_{MP} = P_F(1,0) + P_F(2,0) + P_F(2,1).$$

This approach implicitly assumes that all three outcomes listed above carry the same weight, e.g., $O_F(1,0)$, which corresponds to the case of a single rejection lost after the multiplicity adjustment based on Procedure F, is not distinguishable from $O_F(2,0)$, which corresponds to two lost rejections. It is generally more meaningful to assign different weights to the individual outcomes. For example, it is sensible to assign the same weight to $O_F(1,0)$ and $O_F(2,1)$ and a greater weight to $O_F(2,0)$ to account for the fact that the last outcome should be associated with a more severe multiplicity penalty.

A multiplicity penalty matrix can also be constructed to support a head-to-head comparison of two multiple testing procedures. To perform a head-to-head comparison of Procedures F and H in this case study, a simplified set of outcomes will be considered again. Let h denote the number of null hypotheses of no effect rejected by Procedure H. The (i,j) element of the multiplicity penalty matrix is defined as follows:

$$P_{FH}(i-1, j-1) = P\{f = i-1 \text{ and } h = j-1\}, \ i, j = 1, 2, 3.$$

It is helpful to note that only two non-diagonal cells, namely, $P_{FH}(0,1)$ and $P_{FH}(1,0)$, can be positive in this matrix. The other non-diagonal entries are all equal to zero. This is due to the fact that, for example, there are no configurations of raw p-values for the two null hypotheses that would result in no rejections for Procedure F and two rejections for Procedure H. This means that the sum of the entries above the main diagonal equals $P_{FH}(0,1)$ and the sum of the below-diagonal entries equals $P_{FH}(1,0)$. These sums can be used to measure the degree of superiority of one multiplicity adjustment over the other. For example, the sum of the below-diagonal entries in the matrix P_{FH} is the probability that Procedure F rejects more null hypotheses than the other procedure. This value can be viewed as the probability that Procedure F is superior to Procedure H. Along the same line, the probability of superiority for Procedure H can be defined as the sum of the above-diagonal entries in the matrix P_{FH}.

In addition, it is worth noting that the multiplicity penalty matrix for the head-to-head comparison is closely related to the multiplicity penalty matrices introduced above. It is easy to verify that, in this particular setting with two null hypotheses, the difference between $P_{FH}(0,1)$ and $P_{FH}(1,0)$ is equal to the difference between $P_F(1,0)$ and $P_H(1,0)$.

2.3.2 Qualitative sensitivity assessment

As stated at the beginning of Section 2.3, this case study illustrates the use of sensitivity assessments to select the optimal analysis model (i.e., an analysis model with the most efficient multiplicity adjustment) which is robust with respect to deviations from the main data model assumed in the rheumatoid arthritis clinical trial. The assessments will be performed using the two approaches defined in Chapter 1, i.e., using qualitative and quantitative sensitivity analysis techniques. Qualitative sensitivity assessments assume a fixed number of pre-specified alternative data models whereas quantitative assessments discussed in Section 2.3.3 rely on a large number of alternative data models based on random deviations from the main data model.

A qualitative or pivoting-based approach is aimed at studying the impact of qualitative deviations from a given data model on the candidate analysis models. In this case, the main data model assumes an equal treatment effect at Doses L and H with the ACR20 response rates in the three trial arms given by 30%, 50% and 50%, respectively. The true treatment differences in the two dosing arms are, of course, unknown and it is critical to understand how deviations from the hypothesized dose-response function affect the conclusions based on the main data model. To facilitate the process, two alternative data models introduced in Section 2.3.1 (see Scenarios 2 and 3 Table 2.2) will be utilized as part of a qualitative sensitivity assessment. The performance of Procedures F and H under each data model will be evaluated based on the criteria defined in Section 2.3.1.

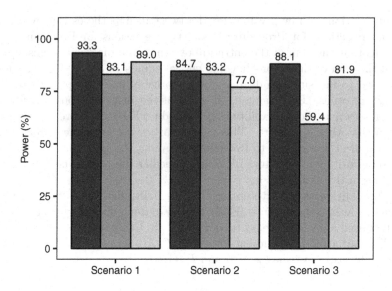

FIGURE 2.2: Disjunctive power for each analysis method (no adjustment, black bars; Procedure F, dark gray bars; Procedure H, light gray bars) under three scenarios in Case study 2.1.

Sensitivity assessments based on disjunctive and weighted power

The first set of qualitative sensitivity assessments focused on the exceedence and expectation evaluation criteria, i.e., disjunctive power, simple weighted power and partition-based weighted power. The basic analysis strategy that relies on testing the hypotheses H_1 and H_2 without a multiplicity adjustment (unadjusted procedure) was included in this comparison to define the best-case scenario for the candidate multiple testing procedures (recall that the value of any success criterion for any multiplicity adjustment cannot exceed that of the unadjusted procedure).

Figure 2.2 provides a summary of disjunctive power under the main data model (Scenario 1) and two pre-specified alternative models (Scenarios 2 and 3). It follows from the figure that disjunctive power of Procedure H was fairly close to that of the unadjusted procedure (89% and 93.3%, respectively) when the main data model was considered, which means that Procedure H provided an efficient multiplicity adjustment. Procedure F performed poorly in this case with a 10% drop in disjunctive power compared to the unadjusted procedure. This finding is a direct consequence of the fact that disjunctive power of Procedure F was driven completely by the test of the hypothesis H_1 (see Section 2.3.1). Even though disjunctive power is supposed to provide an overall assessment of the treatment effect at Doses L and H, it was in reality equal to the marginal probability of detecting a significant effect at the high dose, which resulted in reduced power.

Somewhat different patterns were observed when the monotone and non-monotone dose-response relationships corresponding to Scenarios 2 and 3 were assumed. With a monotone dose-response function (Scenario 2), Procedure F demonstrated a good performance and resulted in a higher probability of success compared to Procedure H. Disjunctive power of Procedures F and H was equal to 83.2% and 77%, respectively. On the other hand, when the last data model (Scenario 3) was considered, Procedure H provided a substantial advantage over Procedure F. The difference in terms of disjunctive power was over 20 percentage points. To understand why Procedure F performed poorly under Scenario 3 compared to Scenario 2, note that the latter represented a favorable set of assumptions for the fixed-sequence testing method. This method is known to perform best when the *monotonicity assumption* is met, i.e., when the treatment effect decreases monotonically along the testing sequence (Dmitrienko and D'Agostino, 2013). In this setting, the monotonicity assumption is equivalent to requiring that the effect size of the Dose H test should be greater than the effect size of the Dose L test. When this assumption is not satisfied, the fixed-sequence testing method needs to be used with great caution due to considerable power loss. Since Procedure H is based on an algorithm with a data-driven testing sequence, it was not that sensitive to the shape of the true dose-response curve and it performed well under the last data model.

A similar set of qualitative sensitivity assessments was performed using the two evaluation criteria derived from weighted power. First of all, a summary of assessments based on simple weighted power is provided in Figure 2.3. Simple weighted power was defined as follows:

$$\psi_W = 0.4P(\text{Reject } H_1) + 0.6P(\text{Reject } H_2),$$

Note that a higher weight ($v_2 = 0.6$) was assigned to the comparison between Dose L and placebo to indicate that it was more important for the trial's sponsor to demonstrate that the novel treatment is effective at the low dose compared to the high dose. A significant effect at Dose H could be accompanied by potentially undesirable safety issues and thus the corresponding test received a smaller weight ($v_1 = 0.4$).

It can be seen from Figure 2.3 that the procedures (unadjusted, Procedure F and Procedure H) were arranged in the same order under the main data model with a flat dose-response (Scenario 1) and non-monotone dose-response (Scenario 3) as in the assessment based on disjunctive power (see Figure 2.2). Procedure H was superior to Procedure F under both data models. This figure also shows that the three procedures were much closer to each other in terms of weighted power under Scenario 2 compared to the similar setting with disjunctive power. This effect was a reflection of an elevated importance of the comparison between Dose L and placebo. Recall that the criterion based on simple weighted power, unlike the disjunctive power

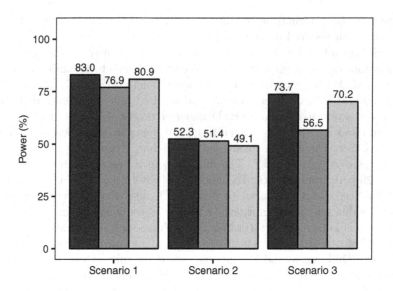

FIGURE 2.3: Simple weighted power with $v_1 = 0.4$ and $v_2 = 0.6$ for each analysis method (no adjustment, black bars; Procedure F, dark gray bars; Procedure H, light gray bars) under three scenarios in Case study 2.1.

criterion, can directly account for the relative importance of the individual dose-placebo comparisons, which led, in this particular case, to higher power for Procedure H.

Figure 2.4 displays partition-based weighted power for the unadjusted procedure and two candidate multiple testing procedures under the same three data models. Partition-based weighted power was defined using a non-additive weighting scheme that recognized the importance of demonstrating a statistically significant treatment effect simultaneously at Dose L and Dose H.

Partition-based weighted power was given by

$$
\begin{aligned}
\psi_{PW} \;=\;& 0.15 P(\text{Reject } H_1 \text{ only}) + 0.25 P(\text{Reject } H_2 \text{ only}) \\
+\;& 0.6 P(\text{Reject } H_1 \text{ and } H_2).
\end{aligned}
$$

It can be checked that $v_{12} = 0.6$ is greater than the sum of $v_1 = 0.15$ and $v_2 = 0.25$, which implies a non-additive weighting scheme. Additionally, the importance of a beneficial treatment effect at Dose H was set to a lower value ($v_1 = 0.15$) compared to Dose L ($v_2 = 0.25$). This approach is similar to the one utilized in the definition of basic weighted power and puts more emphasis on demonstrating treatment-related improvement at the low dose. This approach assumes that the trial's sponsor is interested in selecting a dose with a better safety profile and the low dose is less likely to be associated with safety concerns than the high dose.

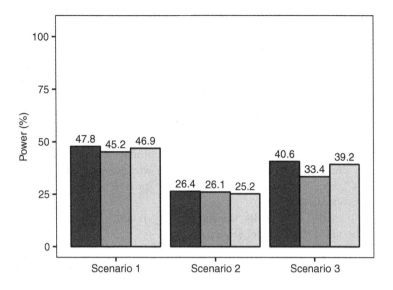

FIGURE 2.4: Partition-based weighted power with $v_1 = 0.15$, $v_2 = 0.25$ and $v_{12} = 0.6$ for each analysis method (no adjustment, black bars; Procedure F, dark gray bars; Procedure H, light gray bars) under three scenarios in Case study 2.1.

The results presented in Figure 2.4 are quite similar to those displayed in Figure 2.3. When partition-based weighted power was computed, Procedure H was very close in terms of its performance to the unadjusted procedure under all three data models. As before, Procedure F performed very poorly under the last data model (Scenario 3) because this procedure relies heavily on the monotonicity assumption which was not met in this case.

Sensitivity assessments based on multiplicity penalties

The evaluation criteria based on disjunctive and weighted power support an indirect comparison of the two candidate multiple testing procedures (Procedures F and H) in the sense that they cannot explicitly differentiate between the cases where the two procedures lead to the same conclusion, e.g., both procedures reject the same null hypothesis of no effect, or different conclusions, i.e., the first procedure rejects one hypothesis whereas the second procedure rejects no hypotheses. A direct approach to defining evaluation criteria was described in Section 2.3.1. This approach relies on overall multiplicity penalties computed from multiplicity penalty matrices for Procedures F and H as well as a matrix for a head-to-head comparison of the two procedures.

A simulation study was performed to compute the overall multiplicity penalties for Procedures F and H under the three treatment effect scenarios used in this case study. Overall multiplicity penalties for Procedures F and H were computed using a simplified approach based on the total number of rejected null hypotheses of no effect. The overall multiplicity penalty for each procedure was defined using an unweighted approach, i.e., the penalty was equal to the sum of the entries below the main diagonal:

$$\psi_{MP} = P(1,0) + P(2,0) + P(2,1).$$

This penalty can be thought of as the probability of rejecting fewer null hypotheses compared to the basic procedure without any multiplicity adjustment. A larger overall multiplicity penalty indicates a less efficient multiple testing procedure.

For illustration, consider the multiplicity penalty matrix for Procedure F under the main data model (Scenario 1):

$$P_F = \begin{bmatrix} P_F(0,0) = 0.067 & P_F(0,1) = 0.000 & P_F(0,2) = 0.000 \\ P_F(1,0) = 0.102 & P_F(1,1) = 0.103 & P_F(1,2) = 0.000 \\ P_F(2,0) = 0.000 & P_F(2,1) = 0.000 & P_F(2,2) = 0.728 \end{bmatrix}.$$

First of all, the sum of the diagonal entries in the matrix, i.e.,

$$P_F(0,0) + P_F(1,1) + P_F(2,2) = 0.898,$$

is the probability that the unadjusted procedure and Procedure F rejected the same number of hypotheses in this clinical trial example. Further, it is easy to see that only one below-diagonal entry is positive in this matrix. This entry corresponds to the case where a single null hypothesis is rejected before Procedure F is applied but this rejection is lost after this multiplicity adjustment. Since $P_F(1,0) = 0.102$, the probability of this outcome was 10.2%. Further, using the definition given above, the overall multiplicity penalty for Procedure F was simply equal to $P_F(1,0)$, i.e., $\psi_{MP} = 0.102$.

Similarly, the multiplicity penalty matrix was computed for Procedure H under the main data model:

$$P_H = \begin{bmatrix} P_H(0,0) = 0.067 & P_H(0,1) = 0.000 & P_H(0,2) = 0.000 \\ P_H(1,0) = 0.043 & P_H(1,1) = 0.162 & P_H(1,2) = 0.000 \\ P_H(2,0) = 0.000 & P_H(2,1) = 0.000 & P_H(2,2) = 0.728 \end{bmatrix}.$$

The pattern of positive entries in the matrix P_H was identical to that in the matrix P_F. The only positive entry below the main diagonal also corresponded to the case of a single rejection by the unadjusted procedure which was lost due to the multiplicity adjustment based on Procedure H. This entry was $P_H(1,0) = 0.043$, which implies that the total number of hypotheses rejected by Procedure H was equal to that of the unadjusted procedure most of the time. The only exception was a single rejection lost due to the Hochberg-based multiplicity adjustment, which occurred only 4.3% of the time. Thus the overall multiplicity penalty for Procedure H was equal to $\psi_{MP} = P_H(1,0) = 0.043$.

To understand why the probability of a single rejection lost due to multiplicity adjustment was much lower for Procedure H compared to Procedure F, it is instructive to compare the values of $P_F(1,1)$ and $P_H(1,1)$. First of all, note that the sum of the entries in the second row is constant between the two multiplicity penalty matrices, i.e.,

$$P_F(1,0) + P_F(1,1) = P_H(1,0) + P_H(1,1),$$

since this sum is equal to the probability that the unadjusted procedure rejects a single null hypothesis. Thus a lower value of $P_H(1,0)$ compared to $P_F(1,0)$ automatically implies that $P_H(1,1)$ is greater than $P_F(1,1)$. In other words, whenever a single hypothesis was rejected by the unadjusted procedure, Procedure H was quite likely to reject a single hypothesis as well and, by contrast, Procedure F tended to reject no hypotheses. This indicates that Procedure F provided a less efficient approach to multiplicity adjustment compared to Procedure H under the main data model.

A summary of the overall multiplicity penalties for Procedures F and H under the three pre-defined scenarios is provided in Figure 2.5. As stated above, Procedure H was superior to Procedure F under the main data model (Scenario 1). When the alternative data models were examined, the overall multiplicity penalty favored Procedure F under Scenario 2 with a positive dose-response relationship. The overall multiplicity penalties for Procedures F and H were equal to 1.5 and 7.7%, respectively. Finally, when the monotonicity assumption was not met due to a large effect size of the Dose L test (Scenario 3), Procedure H was associated with a much lower multiplicity penalty (6.2%) compared to Procedure F (28.7%), which means that a multiplicity adjustment based on Procedure F would result in considerable power loss compared to the unadjusted analysis under this scenario. These general conclusions are consistent with those based on disjunctive and simple weighted power (see Figures 2.2 and 2.3).

To support a head-to-head comparison of the fixed-sequence and Hochberg procedures, the following matrix was computed under the main data model:

$$P_{FH} = \begin{bmatrix} P_{FH}(0,0) = 0.088 & P_{FH}(0,1) = 0.080 & P_{FH}(0,2) = 0.000 \\ P_{FH}(1,0) = 0.022 & P_{FH}(1,1) = 0.081 & P_{FH}(1,2) = 0.000 \\ P_{FH}(2,0) = 0.000 & P_{FH}(2,1) = 0.000 & P_{FH}(2,2) = 0.728 \end{bmatrix}.$$

The non-zero entries below and above the main diagonal, i.e., $P_{FH}(0,1)$ and $P_{FH}(1,0)$, represented the cases where one of the two procedures rejected a single null hypothesis in this multiplicity problem but the other procedure failed to reject any null hypotheses. An illustration of the cases where Procedure H makes more rejections than Procedure F or, alternatively, where Procedure F rejects more hypotheses than Procedure H was provided in Section 2.3.1. It can be shown that all of the other combinations of rejected null

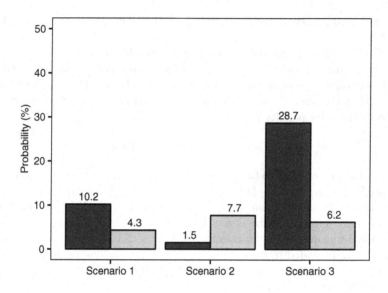

FIGURE 2.5: Overall multiplicity penalty for the two multiple testing procedures (Procedure F, black bars; Procedure H, gray bars) under three scenarios in Case study 2.1.

hypotheses, e.g., two hypotheses rejected by Procedure F and one hypothesis rejected by Procedure H, are impossible and thus all of the remaining non-diagonal entries in the matrix P_{FH} must be equal to 0.

Recall from Section 2.3.1 that the sum of the below-diagonal entries in the matrix P_{FH} can be thought of as the probability that Procedure F is superior to Procedure H. Similarly, the sum of the above-diagonal entries in the matrix P_{FH} can be viewed as the probability that Procedure F is superior to Procedure H. The matrix P_{FH} shows that, under the main model, the probability of superiority for Procedure F was fairly low (2.2%) and the probability of superiority for Procedure H was relatively high (8%). This shows that Procedure H is a more efficient multiplicity adjustment under the assumption of equal response rates at Doses L and H.

The calculations presented above focused on the main data model and Figure 2.6 displays the probabilities of superiority under all three scenarios. The overall pattern observed in this figure is very similar to that in Figure 2.5. Beginning with Scenario 2, the probability of superiority for Procedure H was lower than that for Procedure F (7.0% versus 0.8%) with a linear dose-response function. However, under a slightly non-monotone dose-response relationship (Scenario 3), Procedure H was clearly more attractive than Procedure F. The probability that the former rejects more null hypotheses than the latter was close to 25%. This probability was substantially higher than the probability

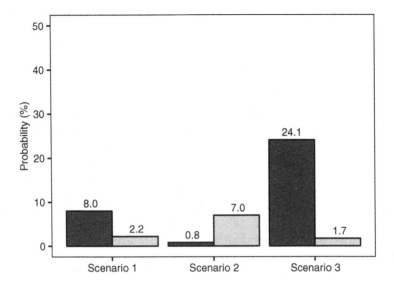

FIGURE 2.6: Head-to-head comparison of the candidate multiple testing procedures (Procedure H is superior to Procedure F, black bars; Procedure F is superior to Procedure H, gray bars) under three scenarios in Case study 2.1.

of superiority for Procedure F, which again demonstrates that Procedure F performs very poorly when the assumption of monotonicity is not satisfied.

2.3.3 Quantitative sensitivity assessment

The overall conclusion presented in Section 2.3.2 was that a multiplicity adjustment based on the Hochberg procedure (Procedure H) was either superior or generally comparable in terms of its performance to the fixed-sequence procedure (Procedure F) based on a broad set of evaluation criteria. What was particularly important was that Procedure H provided a consistent advantage over Procedure F under the main data model which corresponds to Scenario 1 (see Table 2.2). For example, using a head-to-head comparison based on the probability of rejecting more null hypotheses, the probability of superiority for Procedure H was 8.0% and the probability of superiority for Procedure F was only 2.2%. This indicates that Procedure H is substantially more likely to provide a meaningful advantage over the other procedure (i.e., detect more significant dose-placebo contrasts) compared to Procedure F.

This section provides a summary of additional sensitivity assessments. This sensitivity assessment approach will focus on evaluating the characteristics of the two multiple testing procedures under quantitative deviations from the main data model using random perturbations. These assessments will help predict the potential behavior of the candidate procedures if the true ACR20 response rates in the trial arms are somewhat different from those assumed under the selected data model (see Table 2.2).

Parametric bootstrap

Quantitative sensitivity assessments were performed using the general parametric bootstrap algorithm defined in Chapter 1. For more information on the use of parametric bootstrap methods in quantitative assessments; see Section 1.3.3 and a clinical trial example provided in Section 1.4.

The performance of each analysis method (no adjustment, Procedure F and Procedure H) was evaluated by randomly generating a large number of dose-response curves that were slightly different from the flat dose-response function under the main data model. The amount of variability around the hypothesized dose-response function was controlled by the *uncertainty parameter* denoted by c ($c > 0$). A detailed description of the parametric bootstrap algorithm used in this sensitivity assessment is provided below.

- Step 1. Consider the response rates associated with the main data model, i.e., $\pi_1 = 0.3$, $\pi_2 = 0.5$ and $\pi_3 = 0.5$, and generate k sets of response rates in the three trial arms by sampling from the following beta distributions:

$$\pi'_{ij} \sim \text{Beta}(\alpha_i, \beta_i), \ i = 1, 2, 3, \ j = 1, \ldots, k.$$

The parameters of each beta distribution are chosen to ensure that the bootstrap response rates are centered around the corresponding response rates in the main data model. The common coefficient of variation is set to c and, with a larger value of c, the randomly generated response rates will exhibit more variability. As shown in Section 1.4,

$$\frac{\alpha_i}{\alpha_i + \beta_i} = \pi_i, \ \frac{\beta_i}{\alpha_i(\alpha_i + \beta_i + 1)} = c^2.$$

- Step 2. Using each set of bootstrap response rates as the "true" response rates, define appropriate *bootstrap data models*. Evaluate the performance of the candidate multiple testing procedures as well as the unadjusted procedure based on these bootstrap data models using the pre-defined criteria via simulations. Examine empirical distributions of the evaluation criteria computed from the bootstrap data models to help understand how deviations from the assumed dose-response function affect the performance of a particular analysis method.

This algorithm was applied to perform sensitivity assessments for Procedures F and H with the unadjusted procedure serving as a reference. The uncertainty parameter c was set to 0.1. Table 2.3 provides a detailed summary of the assumed distributions of the ACR20 response rates in the three

TABLE 2.3: Assumed distributions of the ACR20 response rates in the three trial arms based on the uncertainty parameter $c = 0.1$ in Case study 2.1.

Trial arm	Distribution	Mean (standard deviation)	95% range
Placebo	Beta(69.7, 162.6)	0.3 (0.03)	(0.24, 0.36)
Dose L	Beta(49.5, 49.5)	0.5 (0.05)	(0.4, 0.6)
Dose H	Beta(49.5, 49.5)	0.5 (0.05)	(0.4, 0.6)

trial arms. This table defines the parameters of the individual beta distributions and, most importantly, the summary includes a 95% range for the true response rate in each arm. The 95% range was computed as the interval between the 2.5th and 97.5th percentiles of the corresponding distribution and helps quantify the amount of uncertainty around the response rate. Even though the coefficient of variation, which serves as the key uncertainty parameter in this setting, was set to a fairly small value ($c = 0.1$), the table shows that the associated 95% ranges for the response rates were quite wide. Focusing, for example, on the response rates at Doses L and H, the response rates in the bootstrap data models would be expected to range between 40% and 60%. It would be fair to describe the associated setting as the case where the original statistical assumptions based on the main data model are considered fairly unreliable.

Quantitative sensitivity assessments with $k = 1,000$ bootstrap data models were performed for all evaluation criteria defined in Section 2.3.1. For compactness, the assessment results for only three criteria (disjunctive power, simple weighted power and overall multiplicity penalty) are presented below.

Sensitivity assessments based on disjunctive and weighted power

Figure 2.7 provides a visual summary of sensitivity assessments based on disjunctive power. This figure uses "violin plots" to display the probability density functions of disjunctive power computed from the bootstrap data models. In addition, each plot includes a standard box plot to show the lower quartile, median and upper quartile of each distribution as well as the mean value.

Figure 2.7 demonstrates the impact of possible deviations from the main set of statistical assumptions on disjunctive power of the selected analysis methods (unadjusted procedure, Procedure F and Procedure H). The distributions were highly skewed with long tails extending down to the bottom of the figure. The shapes of the violin plots for the unadjusted procedure and Procedure H were quite similar to each other. A visual examination of the box plots reveals that disjunctive power for the unadjusted procedure and Procedure H under bootstrap sampling was generally close to the values computed under the main data model (see Figure 2.2). By contrast, the violin plot for Procedure F was quite different from the other two and the corresponding

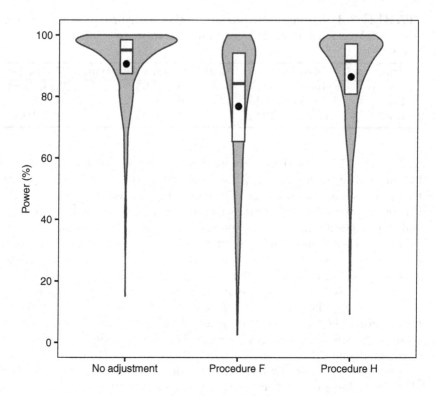

FIGURE 2.7: Distribution of disjunctive power computed from the bootstrap data models in the quantitative sensitivity assessment in Case study 2.1. Each box plot provides a summary of the lower quartile, median and upper quartile of disjunctive power and the black dot is the average level of disjunctive power.

box plot was shifted downward with the mean dropping below 80% and lower quartile approaching 60%.

A more detailed summary of the quantitative sensitivity assessments based on disjunctive power and simple weighted power is presented in Table 2.4. The table displays the values of disjunctive power and simple weighted power based on the original statistical assumptions (Scenario 1) as well as the lower quartile, median and upper quartile of the values computed from the bootstrap data models.

Table 2.4 provides important information on the operating characteristics of Procedures F and H that are to be expected with significant deviations from the original assumptions about the dose-response relationship in the clinical trial. For example, it follows from the top panel of Table 2.4 that the interquartile range for disjunctive power was quite tight for the analysis

TABLE 2.4: Summary of sensitivity assessments based on disjunctive and simple weighted power under the main data model (Scenario 1) in Case study 2.1.

Multiple testing procedure	Power under the main data model (%)	Power computed from bootstrap data models (%)		
		Lower quartile	Median	Upper quartile
Disjunctive power				
No adjustment	93.3	87.5	95.2	98.5
Procedure F	83.1	65.4	84.3	94.2
Procedure H	89.0	80.9	91.7	97.2
Simple weighted power				
No adjustment	83.0	66.1	80.8	90.3
Procedure F	76.9	53.8	73.4	85.9
Procedure H	80.9	62.9	79.3	89.7

strategy without a multiplicity adjustment. The width of the interval between the lower and upper quartiles was about 11 percentage points (from 87.5% to 98.5%). A somewhat wider interquartile range was observed for Procedure H, the width of the corresponding interval was approximately 17 percentage points (from 80.9% to 97.2%). This implies that about 75% of the time disjunctive power of Procedure H would be above the 80% threshold. In other words, using an absolute scale, 75% of the time disjunctive power of this multiple testing procedure would drop by less than 10 percentage points compared to disjunctive power computed under the original assumptions (89%). Further, with Procedure F, the lower quartile for disjunctive power was 65.4%, which indicates that disjunctive power of this procedure was expected to be less than 65% about 25% of the time. It was pointed out in Section 2.3.2 that Procedure F relies heavily on the monotonicity assumption and, if this assumption is violated, it tends to perform very poorly. Deviations from this assumption are generally likely under bootstrap sampling and this explains the lack of robustness and considerable power loss compared to Procedure H which is based on a more flexible algorithm with a data-driven testing sequence.

The bottom panel of Table 2.4 provides a summary of the quantitative sensitivity assessments based on simple weighted power and supports similar conclusions, namely, Procedure H was quite robust against significant deviations from the original statistical assumptions whereas simple weighted power of Procedure F tended to drop well below the value computed under the original data model.

Sensitivity assessments based on multiplicity penalties

Figure 2.8 and Table 2.5 summarize the results of quantitative sensitivity assessments based on the overall multiplicity penalty computed using a simpli-

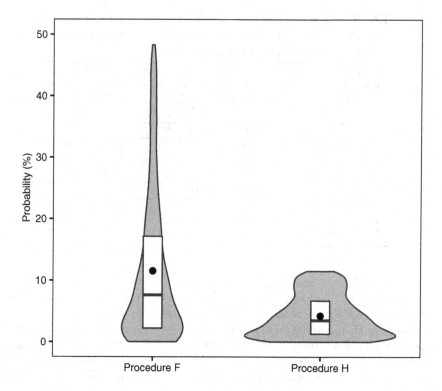

FIGURE 2.8: Distribution of the overall multiplicity penalty for Procedures F and H computed from the bootstrap data models in the quantitative sensitivity assessment in Case study 2.1. Each box plot provides a summary of the lower quartile, median and upper quartile of the multiplicity penalties and the black dot is the average multiplicity penalty.

fied multiplicity penalty matrix (the same definition of the overall multiplicity penalty was used in Figure 2.5).

The violin plots in Figure 2.8 display the probability density functions of the overall multiplicity penalty for Procedures F and H computed from the parametric bootstrap algorithm. As indicated above, the quantitative assessments presented in this section correspond to a setting with a fairly high amount of uncertainty about the efficacy profile of the experimental treatment. Under this assessment scheme, the overall multiplicity penalty for Procedure H was generally much lower than that for Procedure F. Since a higher overall multiplicity penalty is a sign of a less efficient multiplicity adjustment, Procedure H provided a tangible advantage over the other procedure. Figure 2.8 shows that Procedure F tended to perform quite poorly most of the time when

TABLE 2.5: Summary of sensitivity assessments based on the overall multiplicity penalty under the main data model (Scenario 1) in Case study 2.1.

Multiple testing procedure	Multiplicity penalty under the main data model (%)	Multiplicity penalty based on bootstrap data models (%)		
		Lower quartile	Median	Upper quartile
Procedure F	10.2	2.3	8.2	19.6
Procedure H	4.3	1.3	3.5	6.7

the true dose-response curve in the rheumatoid arthritis clinical trial deviated from the assumed flat dose-response.

Key descriptive statistics of the bootstrap distributions displayed in Figure 2.8 are shown in Table 2.5. This includes, as above, the lower quartile, median and upper quartile of the multiplicity penalties for Procedures F and H. The median multiplicity penalty for Procedure F was lower than the overall multiplicity penalty under the main data model (8.2% versus 10.2%). However, the upper quartile was almost twice as large, which indicates that there was a considerable loss of efficiency compared to the unadjusted procedure in a large fraction of the bootstrap data models. This observation needs to be contrasted with an important observation that the upper quartile of the multiplicity penalty distribution for Procedure H was only 6.7%, which was only slightly worse than the overall multiplicity penalty under the main data model shown in Figure 2.5 (4.3%).

Relevant performance loss

The results of sensitivity assessments presented above indicate that random deviations from the main data model resulted in performance loss for both candidate multiple testing procedures. As indicated in Section 1.3.3, it will be of interest to compute the probability of relevant performance loss for these procedures as well as the unadjusted analysis as part of the quantitative sensitivity assessment. Relevant performance loss was defined as a relative reduction in disjunctive power or simple weighted power greater than 10% based on a bootstrap dose-response function compared to the original dose-response function (Scenario 1).

A summary of performance loss evaluations is provided in Figure 2.9. The results presented in this figure provide additional insights into the "robustness profile" of the three analysis strategies. The probability of relevant performance loss based on disjunctive power was generally comparable between the unadjusted procedure and Procedure H (19.6% and 23.4%, respectively). Using Procedure H as an example, disjunctive power under Scenario 1 was 89% (see, for example, Table 2.4). With a 10% relative reduction, disjunctive power of Procedure H under bootstrap sampling dropped below $89 \times 0.9 = 80.1\%$

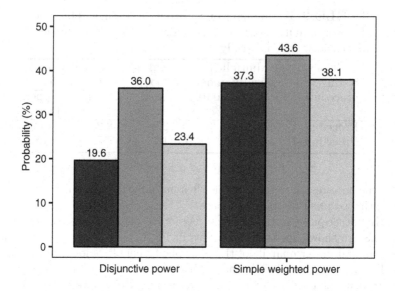

FIGURE 2.9: Probability of relevant performance loss for each analysis method (no adjustment, black bars; Procedure F, dark gray bars; Procedure H, light gray bars) based on disjunctive and simple weighted power in the quantitative sensitivity assessment in Case study 2.1.

only about 23% of the time. A similar conclusion was supported by the results presented in Table 2.4. Disjunctive power of Procedure F was, by contrast, quite likely to decrease by more than 10% on a relative scale. It can be seen from Figure 2.9 that this occurred 36% of the time.

Figure 2.9 also summarizes the results of performance loss assessments for the simple weighted criterion. These results are similar to those based on the disjunctive criterion, namely, Procedure F was again quite sensitive to quantitative deviations from the assumed dose-response function and the probability of performance loss was greater than 40% whereas the probability of performance loss for the unadjusted analysis and Procedure H was between 37% and 38%.

2.3.4   Software implementation

Simulation-based assessments of the candidate multiplicity adjustments presented in this section are easily implemented using the **Mediana** package (for more information on this R package; see Chapter 1). Since the **Mediana** package supports evaluation of trial designs and analysis methods within a general Clinical Scenario Evaluation framework, it is shown below that it is quite straightforward to directly "translate" the data, analysis and evaluation models defined above into R code and run simulations aimed at evaluating the performance of the three analysis methods (unadjusted, fixed-sequence and Hochberg procedures) in the Phase III clinical trial defined in Section 2.3.1.

Data model

The data model defines parameters used for generating patient data in the clinical trial. In this case study, a set of outcome distribution parameters is specified for each of the three samples in the data model to represent different assumptions on the expected proportions of patients who meet the ACR20 response criterion at Week 24. The sets correspond to the three scenarios defined in Table 2.2.

LISTING 2.1: Outcome parameter specifications in Case study 2.1

```
# Outcome parameters - Scenario 1
outcome.placebo.sc1 = parameters(prop = 0.30)
outcome.dose1.sc1 = parameters(prop = 0.50)
outcome.doseh.sc1 = parameters(prop = 0.50)

# Outcome parameters - Scenario 2
outcome.placebo.sc2 = parameters(prop = 0.30)
outcome.dose1.sc2 = parameters(prop = 0.40)
outcome.doseh.sc2 = parameters(prop = 0.50)

# Outcome parameters - Scenario 3
outcome.placebo.sc3 = parameters(prop = 0.30)
outcome.dose1.sc3 = parameters(prop = 0.50)
outcome.doseh.sc3 = parameters(prop = 0.45)
```

The sample size is set to 100 patients per arm and a simplified assumption that all patients complete the trial is made in this case study. In the **Mediana** package, a dropout mechanism can be introduced to model more realistic settings with incomplete outcomes. This can be easily accomplished by specifying the dropout distribution and associated parameters (enrollment distribution, follow-up duration) in a `Design` object. For example, the dropout process can be modeled using an exponential distribution. As the primary endpoint is evaluated at Week 24, the follow-up duration is considered fixed for all patients, i.e., 24 weeks, and the enrollment period is estimated to be approximately 2 years, i.e., 104 weeks.

LISTING 2.2: Specification of dropout parameters

```
# Design parameters (in weeks)
Design(enroll.period = 104,
       followup.period = 24,
       enroll.dist = "UniformDist",
```

```
      dropout.dist = "ExpoDist",
      dropout.dist.par = parameters(rate = 0.01))
```

The data model is initialized using the `DataModel` object and each component of this object can be added one at a time. The outcome distribution is defined using the `OutcomeDist` object with the `BinomDist` distribution, the common sample size per arm is specified in the `SampleSize` object and the outcome distribution parameters for each trial arm are specified in `Sample` objects.

LISTING 2.3: Data model in Case study 2.1

```
# Data model
mult.cs1.data.model =
  DataModel() +
  OutcomeDist(outcome.dist = "BinomDist") +
  SampleSize(100) +
  Sample(id = "Placebo",
         outcome.par = parameters(outcome.placebo.sc1,
                                   outcome.placebo.sc2,
                                   outcome.placebo.sc3)) +
  Sample(id = "Dose L",
         outcome.par = parameters(outcome.dosel.sc1,
                                   outcome.dosel.sc2,
                                   outcome.dosel.sc3)) +
  Sample(id = "Dose H",
         outcome.par = parameters(outcome.doseh.sc1,
                                   outcome.doseh.sc2,
                                   outcome.doseh.sc3))
```

Analysis model

The analysis model is composed of the two statistical tests that will be performed to compare Doses L and H to Placebo as well as the multiplicity adjustment procedures used to control the Type I error rate.

Each dose-placebo comparison will be carried out using a two-sample test for proportions, defined in the `Test` object with the `PropTest` method. Since the statistical tests are one-sided, the order of the two samples in the `samples` argument is important. If a higher numerical value of the endpoint indicates a beneficial effect, which is the case with the ACR20 response rate, the first sample must correspond to the sample expected to have the lower value of the endpoint. Thus `"Placebo"` is included as the first sample in the test specification.

Concerning the multiplicity adjustment procedures, three procedures are defined in this analysis model using the `MultAdjProc` object. First, in order to request a straightforward analysis without any adjustment, an empty object is set up, i.e., `MultAdjProc(proc = NA)`. The fixed-sequence procedure (Procedure F) is defined using a `FixedSeqAdj` method while the Hochberg adjustment procedure (Procedure H) is defined using the `HochbergAdj` method.

LISTING 2.4: Analysis model in Case study 2.1

```
# Analysis model
mult.cs1.analysis.model = AnalysisModel() +
  MultAdjProc(proc = NA) +
  MultAdjProc(proc = "FixedSeqAdj") +
  MultAdjProc(proc = "HochbergAdj") +
  Test(id = "Placebo vs Dose H",
       samples = samples("Placebo", "Dose H"),
       method = "PropTest") +
  Test(id = "Placebo vs Dose L",
       samples = samples("Placebo", "Dose L"),
       method = "PropTest")
```

It is worth noting that, by default, the multiplicity adjustment procedures defined in the analysis model will be applied to all tests included in the `AnalysisModel` object in the order specified. Specifically, the fixed-sequence procedure will begin with the test of Dose H versus Placebo and then examine the test of Dose L versus Placebo.

Evaluation model

The evaluation model specifies the metrics for assessing the performance of the analysis model based on the assumptions defined in the data model. In this case study, several criteria are evaluated to assess the performance of the three analysis methods (no multiplicity adjustment, Procedure F and Procedure H).

First, the disjunctive criterion, ψ_D, is defined as the probability to reject at least one null hypothesis, i.e., the probability of demonstrating a statistically significant effect with at least one dose. This criterion is defined using the `DisjunctivePower` method.

The second criterion is based on simple weighted power, ψ_W, which corresponds to the weighted sum of the marginal power functions of the two dose-placebo tests. This criterion can be defined in the evaluation model using the `WeightedPower` method, where the weights associated with each test are specified in the `par` argument.

Finally, the partition-based weighted criterion is a custom criterion, which is not currently implemented in the **Mediana** package. Nonetheless, a custom criterion function can be created and used within the evaluation model. This custom function includes three arguments. The first argument (`test.result`) is a matrix of p-values associated with the tests defined in the `tests` argument of the `Criterion` object. Similarly, the second argument (`statistic.result`) is a matrix of results corresponding to the statistics defined in the `statistics` argument of the `Criterion` object. In this case study, no `Statistic` objects were specified in the analysis model and this criterion will only use the p-values returned by the tests associated with the two dose-placebo comparisons. Finally, the last argument (`parameter`) contains the optional parameter(s) defined in the `par` argument of the `Criterion` object. For the partition-based weighted power, the `par` argument must contain the weights associated with each of the three outcomes:

- Reject H_1 only.

- Reject H_2 only.

- Simultaneously reject H_1 and H_2.

The `mult.cs1.PartitionBasedWeightedPower` function evaluates the probability of each outcome and then computes the weighted sum.

LISTING 2.5: Custom function for computing partition-based weighted power in Case study 2.1

```
# Custom evaluation criterion based on partition-based
    weighted power
mult.cs1.PartitionBasedWeightedPower =
  function(test.result, statistic.result, parameter) {

  # Parameters
  alpha = parameter$alpha
  weight = parameter$weight

  # Outcomes
  H1_only = ((test.result[,1] <= alpha) & (test.result[,2]
    > alpha))
  H2_only = ((test.result[,1] > alpha) & (test.result[,2]
    <= alpha))
  H1_H2 = ((test.result[,1] <= alpha) & (test.result[,2] <=
    alpha))

  # Weighted power
  power = mean(H1_only) * weight[1] + mean(H2_only) *
    weight[2] + mean(H1_H2) * weight[3]

  return(power)
}
```

It needs to be noted that the order of tests in the `tests` argument of this custom function is important. The first test should be the one corresponding to the comparison of Dose H versus Placebo and the second test is based on the comparison of Dose L versus Placebo.

Finally, the evaluation model can be constructed by specifying each

`Criterion` object. In addition, marginal power of each test can be computed using the `MarginalPower` method.

LISTING 2.6: Evaluation model in Case study 2.1

```
# Evaluation model
mult.cs1.evaluation.model = EvaluationModel() +
  Criterion(id = "Marginal power",
            method = "MarginalPower",
            tests = tests("Placebo vs Dose H",
                          "Placebo vs Dose L"),
            labels = c("Placebo vs Dose H",
                       "Placebo vs Dose L"),
            par = parameters(alpha = 0.025)) +
  Criterion(id = "Disjunctive power",
            method = "DisjunctivePower",
            tests = tests("Placebo vs Dose H",
                          "Placebo vs Dose L"),
            labels = "Disjunctive power",
            par = parameters(alpha = 0.025)) +
  Criterion(id = "Simple weighted power",
            method = "WeightedPower",
            tests = tests("Placebo vs Dose H",
                          "Placebo vs Dose L"),
            labels = "Weighted power (v1 = 0.4, v2 = 0.6)",
            par = parameters(alpha = 0.025,
                             weight = c(0.4, 0.6))) +
  Criterion(id = "Partition-based weighted power",
            method = "mult.cs1.PartitionBasedWeightedPower",
            tests = tests("Placebo vs Dose H",
                          "Placebo vs Dose L"),
            labels = "Partition-based weighted power (v1 =
  0.15, v2 = 0.25, v12 = 0.6)",
            par = parameters(alpha = 0.025,
                             weight = c(0.15, 0.25, 0.6)))
```

Simulation results

Once the data, analysis and evaluation models have been built, the simulation parameters need to be specified as explained in Chapter 1, including the number of simulation runs. Table 2.6 provides a summary of the simulation results based on the CSE models specified above with 100,000 replications. For the purpose of illustration, only one treatment effect scenario (Scenario 1) is included in this table. The simulation results presented in this table are very similar to those displayed in Figures 2.3, 2.4 and 2.5 (the results may be slightly different due to Monte Carlo errors).

TABLE 2.6: Summary of simulation results.

Evaluation criterion	Multiplicity adjustment	Value
Marginal power	No adjustment	Placebo vs Dose H: 83.2%
	No adjustment	Placebo vs Dose L: 83.1%
	Procedure F	Placebo vs Dose H: 83.2%
	Procedure F	Placebo vs Dose L: 72.9%
	Procedure H	Placebo vs Dose H: 81.1%
	Procedure H	Placebo vs Dose L: 81.0%
Disjunctive power	No adjustment	93.5%
	Procedure F	83.2%
	Procedure H	89.1%
Simple weighted power	No adjustment	83.2%
	Procedure F	77.0%
	Procedure H	81.0%
Partition-based weighted power	No adjustment	47.8%
	Procedure F	45.3%
	Procedure H	47.0%

2.3.5   Conclusions and extensions

To summarize the key findings presented in this section, comprehensive qualitative and quantitative sensitivity analyses were presented to assess the performance of two candidate multiplicity adjustments in a traditional setting with a single source of multiplicity. The sensitivity assessments based on several evaluation criteria revealed that the multiple testing procedure that relies on a data-driven testing sequence (Hochberg procedure) outperformed the procedure with a pre-defined hypothesis ordering (fixed-sequence procedure) under the main data model and provided comparable or superior performance under alternative data models. An additional set of quantitative assessments could be performed using compound criteria, i.e., minimum and average criteria, introduced in Chapter 1 (see Section 1.3.3). These criteria support performance assessments under the worst-case scenario as well as under the "average" scenario computed from the pre-defined sets of treatment effect assumptions.

When comparing the evaluation criteria used in the sensitivity analyses, it is helpful to discuss the role of more advanced criteria such as partition-based weighted criteria and more basic criteria derived from simple weighted power. As pointed out in Section 2.2.3, an important advantage of using the partition-based weighted criterion is that this evaluation criterion provides the trial's sponsor with much flexibility. For example, this criterion enables the sponsor to explicitly incorporate outcomes corresponding to regulatory claims pursued in a clinical trial. Using this general criterion may prove advantageous in certain multiplicity problems. However, the conclusions based on simple weighted power and partition-based weighted power were very similar in a straightforward multiplicity problem considered in this section.

2.4 Case study 2.2: Direct selection of optimal procedure parameters

This case study focuses on optimal selection of procedure parameters of candidate multiple testing procedures in a complex multiplicity problem with hierarchically ordered objectives. A direct optimization algorithm with univariate and bivariate parameter search will be utilized. The optimization algorithm will be run using several data models that are based on clinically distinct sets of treatment effects and will thus incorporate qualitative sensitivity assessments. Quantitative sensitivity analyses will also be performed to examine the performance of the optimal multiplicity adjustment under random deviations from an assumed data model.

2.4.1 Clinical trial

The clinical trial example used in this case study is based on a Phase III trial that was conducted to evaluate the efficacy and safety of brexpiprazole, a novel treatment for schizophrenia (Correll et al., 2015). The patient population in the case study will include patients with schizophrenia who experience an acute exacerbation. The patients will be treated for 6 weeks and will be randomly assigned to a low dose of the experimental treatment (Dose L), high dose of the experimental treatment (Dose H) or placebo. An unbalanced design with a 1:2:2 randomization scheme will be employed in the trial. The use of unequal randomization helps provide more information on the treatment's safety profile and facilitates patient enrollment since patients are more likely to be allocated to an active treatment.

The case study presents a multiplicity problem with two sources of multiplicity. The two dose-placebo comparisons (Dose L versus placebo and Dose H versus placebo) will serve as the *first source of multiplicity*. In addition to that, the efficacy of the experimental treatment will be evaluated using two ordered clinical endpoints:

- Primary endpoint: Change from baseline in the Positive and Negative Syndrome Scale (PANSS) total score.

- Key secondary endpoint: Change from baseline in the Clinical Global Impressions Severity Scale (CGI-S) score.

Note that lower values of the PANSS total score and CGI-S score are associated with improvement and thus negative changes indicate a beneficial treatment effect.

The key secondary endpoint provides supportive evidence of treatment efficacy and significant findings based on both endpoints can be presented in the product label. The analysis of the primary and secondary endpoints defines the *second source of multiplicity* in this trial.

TABLE 2.7: Marginal outcome distributions in Case study 2.2.

Sample	Trial arm	Endpoint	Marginal outcome distribution
Sample 1	Placebo	Primary	$N(\mu_{10}, \sigma_1^2)$
	Placebo	Secondary	$N(\mu_{20}, \sigma_2^2)$
Sample 2	Dose L	Primary	$N(\mu_{11}, \sigma_1^2)$
	Dose L	Secondary	$N(\mu_{21}, \sigma_2^2)$
Sample 3	Dose H	Primary	$N(\mu_{12}, \sigma_1^2)$
	Dose H	Secondary	$N(\mu_{22}, \sigma_2^2)$

Data model

To define a data model in this case study, note that, as in Case study 2.1, the number of samples is determined by the number of trial arms, i.e., three samples need to be set up. Further, it is important to recognize that two outcomes based on the selected clinical endpoints will be observed for each patient in the trial. This means that a bivariate outcome distribution is to be specified in each sample. To define the outcome distribution parameters, the changes in the PANSS and CGI-S scores were assumed to follow a bivariate normal distribution. As shown in Table 2.7, μ_{10} and μ_{20} denote the means of the marginal distributions of the primary and secondary endpoints in the placebo arm. The similar parameters in the low-dose arm are denoted by μ_{11} and μ_{21} and in the high-dose arm by μ_{12} and μ_{22}. A reasonable assumption of common endpoint-specific standard deviations across the three arms was made in this trial. The common standard deviations for the primary and secondary endpoints are denoted by σ_1 and σ_2, respectively.

The mean values of the primary and key secondary endpoints in the placebo arm were assumed to be

$$\mu_{10} = -12, \ \mu_{20} = -0.8.$$

As stated above, the negative values imply a beneficial treatment effect on both endpoints. The standard deviations were set to $\sigma_1 = 20$ and $\sigma_2 = 1$. The correlation between the two endpoints, denoted by ρ, was set to 0.5, which indicates a fairly strong correlation between the primary and secondary endpoints. This parameter served as a supportive parameter in the data models considered in this case study.

Further, let θ_i, $i = 1, \ldots, 4$, denote the standardized treatment differences (effect sizes) of the four endpoint tests in this clinical trial. Based on these effect sizes, the mean values are related to each other as follows:

$$\mu_{11} = \mu_{10} - \theta_2 \sigma_1, \ \mu_{21} = \mu_{20} - \theta_4 \sigma_2,$$
$$\mu_{12} = \mu_{10} - \theta_1 \sigma_1, \ \mu_{22} = \mu_{20} - \theta_3 \sigma_2.$$

The four effect sizes define the key data model parameters.

TABLE 2.8: Assumed effect sizes for the four tests under the four data models (scenarios) in Case study 2.2.

Scenario	Primary endpoint		Secondary endpoint	
	Dose H vs Placebo	Dose L vs Placebo	Dose H vs Placebo	Dose L vs Placebo
Scenario 1	$\theta_1 = 0.4$	$\theta_2 = 0.3$	$\theta_3 = 0.3$	$\theta_4 = 0.3$
Scenario 2	$\theta_1 = 0.3$	$\theta_2 = 0.3$	$\theta_3 = 0.3$	$\theta_4 = 0.3$
Scenario 3	$\theta_1 = 0.4$	$\theta_2 = 0.3$	$\theta_3 = 0.4$	$\theta_4 = 0.4$
Scenario 4	$\theta_1 = 0.3$	$\theta_2 = 0.3$	$\theta_3 = 0.4$	$\theta_4 = 0.4$

Several clinically distinct sets of the key data model parameters were considered in this case study. The scenarios that define four data models are listed in Table 2.8. Under Scenario 1, the effect size for the primary endpoint at Dose H was greater than the effect size at Dose L ($\theta_2 < \theta_1$). Further, the two doses were expected to be equally effective based on the secondary endpoint ($\theta_3 = \theta_4$). In addition, it was very important to consider other scenarios, especially the case when the two doses would be equally effective on the primary endpoint. This assumption reflects a general observation that flat dose-response curves are rather common in neuroscience trials. For example, Correll et al. (2015) reported that the primary effect size at the high dose was very close to that at the low dose in the brexpiprazole trial. This set of assumptions was defined in Scenario 2. Finally, Scenarios 3 and 4 were based on Scenarios 1 and 2 but assumed a larger common effect size for the secondary endpoint (θ_3 and θ_4 were both equal to 0.4 rather than 0.3).

It needs to be stressed that Scenario 1 is perceived as the most likely scenario and the associated data model will be referred to as the main model in this case study. The alternative data models corresponding to Scenarios 2, 3 and 4 will need to be taken into account to inform the overall decision-making process in this trial and will play an important part in the clinical trial optimization exercise.

The sample size in the placebo arm was set to 100 patients, which, due to the 1:2:2 randomization scheme, resulted in the total sample size of 500 patients in the trial. This sample size guarantees a high probability of success for the primary endpoint test at Dose H under the main data model (Scenario 1 in Table 2.8). Power of this test before a multiplicity adjustment was 90.1%. Power of the primary endpoint test at Dose L as well as the secondary endpoint tests was much lower (68.3%).

As the final comment related to the data generation process in this clinical trial example, it will be assumed for simplicity that all patients complete the 6-week treatment period. In reality, early discontinuation rates in schizophrenia trials could be quite high. For example, the discontinuation rate ranged between 30% and 40% in the brexpiprazole trial (Correll et al., 2015). The **Mediana** package introduced in Chapter 1 supports multiple options for modeling the patient dropout process; see Section 2.3.4 for examples.

Analysis model

It was indicated in the discussion of data models in this case study that the efficacy evaluation will be performed using the four tests based on the two dose-placebo comparisons and two clinical endpoints of interest. The corresponding four null hypotheses of interest are defined as follows:

- H_1: Null hypothesis of no effect at Dose H with respect to the primary endpoint ($\theta_1 = 0$).

- H_2: Null hypothesis of no effect at Dose L with respect to the primary endpoint ($\theta_2 = 0$).

- H_3: Null hypothesis of no effect at Dose H with respect to the secondary endpoint ($\theta_3 = 0$).

- H_4: Null hypothesis of no effect at Dose L with respect to the secondary endpoint ($\theta_4 = 0$).

A successful outcome will be declared in the trial if at least one primary null hypothesis is rejected, which means that the experimental treatment provides a beneficial effect, at either dose or at both doses, on the primary endpoint. Note that, based on marketing considerations, it may be highly desirable to demonstrate that both doses are effective but, from a regulatory perspective, it will be sufficient to establish a significant effect at a single dose. Rejection of the secondary hypotheses will provide supportive evidence of effectiveness that will be presented in the product label.

The four hypothesis tests can be carried out based on appropriate repeated-measures models. The model for each endpoint can include fixed factors such as treatment, visit and treatment-by-visit interaction as well as the baseline value of the endpoint and baseline-by-visit interaction. The analysis strategy based on the four tests induces multiplicity and a multiplicity adjustment is required to protect the Type I error rate at the nominal level (one-sided $\alpha = 0.025$). Note that the Type I error rate is defined in a global sense with respect to all four null hypotheses as opposed to just the primary null hypotheses. As a result, the multiplicity adjustment will serve as the key component of the analysis model in this trial.

When carrying out the four hypothesis tests, it is critical to take into account relevant clinical information. Based on the hierarchical relationship between the primary and secondary endpoints, the four null hypotheses can be grouped into two families:

- Primary family: Null hypotheses H_1 and H_2.

- Secondary family: Null hypotheses H_3 and H_4.

To explicitly account for this hierarchical structure, it is common to impose the following *logical restrictions* on the four tests in the two families:

- The comparison between Dose H and placebo on the secondary endpoint will be carried out only if a significant treatment effect is demonstrated at the same dose in the primary family. In other words, the hypothesis H_3 cannot be rejected unless the hypothesis H_1 is rejected.

- Similarly, the secondary endpoint test at Dose L is meaningful and the hypothesis H_4 can be tested only if the same test is significant in the primary family, i.e., the hypothesis H_2 is rejected.

The importance of accounting for clinically meaningful restrictions of this kind when setting up multiplicity adjustments was emphasized in several publications; see, for example, O'Neill (1997) and Hung and Wang (2009).

Several classes of multiple testing procedures for multiplicity problems with several families of null hypotheses, known as *gatekeeping procedures*, have been considered in the literature. This case study considers two gatekeeping procedures that belong to the class of nonparametric (Bonferroni-based) chain procedures introduced in Section 2.2.2. A more powerful multiplicity adjustment from a class of semiparametric procedures will be presented in Case study 2.3.

The first Bonferroni-based chain procedure that will be referred to as Procedure B1 utilizes the α-allocation and α-propagation rules based on the following vector of initial hypothesis weights and matrix of transition parameters:

$$W_1 = [1\ 0\ 0\ 0], \quad T_1 = \begin{bmatrix} 0 & g_1 & 1-g_1 & 0 \\ 0 & 0 & 0 & 1 \\ 0 & 0 & 0 & 0 \\ 0 & 0 & 0 & 0 \end{bmatrix}.$$

Here g_1 $(0 \leq g_1 \leq 1)$ is a procedure parameter. The resulting decision rules are visualized in Figure 2.10. As in Figure 2.1, each hypothesis is represented by a circle and the initial hypothesis weights are specified by the α-allocation rule. The arrows are based on the α-propagation rules, i.e., visualize the process of re-distributing the error rate after each rejection.

Figure 2.10 shows that, based on the vector W_1, a positive weight will be initially assigned only to the hypothesis H_1, which means that testing will begin by evaluating the treatment effect on the primary endpoint at Dose H. This test will be carried out at α. Further, as indicated in the transition matrix T_1, if the first hypothesis is rejected, the error rate will be split between the Dose L test for the primary endpoint (hypothesis H_2) and the Dose H test for the secondary endpoint (hypothesis H_3). Based on the outgoing arrows with the transition parameters g_{12} and g_{13} shown in the figure, H_2 will be tested at αg_1 and H_3 at $\alpha(1-g_1)$. If a treatment benefit is demonstrated at Dose L based on the primary endpoint (H_2 is rejected), the hypothesis H_4 will be tested at the same significance level as H_2, i.e., at αg_1.

The decision rules presented in Figure 2.10 clearly demonstrate that the proposed procedure is consistent with the logical restrictions defined above.

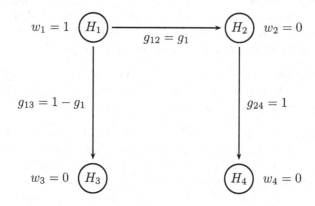

FIGURE 2.10: Basic Bonferroni-based chain procedure (Procedure B1) in Case study 2.2.

Indeed, the null hypothesis H_3 will be tested only if the hypothesis it depends on, i.e., H_1, is rejected, which means that it is impossible to claim a significant treatment effect on the secondary endpoint at Dose H unless a significant effect on the primary endpoint is established at the same dose. Similarly, the null hypothesis H_4 can be tested only if H_2 is rejected and thus the same restriction is valid for the Dose L tests.

Figure 2.10 presents a high-level summary of the α-allocation and α-propagation rules employed in Procedure B1 and it is helpful to review the decision rules that will be applied to test each hypothesis. A detailed visual summary of the decision rules is provided in Figure 2.11. This figure defines the four steps of the testing algorithm based on the following testing sequence:

$$H_1, \ H_3, \ H_2, \ H_4.$$

It is worth pointing out that a testing algorithm can be defined for any sequence of hypotheses and all possible algorithms are mathematically equivalent to each other. This particular testing sequence was selected to achieve compact representation of the decision rules.

As in Figure 2.10, each hypothesis is represented in Figure 2.11 by a circle and the adjusted significance level used in the corresponding test is displayed next to each circle. A solid arrow is used to define the decision path after a hypothesis is rejected and a dashed arrow after a hypothesis is accepted. The four-step testing algorithm is defined as follows:

- Step 1. The first hypothesis in the sequence, i.e., H_1, will be tested at the pre-assigned level α.

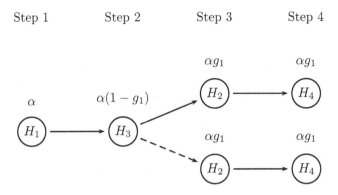

FIGURE 2.11: Decision rules used in the basic Bonferroni-based chain procedure (Procedure B1) in Case study 2.2. A solid arrow defines the decision path after a hypothesis is rejected and a dashed arrow defines the decision path after a hypothesis is accepted. The adjusted significance level used in the corresponding test is shown next to each hypothesis.

- Step 2. If H_1 is rejected in Step 1, the hypothesis H_3 will be tested at $\alpha(1 - g_1)$.

- Step 3. The testing algorithm branches out after Step 2 and both branches lead to the hypothesis H_2. Note that the adjusted significance levels used in the two tests are the same (H_2 is tested at αg_1 if H_3 is rejected and at αg_1 otherwise). This means that the test of this hypothesis is independent of the outcome of the H_3 test.

- Step 4. The last hypothesis in the sequence, i.e., H_4, will be tested at αg_1 after H_2 is rejected.

It is important to note that Procedure B1 represents a rather simplistic approach to performing a multiplicity adjustment in this case study. As explained in Section 2.2.2, the key principle used in multiple testing procedures is the "use it or lose it" principle. According to this principle, the fraction of the overall error rate assigned to a particular hypothesis can be applied to other non-rejected hypotheses after this hypothesis is rejected. However, as shown in Figure 2.10, there are no outgoing connections from the null hypotheses H_3 and H_4. This immediately implies that the fractions of the overall Type I error rate released after the rejection of H_3 and H_4, i.e., $\alpha(1 - g_1)$ and αg_1, will not be applied to other hypotheses in this multiplicity problem and thus they will be "wasted." More formally, the diagrams in Figures 2.10 and 2.11 show that Procedure B1 is not α-exhaustive (see Section 2.2.2). However, as

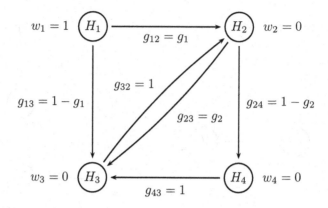

FIGURE 2.12: Advanced Bonferroni-based chain procedure (Procedure B2) in Case study 2.2.

shown below, this multiple testing procedure can be improved by switching to an α-exhaustive testing strategy.

An improved chain procedure that will be referred to as Procedure B2 utilizes the following set of initial hypothesis weights and transition matrix:

$$W_2 = [1\ 0\ 0\ 0], \quad T_2 = \begin{bmatrix} 0 & g_1 & 1 - g_1 & 0 \\ 0 & 0 & g_2 & 1 - g_2 \\ 0 & 1 & 0 & 0 \\ 0 & 0 & 1 & 0 \end{bmatrix},$$

where g_1 and g_2 ($0 \leq g_1 \leq 1$ and $0 \leq g_2 \leq 1$) are pre-defined parameters of the α-propagation rule in this procedure. A visual summary of the decision rules employed by Procedure B2 is presented in Figure 2.12. This procedure serves as an example of an efficient procedure that will provide a power advantage over Procedure B1 by transferring appropriate fractions of the error rate from H_3 and H_4 after their rejection to the hypotheses that have not been rejected yet.

As shown in Figure 2.12, the advanced Bonferroni-based chain procedure (Procedure B2) is similar to Procedure B1 in that it also assigns a positive weight only to the hypothesis H_1. This means that the testing algorithm used in Procedure B2 begins with H_1. This null hypothesis will be tested at the full α level and, if it is rejected, as in Procedure B1, the overall error rate will be divided between H_2 and H_3 according to the parameter g_1. However, after the rejection of H_2, Procedure B2 adds the following additional options. The fraction of the error rate used for testing H_2 will be further split between the hypotheses H_3 and H_4. This splitting rule is governed by another parameter

(g_2). If the hypothesis H_4 is rejected, the significance level used in this test will be transferred to H_3. And, lastly, if H_3 is rejected, the associated fraction of the error rate will be carried over to H_2. Note that H_3 may be tested after the rejection of H_1 and the test of H_2 may not be significant at the level assigned to this hypothesis after H_1 is rejected. Figure 2.12 demonstrates that Procedure B2 is, in fact, α-exhaustive since the error rate after each rejection is applied to one or more non-rejected hypotheses. Also, it is important to note that the final outcome of the procedure, i.e., how many and which hypotheses are rejected, does not depend on the testing order.

Procedure B2 satisfies the logical restrictions imposed on the primary and secondary hypotheses. It follows from Figure 2.12 that the null hypothesis H_3 can be rejected only if the corresponding primary hypothesis (H_1) is rejected and, further, it is impossible to reject H_4 without rejecting H_2. When reviewing the connections between hypotheses in the diagram displayed in Figure 2.12, it is instructive to check if other potential connections would be consistent with the logical restrictions or would be meaningful. For example, a connection from H_1 to H_4 would clearly violate the restrictions since it may enable testing the treatment effect on the secondary endpoint at Dose L without establishing a significant effect on the primary endpoint at the same dose. In other words, it would be possible to reject H_4 without rejecting the corresponding primary hypothesis (H_2). A connection from H_3 to H_4 would lead to the same undesirable situation.

Figure 2.13 provides a detailed summary of the decision rules used in the advanced Bonferroni-based chain procedure. Just like Figure 2.11, it explicitly defines the adjusted significance levels used in each hypothesis test under different scenarios. The four-step testing algorithm presented in this figure relies on the following testing sequence:

$$H_1, \ H_2, \ H_4, \ H_3.$$

As before, the testing sequence was chosen for convenience and a similar algorithm is easily constructed for any other testing sequence.

As shown in Figure 2.13, Procedure B2 utilizes the following testing algorithm:

- Step 1. The first hypothesis in the testing sequence (H_1) will be tested at the full α level.

- Step 2. Following the rejection of H_1, the hypothesis H_2 will be tested at αg_1.

- Step 3. If H_2 is rejected in Step 2, the hypothesis H_4 will be tested at $\alpha g_1(1 - g_2)$. Otherwise, H_4 will not be tested (it will be automatically accepted) and the hypothesis H_3 will be tested at $\alpha(1 - g_1)$.

- Step 4. If H_4 is rejected in Step 3, H_3 will be tested at α. This significance level represents the sum of all connections from the hypotheses H_1, H_2

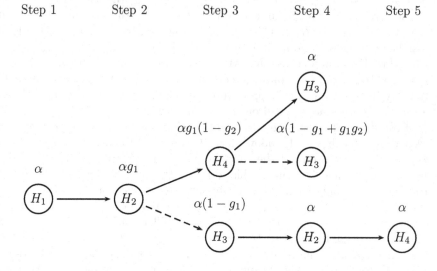

Step 1   Step 2   Step 3   Step 4   Step 5

FIGURE 2.13: Decision rules used in the advanced Bonferroni-based chain procedure (Procedure B2) in Case study 2.2. A solid arrow defines the decision path after a hypothesis is rejected and a dashed arrow defines the decision path after a hypothesis is accepted. The adjusted significance level used in the corresponding test is shown next to each hypothesis.

and H_4 that lead to H_3. On the other hand, if H_4 cannot be rejected in Step 3, the hypothesis H_3 will still be tested but at a lower significance level, namely, at $\alpha(1 - g_1 + g_1 g_2)$. In addition, if H_3 is already rejected in Step 3, H_2 will be tested at α. Note this significance level is equal to the sum of the error rate fractions carried over to H_2 from H_1 and H_3.

- Step 5. If H_2 is rejected in Step 4, H_4 will be tested at the same significance level, i.e., α.

It is easy to see that, whenever Procedure B1 rejects the hypotheses H_1 and H_2, these hypotheses will also be rejected by Procedure B2. A more careful review of the decision rules depicted in Figures 2.11 and 2.13 reveals that the rejection of H_3 by Procedure B1 immediately implies the rejection of this hypothesis by Procedure B2. However, due the splitting rule governed by the g_2 parameter, it is possible for Procedure B2 to fail to reject the hypothesis H_4 after it is rejected by Procedure B1.

Evaluation model

It follows from Figures 2.11 and 2.13 that the numerical values of the procedure parameters, i.e., $g = g_1$ in Procedure B1 and $g = (g_1, g_2)$ in Procedure B2, directly influence the number of hypotheses rejected by each gatekeeping procedure. From a practical perspective, it will be highly desirable to select the parameters to maximize an appropriate success criterion, in which case $g = g_1$ and $g = (g_1, g_2)$ will be treated as the target parameters in an optimization problem. Several criteria that can be utilized in the associated evaluation models are described below.

A large number of options is available when defining evaluation criteria in more complex multiplicity problems with several sources of multiplicity compared to traditional multiplicity problems. When selecting appropriate criteria, it is important to account for the relative importance of the individual families as well as the relative importance of the hypotheses within each family. To define candidate evaluation criteria that will be used in this case study, the notation introduced in Section 2.2.3 will be used, i.e., r_i will denote the rejection indicator for the null hypothesis H_i, $i = 1, \ldots, 4$.

The first evaluation criterion will be based on subset disjunctive power. This criterion is defined as the probability of rejecting at least one primary hypothesis and at least one secondary hypothesis, i.e.,

$$\psi_{SD}(g) = P\{r_1 + r_2 \geq 1 \text{ and } r_3 + r_4 \geq 1\}.$$

Subset disjunctive criteria of this kind were utilized in Brechenmacher et al. (2011) to identify optimal parameters of a Hommel-based gatekeeping procedure designed for a clinical trial with three families of null hypotheses.

The subset disjunctive criterion is conceptually similar to the disjunctive criterion utilized in Case study 2.1 (see Section 2.3.1). Just like the regular disjunctive criterion, the criterion defined above represents a rather simplistic approach to the definition of success in this trial. Indeed, this evaluation criterion does not differentiate between clinically distinct events such as establishing a significant treatment effect at a single dose versus both doses on either endpoint. Additionally, this criterion is symmetric with respect to the primary and secondary families, which leads to the counterintuitive assumption that the rejection of a secondary hypothesis is as important as the rejection of a primary hypothesis.

More flexible criteria that enable the trial's sponsor to account for the utility of demonstrating a beneficial effect on the primary and secondary endpoints can be set up using the general approaches utilized in Case study 2.1. These evaluation criteria are formulated using simple weighted power or partition-based weighted power and enable the trial's sponsor to "fine-tune" the criterion function by upweighting or downweighting the primary and secondary families and, in addition, assigning appropriate weights to the tests within each family.

As in Case study 2.1, the simple weighted criterion is defined as a weighted sum of the marginal probabilities of rejecting each of the four null hypotheses, i.e.,

$$\psi_{SW}(\boldsymbol{g}) = v_1 P\{r_1 = 1\} + v_2 P\{r_2 = 1\} + v_3 P\{r_3 = 1\} + v_4 P\{r_4 = 1\},$$

where v_1 through v_4 are non-negative values that determine the relative importance of a significant outcome for each hypothesis test. By considering different configurations of the importance values, the sponsor can find a desirable balance between the influence of the primary and secondary tests on the criterion. For example, since v_1 and v_2 correspond to the primary hypotheses, it will be natural to focus on the configurations where the importance parameters in the primary family are greater than the importance parameters associated with the secondary hypotheses. However, if much larger values are chosen for v_1 and v_2 compared to v_3 and v_4, the simple weighted criterion will be virtually independent of the secondary tests.

It was pointed out earlier that partition-based weighted criteria enable the sponsor to incorporate outcomes corresponding to specific regulatory claims. This is accomplished by enumerating partitions of the event that defines an overall successful outcome in a given trial. Recall that the schizophrenia trial will be declared successful if at least one hypothesis is rejected in the primary family, i.e., if H_1 or H_2 is rejected. As an extreme case, this event could be partitioned as follows:

- The null hypothesis H_1 is rejected but all other hypotheses are accepted.

- The null hypotheses H_1 and H_2 are rejected but all other hypotheses are accepted.

- The null hypotheses H_1, H_2 and H_3 are rejected but all other hypotheses are accepted, etc.

This approach to defining a partition-based criterion gives the sponsor an option to specify the utility of each individual trial outcome. In practice, the process of eliciting and assigning weights to each outcome will likely be a daunting task. A coarser partition will be more practical and more attractive from an interpretation perspective. As an illustration, a weighted criterion can be set up based on the following partition of the overall successful outcome in the trial:

- Exactly one hypothesis is rejected in the primary family ($r_1 + r_2 = 1$), i.e., one dose is superior to placebo on the primary endpoint and may also be superior to placebo on the secondary endpoint.

- Two hypotheses are rejected in the primary family and fewer than two hypotheses are rejected in the secondary family ($r_1 + r_2 = 2$ and $r_3 + r_4 \leq 1$), i.e., one dose is superior to placebo simultaneously on both endpoints and the other dose only on the primary endpoint.

- Two hypotheses are rejected in the primary family and two hypotheses are rejected in the secondary family ($r_1 + r_2 = 2$ and $r_3 + r_4 = 2$), i.e., both doses are superior to placebo on both endpoints.

The corresponding outcomes are ordered from the least desirable to the most desirable. Specifically, the very first outcome provides very limited information on the efficacy profile of the experimental treatment. By contrast, the last outcome supplies information that helps characterize the dose-response relationship on both endpoints, which may help strengthen the treatment's product label.

The evaluation criterion associated with this partition is given by

$$
\begin{aligned}
\psi_{PW}(\boldsymbol{g}) \;=\; & v_1 P\{r_1 + r_2 = 1\} \\
+ \; & v_2 P\{r_1 + r_2 = 2 \text{ and } r_3 + r_4 \leq 1\} \\
+ \; & v_3 P\{r_1 + r_2 = 2 \text{ and } r_3 + r_4 = 2\}.
\end{aligned}
$$

Again, v_1, v_2 and v_3 represent the relative importance of the three outcomes listed above. Given the underlying hierarchy of the three outcomes, it is most sensible to select the importance parameters to satisfy the following condition:

$$
v_1 < v_2 < v_3.
$$

It is also worth mentioning evaluation criteria based on the general concept of multiplicity penalties introduced in Section 2.2.3. Given that a relatively large number of hypotheses is pre-defined in this multiplicity problem, it is most sensible to consider the simplified approach to defining multiplicity penalty matrices. In other words, an overall multiplicity penalty compared to the reference procedure, e.g., the basic procedure without any adjustment for multiplicity, should be computed using the total number of hypotheses rejected by a procedure of interest. Further, when defining the overall multiplicity penalty, it is recommended to assign weights to the individual probabilities in a multiplicity penalty matrix to account for the fact that outcomes associated with rejecting a primary hypothesis are more important than those associated with rejecting a secondary hypothesis. Criteria based on multiplicity penalties will not be used in this case study.

Optimal selection of the single parameter of Procedure B1 (g_1) based on a univariate grid-search algorithm is discussed in Section 2.4.2. Section 2.4.3 presents a bivariate search algorithm aimed at identifying an optimal configuration of the two parameters of Procedure B2 (g_1 and g_2).

2.4.2 Optimal selection of the target parameter in Procedure B1

An optimization algorithm based on a simple grid search over the $[0, 1]$ interval was applied to identify optimal values of the target parameter (g_1) of the basic chain procedure (Procedure B1) defined in Figure 2.11. This parameter defines the rule for splitting the error rate between the primary endpoint test at Dose L (hypothesis H_2) and secondary endpoint test at Dose H (hypothesis H_3) after a beneficial treatment effect is established in the primary analysis at Dose H (H_1 is rejected). An optimal splitting rule is influenced by the hypothesized effect sizes of the endpoint tests as well as the relative importance of rejecting the hypotheses H_2 and H_3.

Optimization algorithms were applied based on the three evaluation criteria defined above, i.e., the subset disjunctive, simple weighted and partition-based weighted criteria. The evaluation was performed under the four sets of effect sizes of the four hypothesis tests (scenarios) specified in Table 2.8. The first data model (Scenario 1) served as the main data model and the other three models were treated as important supportive models.

Subset disjunctive power

Figure 2.14 displays the criterion functions based on subset disjunctive power corresponding to the four effect size scenarios. The subset disjunctive criterion was a monotonically decreasing function of the target parameter g_1 in each panel of the figure. As a consequence, the "point estimate" of the optimal target parameter, defined as the value that maximizes each criterion function, is easily found in each panel (this value will be denoted by g_1^*). It is important to note that the range of the optimal values across the four scenarios was quite tight. It follows from the figure that g_1^* ranged between 0 (Scenario 1) and 0.12 (Scenario 2).

Figure 2.14 also presents 99% optimal intervals that can be thought of as "confidence intervals" for the optimal target parameter or sets of nearly optimal values. A 99% optimal interval includes all values of the target parameter for which the criterion function is no more than 1% lower than its maximum value. The optimal intervals computed under the four scenarios overlapped, which supports the overall conclusion that an optimal value of the parameter of interest could be set to any value between 0 and 0.25. In other words, based on the subset disjunctive criterion, an optimal approach to constructing the splitting rule in Procedure B1 is to "spend" most of the error rate released after the rejection of the primary hypothesis H_1 on a secondary hypothesis, namely, H_3, rather than on the other primary hypothesis. For example, using the diagram presented in Figure 2.11 with a one-sided $\alpha = 0.025$, if g_1^* is set to 0.2, the hypothesis H_3 will be tested at the significance level of 0.02 in Step 2 and the level of 0.005 will be used to test the hypothesis H_2 in Step 3.

Simple and partition-based power

It is instructive to compare the optimization algorithm based on the subset disjunctive criterion to the algorithms that utilize weighted power, i.e., the simple weighted criterion (ψ_{SW}) and partition-based weighted criterion

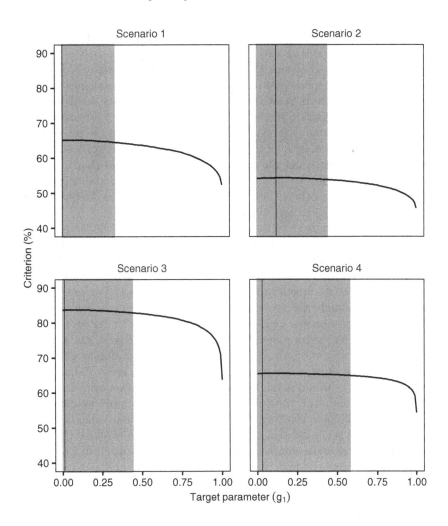

FIGURE 2.14: Subset disjunctive criterion as a function of the target parameter (g_1 parameter of Procedure B1) under four scenarios in Case study 2.2. The vertical lines represent the optimal values of the target parameter and the gray rectangles define the 99% optimal intervals for g_1.

(ψ_{PW}). The weighted criteria were defined as follows:

$$\psi_{SW} = 0.4P\{r_1 = 1\} + 0.4P\{r_2 = 1\} + 0.1P\{r_3 = 1\} + 0.1P\{r_4 = 1\},$$

$$\begin{aligned} \psi_{PW} = {} & 0.2P\{r_1 + r_2 = 1\} \\ & + 0.35P\{r_1 + r_2 = 2 \text{ and } r_3 + r_4 \leq 1\} \\ & + 0.45P\{r_1 + r_2 = 2 \text{ and } r_3 + r_4 = 2\}. \end{aligned}$$

It can be seen from the first definition that 80% of the overall weight in the simple weighted criterion was assigned to the primary family and then split equally between the two primary hypotheses. The rest of the weight was divided equally between the two secondary hypotheses. This weighting scheme reflects the perceived importance of significant outcomes in the two primary endpoint tests relative to the dose-placebo tests on the secondary endpoint. The definition of the partition-based weighted criterion indicates that the first outcome (rejection of a single hypothesis in the primary family and potentially another hypothesis in the secondary family) was treated as much less important than the second and third outcomes that included two significant results in the primary family. As expected, the third outcome (rejection of two hypotheses in both families) was viewed as the most desirable one and received the largest weight.

A graphical summary of the criterion functions based on simple weighted power under the four scenarios is presented in Figure 2.15. The shapes of the criterion functions displayed in this figure are quite different from those shown in Figure 2.14. The criterion functions in all four panels of Figure 2.15 were generally increasing functions of the target parameter. For example, when the simple weighted criterion was evaluated under the main data model (Scenario 1), the criterion was an increasing function of the target parameter when $0 \leq g_1 \leq 0.6$, reached a plateau when $0.6 \leq g_1 \leq 0.9$ and was a decreasing function of g_1 over the remaining short interval. Very similar patterns were observed in the other three panels. These patterns clearly indicated that a larger value of g_1 would maximize the selected evaluation criterion.

To understand why the subset disjunctive and simple weighted criteria resulted in dissimilar conclusions regarding the optimal value of the target parameter in this clinical trial example, it is helpful to examine the structure of the former criterion. Since the testing algorithm utilized in Procedure B1 always begins with the hypothesis H_1 and all other hypotheses can be tested only after H_1 is rejected, the probability of meeting the first condition in the subset disjunctive criterion, i.e., $r_1 + r_2 \geq 1$, did not depend on g_1. However, the probability of meeting the second condition, i.e., $r_3 + r_4 \geq 1$, was generally improved[1] by selecting a smaller value of g_1, which resulted in a higher fraction of α being assigned to the test of H_3. This implies that the subset disjunctive criterion was essentially driven by the goal of maximizing the probability of success in the secondary family and it is not surprising that an optimal value of the target parameter based on this criterion was close to 0. The simple weighted criterion, on the other hand, provided a more balanced treatment of the primary endpoint tests. Since the criterion was based on a weighted sum of the marginal rejection probabilities for all four null hypotheses, it

---

[1]It is worth noting that the relationship between g_1 and $P\{r_3 + r_4 \geq 1\}$ is a bit more complex since a smaller value of g_1 improves the chances of rejecting H_3 but, at the same time, reduces the chances of rejecting H_4, which can be tested only after H_2 is rejected. But it is generally true that the probability of at least one rejection in the secondary family is improved if g_1 is close to 0.

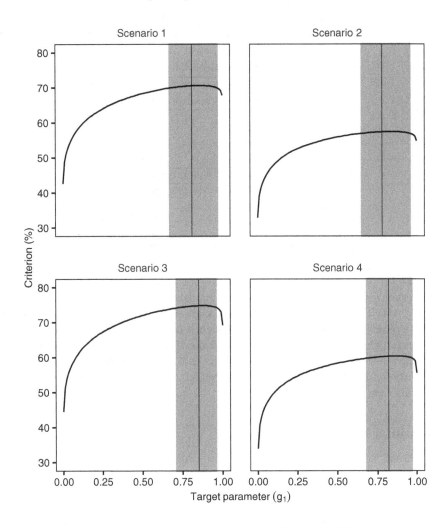

FIGURE 2.15: Simple weighted criterion as a function of the target parameter (g_1 parameter of Procedure B1) under four scenarios in Case study 2.2. The vertical lines represent the optimal values of the target parameter and the gray rectangles define the 99% optimal intervals for g_1.

favored the values of g_1 that were consistent with the goal of increasing the probability of a simultaneous rejection of both primary hypotheses. The goal of improving power of the secondary tests played a less important role in the simple weighted criterion. The optimal value of the target parameter that resulted in a compromise between these two goals turned out to be a value that was fairly close to the upper end of the $[0, 1]$ interval.

Figure 2.16 displays the partition-based weighted criterion as a function

TABLE 2.9: Optimal values of the target parameter (g_1 parameter) and optimal intervals based on simple weighted power and partition-based weighted power in Case study 2.2.

Scenario	Optimal value	99% optimal interval
Simple weighted power		
Scenario 1	0.81	$(0.67, 0.97)$
Scenario 2	0.78	$(0.65, 0.96)$
Scenario 3	0.85	$(0.71, 0.96)$
Scenario 4	0.82	$(0.68, 0.97)$
Partition-based weighted power		
Scenario 1	0.73	$(0.62, 0.92)$
Scenario 2	0.69	$(0.59, 0.90)$
Scenario 3	0.78	$(0.68, 0.94)$
Scenario 4	0.80	$(0.68, 0.93)$

of the target parameter under the same four data models. The shapes of the criterion functions were almost indistinguishable from those shown in Figure 2.15. The two criteria based on weighted power led to a consistent set of recommendations on the optimal values of the target parameter g_1. By contrast, the evaluation criterion based on disjunctive power was "lopsided" in the sense that it was dominated by the goal of maximizing power in the secondary family. For this reason, this criterion would not be considered relevant in this case study.

Optimal intervals

Optimal values of the g_1 parameter in Procedure B1 under the four data models (scenarios) based on the most relevant evaluation criteria (simple and partition-based weighted criteria) are listed in Table 2.9. This table provides a detailed summary of the information presented in Figures 2.15 and 2.16. As discussed above, the optimal values of the target parameter exhibited strong consistency across the data models. For example, the "point estimate" of the optimal value of g_1 was 0.81 under the main data model (Scenario 1) and ranged between 0.78 and 0.85 under the alternative models when the evaluation criterion based on simple weighted power was applied. With partition-based weighted power, the point estimates were somewhat less consistent. They were also slightly shifted to the left compared to the first criterion, e.g., the optimal value of the target parameter was 0.73 under the main data model.

Table 2.9 also shows the 99% optimal intervals for the target parameter. The criterion functions were virtually flat over these intervals and, for all practical purposes, any value from each optimal interval can be treated as an optimal value of g_1 under the corresponding data model. It can be seen

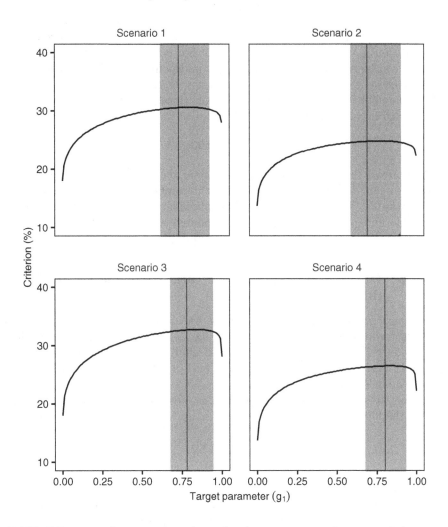

FIGURE 2.16: Partition-based weighted criterion as a function of the target parameter (g_1 parameter of Procedure B1) under four scenarios in Case study 2.2. The vertical lines represent the optimal values of the target parameter and the gray rectangles define the 99% optimal intervals for g_1.

from the table that the optimal intervals were fairly tight and quite consistent across the four scenarios of interest for both evaluation criteria.

Using the four intervals for each evaluation criterion, a joint optimal interval for the target parameter is easily constructed by taking the intersection of the intervals. For example, the joint 99% optimal interval for g_1 based on simple weighted power was given by

$$(0.71, 0.96).$$

By the definition of this interval, Procedure B1 would be expected to exhibit optimal performance under any of the chosen data models whenever the g_1 parameter is selected from this interval. For concreteness, an optimal value of g_1 can be set to a value close to the mid-point of the joint interval, e.g., $g_1^* = 0.8$.

The joint 99% optimal interval for partition-based weighted power can be obtained in a similar way. This joint interval was equal to

$$(0.68, 0.90).$$

An optimal value of the g_1 parameter under the four data models of interest can be again defined by computing the mid-point of the interval, i.e., to g_1^* can be set to 0.8. This indicates that the application of the two evaluation criteria (simple and partition-based weighted power) resulted in the same optimal value of the target parameter in Procedure B1.

2.4.3   Optimal selection of the target parameters in Procedure B2

The next set of optimization algorithms was developed to determine optimal configurations of the target parameters, i.e., g_1 and g_2, of the advanced chain procedure (Procedure B2) that was expected to provide a power advantage over Procedure B1. The evaluation was performed using the same criteria and data models as in Section 2.4.2.

As part of the optimization algorithms, bivariate searches were performed over the following grid:

$$(g_1, g_2) = (i/10, j/10), \ i = 0, \ldots, 10, \ j = 0, \ldots, 10.$$

Three evaluation criteria defined in Section 2.2.3 (subset disjunctive, simple weighted and partition-based weighted criteria) were evaluated for each point on this grid and the results were summarized using heat maps. For example, Figures 2.17, 2.18 and 2.19 present the three criteria as a function of the two target parameters under the main data model (Scenario 1). The heat maps conveniently display the numeric values of the three evaluation criteria, which helps identify an optimal configuration of g_1 and g_2 that corresponds to the highest value of the corresponding criterion function, as well as 99% optimal regions for the two parameters.

Subset disjunctive power

Figure 2.17 defines a heat map that summarizes the impact of the two parameters of interest on subset disjunctive power of Procedure B2. Subset disjunctive power was a monotonically decreasing function of both parameters. The subset disjunctive criterion was maximized when $g_1 = 0$ regardless

g_1											
1	52.6	53.2	53.4	53.6	53.5	53.4	53.2	52.9	52.6	51.9	50.6
0.9	58.9	59.1	59.2	59.2	59.0	59.0	58.8	58.5	58.1	57.6	56.3
0.8	61.0	61.0	61.0	60.9	60.8	60.7	60.5	60.2	59.8	59.3	58.1
0.7	62.3	62.2	62.2	62.1	62.0	61.8	61.6	61.3	61.0	60.4	59.4
0.6	63.2	63.0	63.0	62.9	62.8	62.6	62.4	62.1	61.8	61.3	60.4
0.5	63.9	63.8	63.7	63.6	63.5	63.3	63.1	62.9	62.5	62.1	61.3
0.4	64.4	64.3	64.2	64.1	63.9	63.8	63.6	63.4	63.1	62.7	62.0
0.3	64.7	64.7	64.5	64.5	64.4	64.2	64.0	63.8	63.6	63.2	62.7
0.2	65.1	65.0	64.9	64.8	64.7	64.6	64.5	64.3	64.1	63.9	63.5
0.1	65.2	65.2	65.1	65.1	65.0	64.9	64.8	64.7	64.6	64.5	64.3
0	65.2	65.2	65.2	65.2	65.2	65.2	65.2	65.2	65.2	65.2	65.2
	0	0.1	0.2	0.3	0.4	0.5	0.6	0.7	0.8	0.9	1
						g_2					

FIGURE 2.17: Subset disjunctive criterion as a function of the target parameters (g_1 and g_2 parameters of Procedure B2) under the main model (Scenario 1) in Case study 2.2. The dark-colored cells define a 99% optimal region for the two parameters.

of the value of g_2. For the sake of concreteness, an optimal configuration of the procedure parameters can be defined as follows:

$$g_1^* = 0 \text{ and } g_2^* = 0.$$

The criterion was minimized when the target parameters were both equal to 1.

The dark-colored cells shown in Figure 2.17 define a set of nearly optimal values of g_1 and g_2 that were virtually indistinguishable from the optimal values shown above. This bivariate optimal region is a straightforward extension of optimal intervals considered in the context of univariate optimization problems; see, for example, Section 2.4.2. This 99% optimal region included all points on the pre-defined grid where the subset disjunctive criterion was greater than 99% of the highest value of this criterion over the entire grid, i.e., greater than

$$0.99\psi_{SD}(g_1^*, g_2^*) = 0.99 \times 0.652 = 0.6455.$$

Simple and partition-based weighted power

The performance of Procedure B2 was also assessed using the simple and partition-based weighted criteria that were set up using the same set of im-

g_1	g_2=0	0.1	0.2	0.3	0.4	0.5	0.6	0.7	0.8	0.9	1
1	72.4	72.4	72.4	72.3	72.2	72.1	71.9	71.6	71.3	70.7	67.8
0.9	72.6	72.5	72.5	72.4	72.3	72.2	72.0	71.7	71.4	70.8	68.0
0.8	72.4	72.3	72.2	72.2	72.0	71.9	71.7	71.5	71.2	70.6	67.9
0.7	72.1	72.1	72.0	71.9	71.8	71.7	71.5	71.3	70.9	70.4	67.8
0.6	71.9	71.8	71.7	71.6	71.5	71.4	71.2	71.0	70.7	70.1	67.8
0.5	71.5	71.5	71.4	71.3	71.2	71.0	70.9	70.7	70.4	69.9	67.7
0.4	71.1	71.1	71.0	70.9	70.8	70.7	70.5	70.3	70.0	69.6	67.6
0.3	70.7	70.6	70.5	70.5	70.4	70.3	70.1	69.9	69.7	69.2	67.5
0.2	70.2	70.1	70.0	70.0	69.9	69.8	69.6	69.5	69.3	68.9	67.5
0.1	69.4	69.3	69.3	69.2	69.1	69.0	68.9	68.8	68.6	68.4	67.4
0	67.9	67.9	67.9	67.9	67.9	67.9	67.9	67.9	67.9	67.9	67.9

FIGURE 2.18: Simple weighted criterion as a function of the target parameters (g_1 and g_2 parameters of Procedure B2) under the main model (Scenario 1) in Case study 2.2. The dark-colored cells define a 99% optimal region for the two parameters.

portance values as in Section 2.4.2, i.e., the former was defined based on

$$v_1 = v_2 = 0.4, \ v_3 = v_4 = 0.1,$$

and latter was defined based on

$$v_1 = 0.2, \ v_2 = 0.35, \ v_3 = 0.45.$$

When these evaluation criteria were considered, a completely different configuration of optimal parameter values was selected compared to the subset disjunctive criterion. Figures 2.18 and 2.19 present the heat maps for the simple and partition-based weighted criteria under the assumption that the data are generated from the main data model. The two figures suggest the same optimal configuration of the target parameters. The simple and partition-based weighted criteria were both maximized at the following point on the grid:

$$g_1^* = 1 \text{ and } g_2^* = 0.$$

It is easy to show that, with this set of parameters, Procedure B2 simplifies to a basic fixed-sequence procedure that relies on the decision rules defined in Figure 2.20. This procedure utilizes a *sequentially rejective* testing algorithm applied to the following sequence of null hypotheses:

$$H_1, \ H_2, \ H_4, \ H_3.$$

g_1 \ g_2	0	0.1	0.2	0.3	0.4	0.5	0.6	0.7	0.8	0.9	1
1	32.5	32.4	32.4	32.3	32.2	32.0	31.9	31.7	31.4	30.8	28.0
0.9	32.3	32.2	32.1	32.0	31.9	31.8	31.7	31.4	31.1	30.6	27.9
0.8	32.1	32.0	31.9	31.8	31.7	31.6	31.5	31.3	31.0	30.4	27.9
0.7	31.9	31.8	31.7	31.7	31.6	31.4	31.3	31.1	30.8	30.3	27.9
0.6	31.7	31.6	31.6	31.5	31.4	31.3	31.1	30.9	30.6	30.2	27.9
0.5	31.5	31.5	31.4	31.3	31.2	31.1	31.0	30.8	30.5	30.1	28.0
0.4	31.3	31.3	31.2	31.1	31.0	30.9	30.8	30.6	30.4	29.9	28.0
0.3	31.1	31.1	31.0	30.9	30.8	30.7	30.6	30.4	30.2	29.8	28.2
0.2	30.9	30.9	30.8	30.7	30.6	30.5	30.4	30.3	30.1	29.7	28.4
0.1	30.6	30.5	30.5	30.4	30.4	30.3	30.2	30.1	29.9	29.7	28.7
0	30.7	30.7	30.7	30.7	30.7	30.7	30.7	30.7	30.7	30.7	30.7

FIGURE 2.19: Partition-based weighted criterion as a function of the target parameters (g_1 and g_2 parameters of Procedure B2) under the main model (Scenario 1) in Case study 2.2. The dark-colored cells define a 99% optimal region for the two parameters.

The four hypotheses are tested sequentially beginning with H_1 and each test is carried out at the full α level provided all hypotheses placed earlier in the sequence are rejected. Figure 2.20 shows that the optimal procedure recognizes the importance of carrying out the primary tests before proceeding to the secondary tests. Note that nearly optimal procedures associated with the parameters from the optimal regions defined in Figures 2.18 and 2.19 utilize less straightforward decision rules but share the same key features.

It is interesting that the values of the simple and partition-based weighted criteria were very low at the point on the grid where the subset disjunctive criterion was maximized, i.e., at $g_1 = 0$ and $g_2 = 0$. This is due to the same property of the latter criterion that was discussed in Section 2.4.2. Briefly, it is impossible to balance the influence of the primary and secondary tests when the criterion based on subset disjunctive power is applied. In this setting, this criterion favored the secondary tests over the primary tests, which was not consistent with the clinical objective of this trial. The criteria based on weighted power generally provide more reliable guidance in optimization problems than the subset disjunctive criterion. In this clinical trial example, it is recommended to focus on the conclusions presented in Figures 2.18 and 2.19, including the optimal configuration of the two procedure parameters as well as sets of nearly optimal parameters.

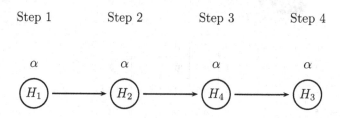

FIGURE 2.20: Fixed-sequence procedure corresponding to Procedure B2 with $g_1 = 1$ and $g_2 = 0$. A solid arrow defines the decision path after each hypothesis is rejected. Each test is carried out at the full α level.

The simple and partition-weighted criterion functions summarized in Figures 2.18 and 2.19 also help assess the impact of utilizing α-exhaustive testing strategies in this clinical trial example. As stated in Section 2.4.1, Procedure B2 was introduced as a more efficient alternative to Procedure B1 that transferred the error rate released after the rejection of each hypothesis to another hypothesis that was yet to be rejected. It is known that α-exhaustive approaches to defining multiple testing procedures lead to a power gain compared to procedures that are not α-exhaustive. The two figures show that an optimal multiplicity adjustment based on Procedure B2 with $g_1 = 1$ and $g_2 = 0$ increased simple weighted power to 72.4% and partition-based weighted power to 32.5%. By contrast, it follows from Figures 2.15 and 2.16 that the highest levels of simple and partition-based weighted power for Procedure B1 under the same data model were equal to 70.6% and 30.6%, respectively. This shows that Procedure B2 resulted in a more efficient multiplicity adjustment compared to Procedure B1 based on the two evaluation criteria and the power gain on a relative scale was equal to 3 and 6 percentage points, respectively.

Joint optimal regions

The optimization algorithms considered so far in the bivariate optimization problem focused on a single data model, namely, the main data model. Given the importance of the alternative data models, it will be critical to apply similar optimization algorithms to the other three data models. This can be accomplished by generating heat maps similar to those displayed in Figures 2.17, 2.18 and 2.19 under Scenario 2, 3 and 4 and identifying the optimal values of the two parameters of Procedure B2 (g_1 and g_2) along with the associated 99% optimal regions for each scenario. It would be generally more informative to combine the findings across the data models by computing a joint 99% optimal region for the target parameters across the four scenarios.

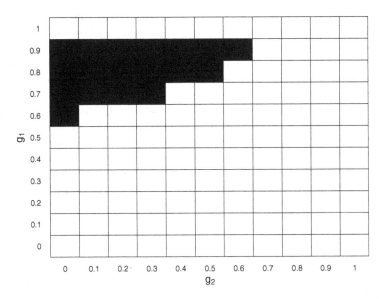

FIGURE 2.21: Joint 99% optimal region for the target parameters (g_1 and g_2 parameters of Procedure B2) based on the simple weighted criterion under the four data models in Case study 2.2.

An advantage of this approach is that it provides a compact summary of the configurations of g_1 and g_2 that result in an optimal performance of this multiple testing procedure under all anticipated sets of effect sizes of the primary and key secondary tests.

As an illustration, Figure 2.21 displays a joint 99% optimal region for the target parameters based on the simple weighted criterion. The dark-colored cells in the upper-left corner of this heat map identify the values of g_1 and g_2 that fell within the joint optimal region. It follows from this figure that a chain procedure which is very close to the fixed-sequence procedure with $g_1 = 1$ and $g_2 = 0$ (see Figure 2.20) as well as related procedures with a more complex set of decision rules will be expected to perform optimally under any of the pre-defined data models. A joint 99% optimal region for the partition-based weighted criterion included the fixed-sequence procedure and several procedures with similar sets of the target parameters.

2.4.4 Sensitivity assessments

Comprehensive sensitivity assessments are an integral part of any clinical trial optimization exercise and include, as explained in Chapter 1, qualitative and quantitative sensitivity analyses. In this case study, the optimization algorithms discussed in Sections 2.4.2 and 2.4.3 already incorporated a straightforward qualitative sensitivity assessment based on the three alternative data models defined in Table 2.8. The assessment results were used to compute a joint optimal interval or optimal region for the target parameters and select the values of the procedure parameters that resulted in nearly optimal performance under all plausible sets of effect sizes in the schizophrenia clinical trial.

This section discusses quantitative sensitivity assessments to study the impact of random perturbations on the optimal multiple testing procedures. These assessments can be conducted with respect to the unknown values of the mean treatment effects at Doses L and H that serve as the key data model parameters in this case study. Additionally, a sensitivity assessment can focus on the supportive parameter of the main data model, i.e., the correlation between the primary and secondary endpoints. Both types of quantitative sensitivity assessments can be performed using parametric bootstrap algorithms very similar to that used in Section 2.3.3.

Quantitative sensitivity assessment based on the key data model parameters

When examining the optimal values of the target parameters identified in Sections 2.4.2 and 2.4.3, it is important to remember that they were found using a *local* optimization approach, i.e., they were derived based on a certain set of statistical assumptions. The key idea behind sensitivity assessments is to assess the impact of possible deviations from the assumed data model on the performance of the optimal multiple testing procedures. The assessments can be performed based on the main data model (Scenario 1) or any of the alternative models.

A general approach to performing sensitivity assessments for key data model parameters was illustrated in Case study 2.1 (see Section 2.3.3). This section will provide a quick outline of the approaches that could be used to perform sensitivity assessments with respect to the outcome distribution parameters defined in Table 2.7. This includes the means of the two marginal distributions in the three pre-defined samples, i.e., μ_{i0}, μ_{i1}, and μ_{i2}, where $i = 1, 2$, as well as the standard deviations σ_1 and σ_2. For compactness, the six means will be denoted by μ_1 through μ_6, i.e.,

$$\mu_1 = \mu_{10}, \ \mu_2 = \mu_{20}, \mu_3 = \mu_{11}, \ \mu_4 = \mu_{21}, \mu_5 = \mu_{12}, \ \mu_6 = \mu_{22}.$$

To run sensitivity analyses based on a parametric bootstrap approach, bootstrap distributions need to be assigned to all parameters of interest. A natural choice for the distribution of μ_i, $i = 1, \ldots, 6$, is a normal distribution centered around the assumed value of the corresponding parameter, i.e., bootstrap data models can be defined based on the following parameters:

$$\mu'_{ij} \sim N(\mu_i, \tau_i^2), \ j = 1, \ldots, k,$$

where k is the number of bootstrap data models. The standard deviations of the bootstrap distributions can be computed by assuming a common coefficient of variation across the samples included in the data model, i.e., $\tau_i = c\mu_i$, $i = 1, \ldots, 6$. This approach assumes that a larger value of the mean effect is associated with higher variability in the bootstrap data models. Alternatively, a constant standard deviation can be assumed for the six bootstrap distributions, i.e., $\tau_i = c$, $i = 1, \ldots, 6$. In both cases c is the uncertainty parameter that quantifies the expected magnitude of deviations from the means assumed under the main data model.

Secondly, considering the standard deviations σ_1 and σ_2, gamma distributions with large variances are appropriate for modeling quantitative deviations from the specified values of σ_1 and σ_2. The standard deviations of these distributions are proportional to the uncertainty parameter c. The last data model parameter, i.e., the correlation between the primary and secondary endpoints, is a supportive parameter of the data model and its value is fixed.

To perform sensitivity assessments, a large number of bootstrap data models, say, $k = 1,000$, need to be generated. The parameters of Procedures B1 and B2 need to be set to their optimal values and empirical distributions of the recommended evaluation criteria (simple weighted and partition-based weighted criteria) can be computed from the bootstrap data models. The distributions can be plotted or key descriptive statistics can be found, as was done in Section 2.3.3, to understand the impact of random deviations from the pre-specified data model on the performance of the two optimal multiple testing procedures based on the selected criteria. It is advisable to consider several values of the uncertainty parameter c to cover medium-uncertainty and high-uncertainty settings.

Quantitative sensitivity assessment based on the supportive data model parameter

In addition to sensitivity assessments based on key data model parameters, it is worth considering similar sensitivity analyses with respect to supportive parameters. In this section, stress testing techniques will be applied to the optimal multiple testing procedures by introducing variability around the assumed value of the correlation between the primary and secondary endpoints. The key data model parameters will be considered fixed and set to the values corresponding to the main data model.

A parametric bootstrap approach was applied and a distribution was selected for the correlation coefficient ρ. Based on historical data, the correlation coefficient was assumed to be positive and follow a beta distribution. The beta distribution was centered around the assumed value of $\rho = 0.5$ and a large coefficient of variation was selected to support an aggressive sensitivity analysis. This analysis was aimed at evaluating the impact of extreme values of ρ on the performance of the optimal multiple testing procedures. The coefficient of variation was set to $c = 0.5$ and the 95% range of the resulting beta

TABLE 2.10: Descriptive statistics of partition-based weighted power in the quantitative sensitivity assessment under the main data model (Scenario 1) in Case study 2.2.

Multiple testing procedure	Power under the main data model (%)	Power computed from bootstrap data models (%)		
		2.5th percentile	Median	97.5th percentile
No adjustment	32.8	32.2	32.9	33.8
Procedure B1	30.6	30.0	30.6	31.3
Procedure B2	32.5	31.3	32.0	33.0

distribution, i.e., the 2.5th and 97.5th percentiles, was given by

$$(0.06, 0.94).$$

In other words, the correlation coefficient was nearly uniformly distributed over the $[0, 1]$ interval.

One thousand bootstrap data models were constructed from the main data model with the correlation coefficient following the selected beta distribution. Partition-based weighted power for Procedures B1 and B2 was computed for each bootstrap data model. The procedure parameters were set to $g_1^* = 0.8$ (Procedure B1) and $g_1^* = 1$ and $g_2^* = 0$ (Procedure B2). As in Case study 2.1, the basic analysis method that uses no adjustment in this multiplicity problem (unadjusted procedure) was included as a reference. As a quick note, the sensitivity assessment presented below was performed based on a single evaluation criterion (partition-based weighted power was selected as the criterion of interest) and sensitivity checks based on other evaluation criteria can be run in a similar way.

Descriptive statistics computed from the empirical distribution of partition-based weighted power for the three analysis method (unadjusted procedure, Procedure B1 and Procedure B2) are listed in Table 2.10. This table gives the 95% range for partition-based weighted power and shows that, despite a high amount of variability around the assumed correlation coefficient, partition-based weighted power for each procedure clustered fairly tightly around the power level corresponding to the original data model.

The results of the bootstrap-based assessments presented in Table 2.10 demonstrate that the optimal multiple testing procedures identified in Sections 2.4.2 and 2.4.3 were very robust against violations of the statistical assumptions about the supportive parameter of the main data model. Procedures B1 and B2 performed well regardless of the true value of the correlation between the two endpoints in this clinical trial example.

2.4.5 Software implementation

The data, analysis and evaluation models defined in Section 2.4.1 can be easily implemented in R code to perform simulations in the schizophrenia clinical trial using an approach very similar to that utilized in Case study 2.1 (see Section 2.3.4).

Data model

In this case study, two clinical endpoints are evaluated for each patient (change from baseline in the PANSS total score and change from baseline on the CGI-S score) and thus a bivariate distribution needs to be specified for each patient's outcome in the data model. A bivariate normal distribution is defined using the MVNormalDist method in the OutcomeDist object. For each sample and each treatment effect scenario, the parameters of this bivariate distribution as well as the correlation matrix need to be defined. For the purpose of illustration, only parameters corresponding to Scenario 1 given in the Table 2.8 are listed below. Recall that the mean values of the primary and key secondary endpoints in the placebo arm are given by

$$\mu_{10} = -12, \ \mu_{20} = -0.8.$$

The common standard deviations for the primary and secondary endpoints are equal to $\sigma_1 = 1$ and $\sigma_2 = 20$ and the mean values of the endpoints in the two dosing arms under Scenario 1 are computed as follows:

$$\mu_{11} = \mu_{10} - \theta_2\sigma_1 = -18, \ \mu_{21} = \mu_{20} - \theta_4\sigma_2 = -1.1,$$
$$\mu_{12} = \mu_{10} - \theta_1\sigma_1 = -20, \ \mu_{22} = \mu_{20} - \theta_3\sigma_2 = -1.1.$$

Finally, the correlation between the two endpoints is $\rho = 0.5$.

LISTING 2.7: Outcome parameter specifications in Case study 2.2

```
# Correlation matrix
corr.matrix = matrix(c(1.0, 0.5,
                       0.5, 1.0), 2, 2)


# Outcome parameters  - Scenario 1
outcome.placebo.sc1 =
parameters(par = parameters(parameters(mean = -12,
                                       sd = 20),
                            parameters(mean = -0.8,
                                       sd = 1)),
           corr = corr.matrix)

outcome.dose1.sc1 =
parameters(par = parameters(parameters(mean = -18,
                                       sd = 20),
```

```
                              parameters(mean = -1.1,
                                          sd = 1)),
          corr = corr.matrix)

outcome.doseh.sc1 =
parameters(par = parameters(parameters(mean = -20,
                                        sd = 20),
                             parameters(mean = -1.1,
                                        sd = 1)),
          corr = corr.matrix)
```

Similar sets of parameters can be set up for Scenarios 2, 3 and 4 and then combined within each `Sample` object. Also, unlike Case study 2.1, this case study utilized an unbalanced design with a 1:2:2 randomization scheme. The number of patients in each trial arm, i.e., in each sample, is specified within each `Sample` object.

LISTING 2.8: Data model in Case study 2.2

```
# Data model
mult.cs2.data.model = DataModel() +
  OutcomeDist(outcome.dist = "MVNormalDist") +
  Sample(id = c("Placebo - E1", "Placebo - E2"),
         outcome.par = parameters(outcome.placebo.sc1,
                                   outcome.placebo.sc2,
                                   outcome.placebo.sc3,
                                   outcome.placebo.sc4),
         sample.size = 100) +
  Sample(id = c("Dose L - E1", "Dose L - E2"),
         outcome.par = parameters(outcome.dosel.sc1,
                                   outcome.dosel.sc2,
                                   outcome.dosel.sc3,
                                   outcome.dosel.sc4),
         sample.size = 200) +
  Sample(id = c("Dose H - E1", "Dose H - E2"),
         outcome.par = parameters(outcome.doseh.sc1,
                                   outcome.doseh.sc2,
                                   outcome.doseh.sc3,
                                   outcome.doseh.sc4),
         sample.size = 200)
```

As in Case study 2.1, it is assumed that all patients complete the 6-week treatment period but, as shown in Section 2.3.4, a dropout process can be easily incorporated into the data model.

Analysis model

The statistical tests carried out in the trial as well as the candidate multiplicity adjustments are specified in the analysis model. As both endpoints follow a normal distribution, the two treatment comparisons for each endpoint will be carried out based on a two-sample t-test. This means that four `Test` objects need to be defined in the `AnalysisModel` object.

Both multiplicity adjustments are based on Bonferroni-based chain procedures, and each procedure is uniquely defined by the α-allocation and α-propagation rules. The difference between Procedure B1 and Procedure B2 lies in the specification of the α-propagation rule, i.e., the set of transition parameters. To specify the procedure-specific α-propagation rules, two objects are introduced below to pass the hypothesis weights and transition parameters to the multiplicity adjustment procedures:

- `chain.weight` defines a vector of initial hypothesis weights, i.e., W_1 in Procedure B1 and W_2 in Procedure B2.

- `chain.transition` defines a matrix of transition parameters, i.e., T_1 in Procedure B1 and T_2 in Procedure B2.

Note that the transition parameters used in these procedures are computed using the optimal values of the target parameters, i.e., $g_1 = 0.8$ in Procedure B1 and $g_1 = 1$ and $g_2 = 0$ in Procedure B2.

LISTING 2.9: Specification of Procedures B1 and B2 in Case study 2.2

```
# Parameters of Procedure B1
# Vector of initial hypothesis weights
chain.weight = c(1, 0, 0, 0)

# Matrix of transition parameters
chain.transition = matrix(c(0, 0.8, 0.2, 0,
                            0, 0, 0, 1,
                            0, 0, 0, 0,
                            0, 0, 0, 0), 4, 4, byrow = TRUE)

mult.adj1 = MultAdjProc(proc = "ChainAdj",
                par = parameters(weight = chain.weight,
                        transition = chain.transition))

# Parameters of Procedure B2
# Vector of initial hypothesis weights
chain.weight = c(1, 0, 0, 0)

# Matrix of transition parameters
chain.transition = matrix(c(0, 1, 0, 0,
                            0, 0, 0, 1,
                            0, 0, 0, 0,
                            0, 0, 1, 0), 4, 4, byrow = TRUE)

mult.adj2 = MultAdjProc(proc = "ChainAdj",
                par = parameters(weight = chain.weight,
                        transition = chain.transition))
```

It is important to note that, as before, the test order in the `AnalysisModel` object is important to ensure that the α-allocation and α-propagation rules are applied correctly.

LISTING 2.10: Analysis model in Case study 2.2

```
# Analysis model
mult.cs2.analysis.model =
  AnalysisModel() +
  MultAdj(mult.adj1,mult.adj2) +
  Test(id = "Placebo vs Dose H - E1",
       samples = samples("Dose H - E1", "Placebo - E1"),
       method = "TTest") +
  Test(id = "Placebo vs Dose L - E1",
       samples = samples("Dose L - E1", "Placebo - E1"),
       method = "TTest") +
  Test(id = "Placebo vs Dose H - E2",
       samples = samples("Dose H - E2", "Placebo - E2"),
       method = "TTest") +
  Test(id = "Placebo vs Dose L - E2",
       samples = samples( "Dose L - E2", "Placebo - E2"),
       method = "TTest")
```

Evaluation model

The marginal, weighted and disjunctive power criteria utilized in this case study are specified in the `EvaluationModel` object using built-in functions. However, two custom functions need to be developed for the subset disjunctive power criterion, ψ_{SD}, and partition-based weighted criterion, ψ_{PW}, as shown below.

LISTING 2.11: Custom functions for computing subset disjunctive power and partition-based weighted power in Case study 2.2

```
# Custom evaluation criterion based on subset disjunctive
    power
mult.cs2.SubsetDisjunctivePower = function(test.result,
  statistic.result, parameter) {

  alpha = parameter$alpha

  # Outcome: Reject (H1 or H2) and (H3 or H4)
  power = mean(((test.result[,1] <= alpha) | (test.result
    [,2] <= alpha)) & ((test.result[,3] <= alpha) | (test.
    result[,4] <= alpha)))

  return(power)
}
```

```
# Custom evaluation criterion based on partition-based
    weighted power
mult.cs2.PartitionBasedWeightedPower = function(test.result
    , statistic.result, parameter) {

  # Parameters
  alpha = parameter$alpha
  weight = parameter$weight

  # Outcome 1: Reject exactly one hypothesis in the primary
    family
  outcome1 = ((test.result[,1] <= alpha) + (test.result[,2]
    <= alpha)) == 1
  # Outcome 2: Reject both hypotheses in the primary family
    and less than two in the secondary family
  outcome2 = (((test.result[,1] <= alpha) + (test.result
    [,2] <= alpha)) == 2) & (((test.result[,3] <= alpha) +
    (test.result[,4] <= alpha)) < 2)
  # Outcome 3: Reject both hypotheses in the primary and
    secondary families
  outcome3 = ((test.result[,1] <= alpha) & (test.result[,2]
    <= alpha) & (test.result[,3] <= alpha) & (test.result
    [,4] <= alpha))

  # Weighted power
  power = mean(outcome1) * weight[1] + mean(outcome2) *
    weight[2] + mean(outcome3) * weight[3]

  return(power)
}
```

Finally, the built-in and custom criterion functions are incorporated into the EvaluationModel object.

LISTING 2.12: Evaluation model in Case study 2.2

```
mult.cs2.evaluation.model = EvaluationModel() +
  Criterion(id = "Marginal power",
            method = "MarginalPower",
            tests = tests("Placebo vs Dose H - E1",
                          "Placebo vs Dose L - E1",
                          "Placebo vs Dose H - E2",
                          "Placebo vs Dose L - E2"),
            labels = c("Placebo vs Dose H - E1",
                       "Placebo vs Dose L - E1",
                       "Placebo vs Dose H - E2",
                       "Placebo vs Dose L - E2"),
            par = parameters(alpha = 0.025)) +
  Criterion(id = "Subset disjunctive power",
            method = "mult.cs2.SubsetDisjunctivePower",
```

```
          tests = tests("Placebo vs Dose H - E1",
                        "Placebo vs Dose L - E1",
                        "Placebo vs Dose H - E2",
                        "Placebo vs Dose L - E2"),
          labels = "Subset disjunctive power",
          par = parameters(alpha = 0.025)) +
  Criterion(id = "Weighted power",
            method = "WeightedPower",
            tests = tests("Placebo vs Dose H - E1",
                          "Placebo vs Dose L - E1",
                          "Placebo vs Dose H - E2",
                          "Placebo vs Dose L - E2"),
            labels = "Weighted power (v1 = 0.4, v2 = 0.4,
    v3 = 0.1, v4 = 0.1)",
            par = parameters(alpha = 0.025,
                      weight = c(0.4, 0.4, 0.1, 0.1))) +
  Criterion(id = "Partition-based weighted power",
            method = "mult.cs2.PartitionBasedWeightedPower",
            tests = tests("Placebo vs Dose H - E1",
                          "Placebo vs Dose L - E1",
                          "Placebo vs Dose H - E2",
                          "Placebo vs Dose L - E2"),
            labels = "Partition-based weighted power (v1 =
    0.20, v2 = 0.35, v3 = 0.45)",
            par = parameters(alpha = 0.025,
                      weight = c(0.20, 0.35, 0.45)))
```

Simulation results

Simulation results for Scenario 1 based on 100,000 replications are presented in Table 2.11. The simulation results are very similar to those presented earlier in this section but may be slightly different due to Monte Carlo errors.

2.4.6   Conclusions and extensions

This section considered the problem of optimal selection of multiplicity adjustments in clinical trials with several sources of multiplicity. The optimization algorithm presented in this case study served as an extension of that utilized in Case study 2.1. Also, more sophisticated evaluation criteria were employed in the current case study to account for the underlying hierarchical structure of endpoint tests in the schizophrenia clinical trial.

It is important to mention that similar optimization problems arise in clinical trials with seemingly different goals and the general optimization approach discussed in this section is easily extended to many other settings. To give an example, an identical optimization problem can be formulated in clinical trials designed to perform non-inferiority and superiority assessments of mul-

TABLE 2.11: Summary of simulation results.

Evaluation criterion	Multiplicity adjustment	Value
Marginal power	Procedure B1	Placebo vs Dose H - E1: 90.2%
	Procedure B1	Placebo vs Dose L - E1: 63.4%
	Procedure B1	Placebo vs Dose H - E2: 43.0%
	Procedure B1	Placebo vs Dose L - E2: 48.5%
	Procedure B2	Placebo vs Dose H - E1: 90.2%
	Procedure B2	Placebo vs Dose L - E1: 66.6%
	Procedure B2	Placebo vs Dose H - E2: 44.7%
	Procedure B2	Placebo vs Dose L - E2: 52.5%
Subset disjunctive power	Procedure B1	60.6%
	Procedure B2	52.5%
Weighted power	Procedure B1	70.6%
	Procedure B2	72.4%
Partition-based weighted power	Procedure B1	30.6%
	Procedure B2	32.5%

tiple doses of an experimental treatment compared to an active control. For instance, using a case study from Dmitrienko et al. (2011), consider a clinical trial for the treatment of Type II diabetes. Two doses of an experimental treatment (labeled Dose L and Dose H) are compared to a control to assess the treatment effects on the reduction in hemoglobin A1c. The dose-control comparisons are carried out based on non-inferiority and superiority tests. The null hypotheses of interest in this clinical trial are defined as follows:

- H_1: Null hypothesis of inferiority of the experimental treatment to the active control at Dose H.

- H_2: Null hypothesis of inferiority of the experimental treatment to the active control at Dose L.

- H_3: Null hypothesis of lack of superiority of the experimental treatment to the active control at Dose H.

- H_4: Null hypothesis of lack of superiority of the experimental treatment to the active control at Dose L.

The most important goal of the trial is to establish non-inferiority of the experimental treatment to the active control on at least one dose and thus it is natural to place the first two hypotheses (H_1 and H_2) in the primary family. The remaining hypotheses (H_3 and H_4) are included in the secondary family. The logical relationships among these four hypotheses are identical to those presented at the beginning of this section. Since it is no longer relevant to carry out a superiority test if non-inferiority is not established, it is meaningful to test H_3 only if H_1 is rejected and, along the same line, H_4 should be tested only after H_2 is rejected. This implies that a multiplicity adjustment can be defined using either chain procedure introduced in this section and optimal selection of procedure parameters can be performed as shown above.

2.5 Case study 2.3: Tradeoff-based selection of optimal procedure parameters

This case study deals with an optimization problem that is conceptually similar to that considered in Case study 2.2. Using the same clinical trial example, a problem of selecting an optimal parameter of a multiple testing procedure in a "bivariate" problem with two sources of multiplicity will be considered. The key difference between the two case studies is that the current case study will be used to illustrate an alternative optimization algorithm, known as a *tradeoff-based optimization algorithm*, that will be applied in conjunction with a qualitative sensitivity assessment.

2.5.1 Clinical trial

Data model

The schizophrenia clinical trial with two dose-placebo comparisons on two clinical endpoints used in Case study 2.2 will be utilized in this case study. The four sets of statistical assumptions listed in Table 2.8 will be re-used and, as before, the data model corresponding to Scenario 1 will be treated as the main model whereas the other three scenarios will be used to define alternative models. The alternative data models will play an important role in the optimization problem considered in this case study.

Analysis model

The analysis model defined in Section 2.4.1 will also be re-used in the sense that the same set of null hypotheses tests based on the dose-placebo comparisons and primary/secondary endpoints will be considered:

- H_1: Null hypothesis of no effect at Dose H with respect to the primary endpoint.

- H_2: Null hypothesis of no effect at Dose L with respect to the primary endpoint.

- H_3: Null hypothesis of no effect at Dose H with respect to the secondary endpoint.

- H_4: Null hypothesis of no effect at Dose L with respect to the secondary endpoint.

The four null hypotheses will be again grouped into two families. The first two hypotheses (H_1 and H_2) will be placed in the primary family and the other two hypotheses (H_3 and H_4) will be placed in the secondary family. However, a more advanced multiplicity adjustment, which serves as the key component of the analysis model, will be utilized in this case study to address multiplicity induced by the four hypotheses. This adjustment will be based on a gatekeeping procedure derived from the Hochberg-type tests applied to the primary and secondary hypotheses and will be referred to as Procedure H.

The general testing algorithm used in Procedure H is depicted in Figure 2.22. This gatekeeping procedure serves as an example of mixture-based gatekeeping procedures introduced in Section 2.2.2. The gatekeeping procedure is constructed using two *component procedures*. Testing begins with the primary family and the first component procedure (*truncated* version of the Hochberg procedure) is applied to test the hypotheses H_1 and H_2. This procedure is indexed by the parameter γ and, for compactness, it will be denoted by Hochberg(γ). The trial's key objective is to reject at least one hypothesis in the primary family. After this objective is met, the secondary hypotheses will be tested by applying the regular Hochberg procedure, which serves as the second component procedure.

It is important to note that the logical restrictions introduced in Case study 2.2 will be imposed on the testing algorithm to ensure clinical relevance of the results. A hypothesis will be "testable" in the secondary family only if the primary hypothesis associated with the same dose level is rejected. A "non-testable" hypothesis is accepted without testing. To illustrate, assume that a significant treatment effect is established at Dose H on the primary endpoint (H_1 is rejected) but there is no evidence of a significant effect at Dose L on the same endpoint (H_2 cannot be rejected). In this case, only one hypothesis will be testable in the secondary family, i.e., H_3, and the other hypothesis, i.e., H_4, will not be examined as it is no longer clinically relevant.

A detailed description of the two-step testing algorithm used in Procedure H is provided below. To define this algorithm, let p_1 and p_2 denote the raw p-values for testing the hypotheses H_1 and H_2. The ordered p-values in the primary family are denoted by $p_{(1)} < p_{(2)}$ and associated ordered hypotheses are denoted by $H_{(1)}$ and $H_{(2)}$. Further, p_3 and p_4 will denote the raw p-values in the secondary family and the ordered p-values as well as ordered hypotheses will be defined as in the primary family.

- Step 1. The primary hypotheses will be tested using the truncated Hochberg procedure with a pre-defined truncation parameter γ, i.e., Hochberg(γ). The truncated procedure must be applied in this family since, as shown in Dmitrienko, Tamhane and Wiens (2008), the regular Hochberg procedure is a "greedy" procedure, formally known as a *non-separable* procedure, and will use up all available α in the primary family unless both H_1 and H_2 are rejected. To enable the decision rules defined in Figure 2.22, the regular Hochberg procedure needs to be modified by applying *truncation* and the resulting truncated procedure can be used in the primary

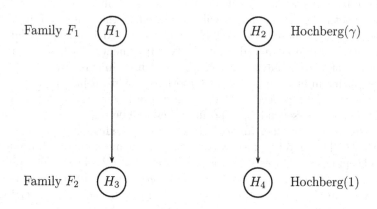

FIGURE 2.22: Hochberg-based gatekeeping procedure (Procedure H) in Case study 2.3.

family if $0 \leq \gamma < 1$. Note that, when $\gamma = 1$, the truncated Hochberg procedure simplifies to the regular Hochberg procedure. With the truncated Hochberg procedure, both hypotheses will be rejected in the primary family if $p_{(2)} \leq \alpha(1 + \gamma)/2$. Alternatively, only $H_{(1)}$ will be rejected if $p_{(1)} \leq \alpha/2$ and $p_{(2)} > \alpha(1 + \gamma)/2$.

- Step 2. The hypotheses in the secondary family will be tested using regular Hochberg procedure, i.e., Hochberg(1), since this is the last family in this multiplicity problem. As shown below, the secondary tests will be carried out at the full α level if both primary hypotheses are rejected and a penalty will be imposed if only one rejection is made in the primary family. This penalty is a consequence of the "use it or lose it" principle discussed in Section 2.4.1 which implies, in this setting, that a certain fraction of the overall Type I error rate will be lost due to the failure to reject one of the primary hypotheses. Specifically, if two rejections are made in the primary family, both secondary hypotheses will be rejected if $p_{(4)} \leq \alpha$ or only $H_{(3)}$ will be rejected if $p_{(3)} \leq \alpha/2$ but $p_{(4)} > \alpha$. However, if only H_1 is rejected in Step 1, H_3 will be rejected if $p_3 \leq \alpha(1 - \gamma)/2$ and H_4 will be automatically accepted. Similarly, if H_2 is the only hypothesis rejected in the primary family, H_4 will be rejected if $p_4 \leq \alpha(1 - \gamma)/2$ and H_3 will be accepted without testing.

In general, a higher value of the truncation parameter γ used in the truncated Hochberg procedure helps improve power in the primary family. At the same time, power in the secondary family will generally be reduced with an increasing truncation parameter. The truncation parameter will serve as the target parameter in this optimization problem and optimal selection of γ will be discussed in Section 2.5.2.

It is worth pointing out that Procedure H can be potentially extended using a re-testing approach. The extended procedure employs a three-step algorithm where the first two steps are identical to those in Procedure H and the third step includes the following tests. The extended procedure will re-test the hypothesis H_1 at the full α level in Step 3 if H_4 is rejected in Step 2 provided H_1 is not rejected in Step 1. Similarly, the hypothesis H_2 will be re-tested at the full α level in Step 3 if H_3 is rejected in Step 2 but the test of H_2 is not significant in Step 1. The testing algorithm used in the extended procedure is defined in Dmitrienko et al. (2011).

A key property of Procedure H is that it is derived from the Hochberg-type tests and, by contrast, the two gatekeeping procedures considered in Case study 2.2, i.e., Procedures B1 and B2, were based on the Bonferroni tests. As shown in Section 2.2.2, the Hochberg procedure is an example of semiparametric multiple testing procedures that are known to be uniformly more powerful than nonparametric procedures such as the Bonferroni. This means that the former will reject all hypotheses rejected by the latter and potentially more. As a result, Procedure H is expected to be more powerful than Procedures B1 and B2.

The test statistics within each family follow a bivariate normal distribution with a positive correlation coefficient due to the simple fact that the two dose-placebo contrasts share the placebo arm. This implies, as indicated in Section 2.2.2, that the truncated and regular Hochberg procedures provide *local control* of the Type I error rate. This means that the truncated Hochberg procedure protects the Type I error rate within the primary family and, similarly, the regular Hochberg procedure preserves the error rate within the second family. As shown in Dmitrienko and Tamhane (2011, 2013), the gatekeeping procedure built from these two components controls the Type I error rate in a global sense, i.e., with respect to all four hypotheses, at a one-sided $\alpha = 0.025$ in this multiplicity problem.

Evaluation model

Optimal values of the target parameter γ in the gatekeeping procedure (Procedure H) can be chosen using a broad set of evaluation criteria. This includes, as in Case study 2.2, exceedence criteria such as the subset disjunctive criterion and expectation criteria such as the simple and partition-based weighted criteria. As in the other case studies, the available evaluation criteria need to be compared in terms of their relevance and optimal selection of the target parameter is to be performed using criteria that are most relevant in the context of this particular clinical trial example.

An important feature of the approach considered in this case study is that the selected evaluation criteria will be incorporated into a tradeoff-based optimization algorithm. The optimal choice of the target parameter γ in this problem will be defined as the value or set of values that provide a balance between two *competing goals*. It will be shown in Section 2.5.2 that most commonly used criteria, including the disjunctive and weighted criteria, turn out to be increasing functions of the target parameter when applied to the primary family and decreasing functions of the parameter when applied to the secondary family. In other words, selecting a larger value of γ leads to a higher probability of meeting the primary objectives in this trial but the probability of meeting the secondary objectives will be lower and vice versa. An optimal value of γ can thus be chosen as the value that leads to a desirable balance of power between the families or, in other words, a meaningful compromise between the competing goals of improving the probability of success for the trial's primary and secondary objectives.

More formally, as explained in Chapter 1, an additive tradeoff-based criterion can be constructed based on a weighted sum of the appropriate evaluation criteria in the two families, e.g.,

$$\psi(\gamma) = v_1\psi_1(\gamma) + v_2\psi_2(\gamma),$$

where v_1 and v_2 are pre-specified non-negative values that define the relative importance of the primary and secondary objectives. These quantities play the same role as the importance values in the weighted criteria used in Case studies 2.1 and 2.2. Since the trial's overall outcome is driven by the primary endpoint and the secondary endpoint provides supportive evidence of treatment effectiveness, the primary family is clearly more important than the secondary one. It is therefore natural to assign a higher importance value to the primary family, i.e., $v_1 > v_2$.

Further, $\psi_1(\gamma)$ and $\psi_2(\gamma)$ denote the components of the criterion that are based on pre-defined criteria evaluated in the primary and secondary families, respectively, for Procedure H with the truncation parameter γ. A tradeoff-based algorithm is aimed at identifying the value of the target parameter that maximizes this optimization criterion.

To illustrate the tradeoff-based approach, the criterion $\psi(\gamma)$ will be defined based on the components derived from disjunctive and weighted power. The components of the disjunctive criterion are defined using disjunctive power in the primary and secondary families, i.e.,

$$\psi_1(\gamma) = P(\text{Reject } H_1 \text{ or } H_2|\gamma), \quad \psi_2(\gamma) = P(\text{Reject } H_3 \text{ or } H_4|\gamma).$$

The resulting tradeoff-based criterion as a function of the target parameter is then simply equal to

$$\psi_D(\gamma) = v_1 P(\text{Reject } H_1 \text{ or } H_2|\gamma) + v_2 P(\text{Reject } H_3 \text{ or } H_4|\gamma).$$

This disjunctive criterion can be viewed as an extension of the subset disjunctive criterion used in Case study 2.2. Recall from that case study that the subset disjunctive criterion was defined as the probability of simultaneously rejecting at least one hypothesis in the primary family and at least one hypothesis in the secondary family. A key limitation of this approach to setting up an evaluation criterion is that it does not support an option to assign weights to the two families to account for the fact that the hypotheses based on the primary endpoint are obviously more important than the secondary ones. By contrast, the tradeoff-based criterion defined above enables the trial's sponsor to incorporate family-specific weights.

The simple weighted criterion utilizes the components based on simple weighted power in the two families:

$$
\begin{aligned}
\psi_1(\gamma) &= v_{11}P(\text{Reject } H_1|\gamma) + v_{12}P(\text{Reject } H_2|\gamma), \\
\psi_2(\gamma) &= v_{21}P(\text{Reject } H_3|\gamma) + v_{22}P(\text{Reject } H_4|\gamma),
\end{aligned}
$$

where v_{11} and v_{12} are non-negative quantities that define the relative importance of establishing a significant effect at Doses H and L on the primary endpoint after a multiplicity adjustment based on Procedure H, and v_{21} and v_{22} play similar roles in the secondary family. As before, it is often convenient to assume that $v_{11} + v_{12} = 1$ and $v_{21} + v_{22} = 1$.

It is easy to show that the tradeoff-based criterion, to be denoted by $\psi_{SW}(\gamma)$, is equal to a weighted sum of the four marginal power functions, i.e.,

$$
\begin{aligned}
\psi_{SW}(\gamma) &= v_1 v_{11}P(\text{Reject } H_1|\gamma) + v_1 v_{12}P(\text{Reject } H_2|\gamma), \\
&+ v_2 v_{21}P(\text{Reject } H_3|\gamma) + v_2 v_{22}P(\text{Reject } H_4|\gamma).
\end{aligned}
$$

Therefore, this tradeoff-based criterion is equivalent to the evaluation criterion based on simple weighted power that was introduced in Case study 2.2.

In general, any meaningful evaluation criterion can be used as a component of the optimization criterion in a tradeoff-based optimization algorithm, including more advanced criteria based on multiplicity penalties introduced in Section 2.2.3.

2.5.2 Optimal selection of the target parameter in Procedure H

The two tradeoff-based criteria (disjunctive and simple weighted criteria) were applied to identify the optimal value of the target parameter, i.e., the truncation parameter γ in Procedure H, in this optimization problem. As in Case study 2.2, the optimization exercise focused on finding the "point estimate" of the optimal parameter by maximizing the appropriate criterion function as well as an optimal interval which includes nearly optimal values of γ. Optimal values of the target parameter were found using a straightforward grid search over the $[0, 1)$ interval. Note that the truncation parameter was strictly less than 1 to guarantee that the truncated Hochberg test applied in the primary family was separable.

Before applying the tradeoff-based criteria, it is instructive to examine the

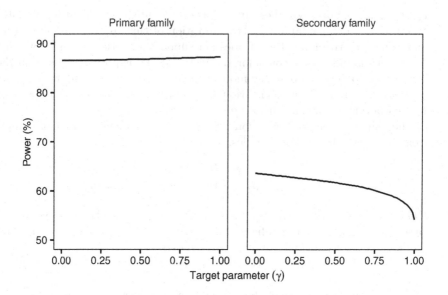

FIGURE 2.23: Disjunctive power as a function of the target parameter (γ) in the primary and secondary families under Scenario 1 in Case study 2.3.

components of each criterion as functions of the target parameter. Figure 2.23 displays the disjunctive power functions in the primary and secondary families under the main data model (Scenario 1). It follows from the left-hand panel that disjunctive power increased with γ in the primary family and the right-hand panel shows that disjunctive power was a decreasing function of the target parameter in the secondary family. It is worth noting that, as the target parameter increased from 0 to 1, the power gain in the primary family was rather trivial and disjunctive power improved by less than one percentage point compared to a power loss of 9 percentage points in the secondary family. This was due to a key property of disjunctive power that was mentioned multiple times throughout this chapter. It could be easily checked that there was a tangible increase in the probabilities of rejecting the individual hypotheses H_1 and H_2 as γ changed from 0 to 1; however, the probability of at least one rejection (disjunctive power) was fairly insensitive to this change.

To summarize, Figure 2.23 confirms that the goals of maximizing disjunctive power in each family were indeed competing goals in the schizophrenia clinical trial and it is natural to consider a tradeoff-based approach to find a value of γ that provides a balance between the two goals. Two definitions of the tradeoff-based disjunctive criterion were examined in this case study. First, the tradeoff-based criterion was computed under the assumption that the two clinical endpoints were equally important, i.e., $v_1 = v_2 = 0.5$. This

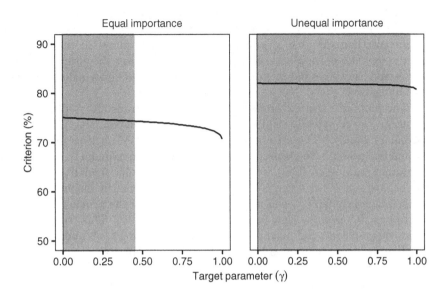

FIGURE 2.24: Disjunctive criterion as a function of the target parameter (γ) under Scenario 1 in Case study 2.3. The criterion is evaluated under the assumption of equal importance of the two families ($v_1 = 0.5$ and $v_2 = 0.5$) as well as unequal importance ($v_1 = 0.8$ and $v_2 = 0.2$). The vertical lines represent the optimal values of the target parameter and the gray rectangles define the 99% optimal intervals for the target parameter.

resulted in the following criterion:

$$\psi_D(\gamma) = 0.5P(\text{Reject } H_1 \text{ or } H_2|\gamma) + 0.5P(\text{Reject } H_3 \text{ or } H_4|\gamma).$$

In addition, a more realistic definition of the disjunctive criterion with unequally weighted families was considered ($v_1 = 0.8$ and $v_2 = 0.2$) and the tradeoff-based criterion was given by

$$\psi_D(\gamma) = 0.8P(\text{Reject } H_1 \text{ or } H_2|\gamma) + 0.2P(\text{Reject } H_3 \text{ or } H_4|\gamma).$$

With this set of importance values, the goal of improving power in the primary family was deemed much more important than the corresponding goal in the secondary family.

Using the main data model, the tradeoff-based disjunctive criterion with the two sets of importance values are plotted in Figure 2.24. The shapes of the two criterion functions in the left-hand panel (equal importance) and right-hand panel (unequal importance) were generally similar. Both functions were quite flat and both functions were maximized when γ was equal to 0. Consequently, the optimal value of the target parameter was $\gamma^* = 0$ but, as shown in the figure, the sets of nearly optimal values of γ based on 99%

optimal intervals were quite wide. For example, in the case where the goal of improving disjunctive power in the primary family was considered more important than the goal of maximizing disjunctive power in the secondary family, the 99% optimal interval extended virtually over the entire range of γ values and the target parameters as large as 0.95 could be formally considered optimal as well.

The plots in Figure 2.24 clearly show that the tradeoff-based disjunctive criterion was completely dominated by the goal of maximizing power in the secondary family. The criterion was maximized at $\gamma^* = 0$ simply because disjunctive power in the secondary family achieved a maximum at this value of the target parameter. The choice of the importance values had little impact on the behavior of the criterion and it was heavily influence by disjunctive power in the secondary family even when the importance of the primary family was set to $v_1 = 0.8$ (see the right-hand panel of Figure 2.24). This criterion failed to provide a meaningful balance between the competing goals and thus it may not be considered relevant in this clinical trial example.

Alternatively, the criterion in a tradeoff-based algorithm can be set up based on simple weighted power. Under this criterion, the probability of success is measured within each family using weighted power. To define this criterion, it was assumed that demonstrating a beneficial treatment effect at Dose L was as important as demonstrating a beneficial treatment effect at Dose H on either clinical endpoint in this schizophrenia clinical trial. In other words, simple weighted power was computed in the primary and secondary families as follows:

$$\psi_1(\gamma) = 0.5P(\text{Reject } H_1|\gamma) + 0.5P(\text{Reject } H_2|\gamma),$$
$$\psi_2(\gamma) = 0.5P(\text{Reject } H_3|\gamma) + 0.5P(\text{Reject } H_4|\gamma),$$

Figure 2.25 plots the two component functions over the range of γ values under the main data model. The left-hand panel of this figure demonstrates that the first component (simple weighted power in the primary family) increased monotonically with the increasing target parameter. Note that the gain in simple weighted power was much larger than the gain in disjunctive power (see Figure 2.23); specifically, simple weighted power increased by 6 percentage points over the $[0, 1]$ interval compared to a gain of approximately one percentage point when disjunctive power was considered. This observation is consistent with earlier observations that weighted power is a more sensitive tool for assessing the probability of success than disjunctive power. Further, it follows from the right-hand panel of the figure that the second component generally decreased with the target parameter (however, it was not a monotonically decreasing function of γ) and thus the goal of increasing power in the primary family conflicted with the goal of increasing power in the secondary family. As shown in Figure 2.25, selecting a larger γ would help improve the probability of success in the primary family at the price of reduced power in the secondary family. On the other hand, with a smaller γ,

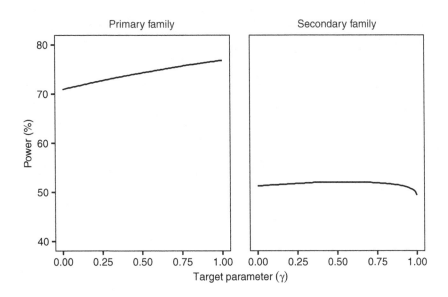

FIGURE 2.25: Simple weighted power as a function of the target parameter (γ) in the primary and secondary families under Scenario 1 in Case study 2.3.

the second component would improve but power of the primary analyses may be unacceptably low.

To address the competing nature of the goals of maximizing power in the two families, the tradeoff-based criterion based on simple weighted power was derived under the assumption that the two goals were equally important ($v_1 = 0.5$ and $v_2 = 0.5$) as well as the assumption that the first goal was considerably more important than the second one ($v_1 = 0.8$ and $v_2 = 0.2$). Using the component functions defined above, the corresponding criterion functions were computed as follows:

$$\psi_{SW}(\gamma) = 0.5\psi_1(\gamma) + 0.5\psi_2(\gamma), \ \psi_{SW}(\gamma) = 0.8\psi_1(\gamma) + 0.2\psi_2(\gamma).$$

The effect of the target parameter γ on the tradeoff-based criterion under the two sets of assumptions is depicted in Figure 2.26. In both cases the criterion achieved a maximum when the target parameter was close to 1. The optimal values of the target parameter that provided a tradeoff between maximizing weighted power in the two families were $\gamma^* = 0.8$ when the two families were deemed to be of equal importance and $\gamma^* = 0.93$ when the first family was deemed to be more important. These conclusions need to be contrasted with those based on the disjunctive criterion presented in Figure 2.24. The value of γ that appeared optimal based on the disjunctive criterion, i.e., $\gamma^* = 0$, resulted in the worst possible performance when the simple weighted criterion was applied. Unlike the disjunctive criterion, the weighted criterion

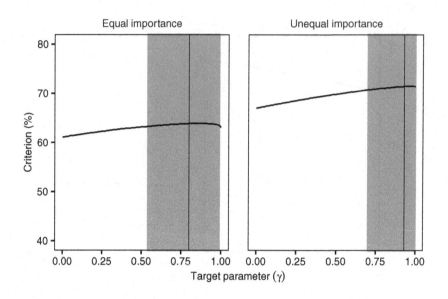

FIGURE 2.26: Simple weighted criterion as a function of the target parameter (γ) under Scenario 1 in Case study 2.3. The criterion is evaluated under the assumption of equal importance of the two families ($v_1 = 0.5$ and $v_2 = 0.5$) as well as unequal importance ($v_1 = 0.8$ and $v_2 = 0.2$). The vertical lines represent the optimal values of the target parameter and the gray rectangles define the 99% optimal intervals for the target parameter.

provided a better balance between the competing goals and thus appeared to be more relevant than the disjunctive criterion in this case study.

Figure 2.26 focused on the tradeoff-based simple weighted criterion under the main data model (Scenario 1) and Figure 2.27 presents the results of a qualitative assessment for this tradeoff-based criterion. This figure includes plots of the tradeoff-based criteria across all plausible data models considered in the schizophrenia clinical trial. The criteria were computed under the assumption that the goal of maximizing the probability of success in the primary family was more important compared to the secondary family. In general, similar overall patterns were observed in the four panels of this figure. The optimal values of the target parameter for each of the four data models were quite consistent and the figure also shows a considerable overlap among the 99% optimal intervals across the data models.

Table 2.12 provides a detailed summary of the optimal values and associated 99% optimal intervals for the target parameter γ under the four data models. As stated above, the optimal values exhibited a good degree of consistency across the effect size scenarios (the scenario-specific optimal value ranged between 0.88 and 0.97). Using the 99% optimal intervals computed

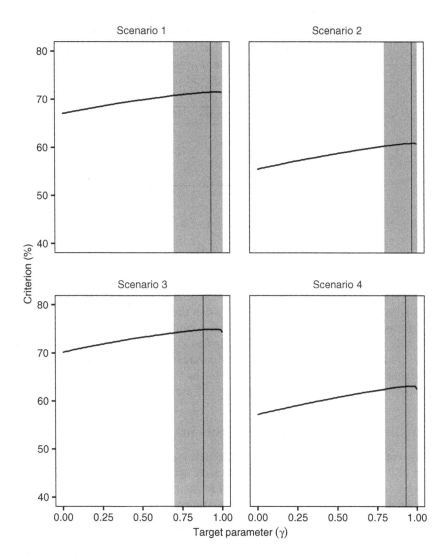

FIGURE 2.27: Simple weighted criterion as a function of the target parameter (γ) under four scenarios in Case study 2.3. The criterion assumes that the primary family is more important than the secondary family ($v_1 = 0.8$ and $v_2 = 0.2$). The vertical lines represent the optimal values of the target parameter and the gray rectangles define the 99% optimal intervals for the target parameter.

under the individual data models, it is easy to find the joint 99% optimal

TABLE 2.12: Optimal values of the target parameter (γ) and optimal intervals based on the simple weighted criterion under the assumption that the primary family is more important than the secondary family ($v_1 = 0.8$ and $v_2 = 0.2$) in Case study 2.3.

Scenario	Optimal value	99% optimal interval
Scenario 1	0.93	$(0.70, 1.00)$
Scenario 2	0.97	$(0.80, 1.00)$
Scenario 3	0.88	$(0.70, 1.00)$
Scenario 4	0.93	$(0.80, 1.00)$

interval for the target parameter:

$$(0.8, 1).$$

An optimal value of γ can be set to the mid-point of the joint interval, e.g., $\gamma^* = 0.9$. The results of the qualitative assessment indicate that the multiplicity adjustment based on Procedure H with the truncated parameter $\gamma = 0.9$ is expected to provide optimal performance under all pre-specified data models in this clinical trial example. In other words, with the optimal procedure, the trial's sponsor can strike a proper balance between the competing goals of maximizing the probability of success in the families of primary and secondary tests under all plausible sets of statistical assumptions.

Quantitative sensitivity assessment

The tradeoff-based optimization approach has been applied so far to a small set of data models as part of a qualitative sensitivity assessment. It is highly recommended to perform an extended sensitivity assessment using a quantitative approach. Since the data model assumed in this case study is identical to that used in Case study 2.2, the permutation-based algorithms considered in Section 2.4.4 can be applied without any modifications to examine the impact of random deviations from an assumed data model, e.g., the main data model, on an optimal multiplicity adjustment based on Procedure H.

2.5.3   Software implementation

As in the other case studies, software implementation of the CSE-based simulation framework in this case study, including the specification of tradeoff-based optimization criteria, is provided below using the **Mediana** package.

Data model

Data model specifications in this case study are identical to those in Case study 2.2 (see Section 2.4.5) since the two case studies share the same clinical trial example.

Analysis model

The analysis model includes the same four statistical tests as in Case study 2.2 and the Hochberg-based gatekeeping procedure. The statistical tests are defined in exactly the same way as in Case study 2.2. However, the specification of the multiple testing procedure is different and necessitates the specification of the following three parameters:

- `family` defines the allocation of the null hypotheses to the families, i.e., the first and second hypotheses are included in the primary family and the other two in the secondary family.

- `component.procedure` defines the component procedures used within the gatekeeping procedure (Hochberg procedures are applied to both families).

- `gamma` specifies the truncation parameters used in the two families (γ is set to 0.9 in the primary family and to 1 in the secondary family since the regular Hochberg procedure is used in the last family). These truncation parameters define an optimal gatekeeping procedure derived in this section.

These parameters are then included in the `MultAdjProc` object and the Hochberg-based gatekeeping procedure is defined using the `MultipleSequenceGatekeepingAdj` method.

LISTING 2.13: Specification of the Hochberg-based gatekeeping procedure in Case study 2.3

```
# Parameters of the Hochberg-based gatekeeping procedure
family = families(family1 = c(1, 2),
                  family2 = c(3, 4))

component.procedure = families(family1="HochbergAdj",
                               family2="HochbergAdj")

gamma = families(family1 = 0.9,
                 family2 = 1)

mult.adj =
  MultAdjProc(proc = "MultipleSequenceGatekeepingAdj",
              par = parameters(family = family,
                               proc = component.procedure,
                               gamma = gamma),
```

```
tests = tests("Placebo vs Dose H - E1",
              "Placebo vs Dose L - E1",
              "Placebo vs Dose H - E2",
              "Placebo vs Dose L - E2"))
```

The `mult.adj` object is then added to the analysis model as in Case study 2.2.

Evaluation model

This case study utilizes tradeoff-based optimization criteria based on disjunctive power, $\phi_D(\gamma)$, and on simple weighted power, $\phi_{SW}(\gamma)$. The latter can be directly specified in the evaluation model using the `WeightedPower` method with the hypothesis weights set to $v_1 v_{11}$, $v_1 v_{12}$, $v_2 v_{21}$ and $v_2 v_{22}$, respectively. As for the tradeoff-based disjunctive criterion, it is not implemented by default in the **Mediana** package and a custom function needs to be written and incorporated into the evaluation model.

The `mult.cs3.TradeoffDisjunctivePower` function, defined below, calculates the probability of rejecting at least one hypothesis in the primary family and at least one hypothesis in the secondary family and then returns a weighted sum of these probabilities.

LISTING 2.14: Custom function for computing the tradeoff-based disjunctive criterion in Case study 2.3

```
# Custom evaluation criterion
mult.cs3.TradeoffDisjunctivePower = function(test.result,
    statistic.result, parameter) {

  alpha = parameter$alpha
  weight = parameter$weight

  family1 = ((test.result[,1] <= alpha) | (test.result[,2]
    <= alpha))
  family2 = ((test.result[,3] <= alpha) | (test.result[,4]
    <= alpha))

  power = weight[1] * mean(family1) + weight[2] * mean(
    family2)

  return(power)
}
```

The resulting `Criterion` objects for the simple weighted criterion and for the tradeoff-based criterion derived from disjunctive power are included in the evaluation model. The criteria are evaluated based on two sets of importance parameters, i.e., parameters that define an equal-importance scenario ($v_1 = v_2 = 0.5$) and unequal-importance scenario ($v_1 = 0.8$, $v_2 = 0.2$).

LISTING 2.15: Evaluation model in Case study 2.3

```
# Evaluation model
mult.cs3.evaluation.model = EvaluationModel() +
  Criterion(id = "Tradeoff-based disjunctive power (v1 =
    0.5, v2 = 0.5)",
            method = "mult.cs3.TradeoffDisjunctivePower",
            tests = tests("Placebo vs Dose H - E1",
                          "Placebo vs Dose L - E1",
                          "Placebo vs Dose H - E2",
                          "Placebo vs Dose L - E2"),
            labels = "Tradeoff-based disjunctive power",
            par = parameters(alpha = 0.025,
                             weight = c(0.5, 0.5))) +
  Criterion(id = "Tradeoff-based disjunctive power (v1 =
    0.8, v2 = 0.2)",
            method = "mult.cs3.TradeoffDisjunctivePower",
            tests = tests("Placebo vs Dose H - E1",
                          "Placebo vs Dose L - E1",
                          "Placebo vs Dose H - E2",
                          "Placebo vs Dose L - E2"),
            labels = "Tradeoff-based disjunctive power",
            par = parameters(alpha = 0.025,
                             weight = c(0.8, 0.2))) +
  Criterion(id = "Weighted power (v1 = 0.5, v2 = 0.5)",
            method = "WeightedPower",
            tests = tests("Placebo vs Dose H - E1",
                          "Placebo vs Dose L - E1",
                          "Placebo vs Dose H - E2",
                          "Placebo vs Dose L - E2"),
            labels = "Weighted power",
            par = parameters(alpha = 0.025,
         weight = c(0.5*0.5, 0.5*0.5, 0.5*0.5, 0.5*0.5))) +
  Criterion(id = "Weighted power (v1 = 0.8, v2 = 0.2)",
            method = "WeightedPower",
            tests = tests("Placebo vs Dose H - E1",
                          "Placebo vs Dose L - E1",
                          "Placebo vs Dose H - E2",
                          "Placebo vs Dose L - E2"),
            labels = "Weighted power",
            par = parameters(alpha = 0.025,
         weight = c(0.8*0.5, 0.8*0.5, 0.2*0.5, 0.2*0.5))))
```

Simulation results

The simulation results for Scenario 1 based on 100,000 replications are presented in Table 2.13.

TABLE 2.13: Summary of simulation results.

Evaluation criterion	Value
Tradeoff-based disjunctive power (v1 = 0.5, v2 = 0.5)	72.5%
Tradeoff-based disjunctive power (v1 = 0.8, v2 = 0.1)	81.3%
Weighted power (v1 = 0.5, v2 = 0.5)	63.7%
Weighted power (v1 = 0.8, v2 = 0.2)	71.3%

2.5.4   Conclusions and extensions

Using a clinical trial example defined in Case study 2.2, this section focused on optimal selection of efficient gatekeeping procedures derived from semiparametric components in "bivariate" multiplicity problems with two sources of multiplicity. Tradeoff-based optimization strategies were utilized to build an analysis model with an optimal multiplicity adjustment.

The multiple testing procedure studied in this section (Procedure H) belongs to the class of gatekeeping procedures known as *multiple-sequence gatekeeping procedures* (Dmitrienko, Kordzakhia and Brechenmacher, 2016). Hochberg-based and similar semiparametric gatekeeping procedures (e.g., Hommel-based gatekeeping procedure) from this class are more powerful than basic Bonferroni-based procedures and can be developed for very general multiplicity problems with multiple branches. This includes bivariate multiplicity problems with multiple clinical endpoints or multiple patient populations and several dose-control comparisons as well as problems with multiple dose-control comparisons and non-inferiority/superiority tests mentioned at the end of Case study 2.2.

3

Subgroup Analysis in Clinical Trials

Alex Dmitrienko

Mediana Inc.

Gautier Paux

Institut de Recherches Internationales Servier

3.1 Introduction

A broad class of issues and considerations related to subgroup analysis in clinical trials have attracted attention across the clinical trial community. Multiple research and review papers on this topic have been published in clinical trial and biostatistical journals over the past ten years. To give a few examples, a review of recent publications and regulatory considerations related to the evaluation of subgroup effects in confirmatory trials was provided in Dmitrienko et al. (2016). Further, Ondra et al. (2016) presented a comprehensive survey of statistical methods used in the assessment of patient subgroups in Phase II and Phase III clinical trials. The U.S. Food and Drug Administration (FDA) and European Medicines Agency (EMA) have recently released draft guidance documents that deal with subgroup analysis and related topics (FDA, 2012; EMA, 2014).

The interest in subgroup analysis reflects the fact that much progress has been made in the general area of personalized/precision medicine. Clinical trials with several patient populations that include the overall population as well as pre-defined focused subgroups based on baseline patient characteristics play a key role in the development of tailored therapies. These biomarker-driven trial designs are known as multi-population tailoring designs. There are numerous examples of novel treatments that were developed as molecularly targeted agents to benefit a subset of the general population of patients but may also have an attractive efficacy profile in the broad population. This includes anti-cancer therapies, e.g., treatments studied in the SATURN trial (Cappuzzo et al., 2010) in patients with advanced non-small cell lung cancer or CRYSTAL trial (Van Cutsem et al., 2009) in patients with metastatic colorectal cancer, as well as treatments for other conditions. Most of the time a single subpopulation is pre-specified in multi-population trials but examples of confirmatory Phase III clinical trials with two subpopulations can also be found. For instance, two subgroups of patients who were expected to experience enhanced treatment benefit were pre-defined in the APEX trial (Cohen et al., 2013; Cohen et al., 2014).

There are multiple types of subgroup assessments performed in clinical trials. Grouin, Coste and Lewis (2005) made one of the first attempts to create a classification of general goals of subgroup evaluation in confirmatory Phase III trials, e.g.,

- Consistency assessments to confirm efficacy benefits in the trial population across relevant subgroups.

- Subgroup analyses to identify patient subgroups with desirable characteristics such as a larger treatment effect or reduced treatment effect in a clinical trial with a positive overall effect.

- Subgroup analyses to select subgroups with a beneficial effect when the overall effect is negative (these subgroups can be used to define the patient population in other Phase III trials).

- Subgroup analyses to find subgroups with safety problems (these subgroups will be excluded from subsequent analyses).

A modified version of this classification scheme was later included in the EMA guidance on the investigation of subgroups in confirmatory clinical trials (EMA, 2014). Similar and extended classification schemes were presented in other publications; see, for example, Lipkovich, Dmitrienko and D'Agostino (2017), Dmitrienko, Millen and Lipkovich (2017) and Alosh et al. (2017). These schemes dealt with subgroup evaluation and subgroup search strategies in confirmatory subgroup assessments with a few pre-specified subpopulations or exploratory subgroup analysis in clinical trial databases with a very large number of potential patient subgroups.

This chapter will approach the topic of subgroup analysis in Phase III trials from a general Clinical Scenario Evaluation (CSE) perspective and introduce practical approaches to clinical trial optimization in a *confirmatory subgroup analysis* setting, i.e., in Phase III clinical trials with pre-defined patient subpopulations. Subpopulations are assumed to be defined based on binary classifiers derived from baseline factors such as demographic variables, gene or protein expression markers, etc. These classifiers will be referred to as *biomarkers*. For each binary biomarker, patients in the *biomarker-positive* subgroup are expected to experience improved treatment effect whereas patients in the complementary subgroup, termed the *biomarker-negative* subgroup, may not experience beneficial effect or the magnitude of beneficial effect may be reduced compared to the other subgroup. As mentioned earlier, it is quite uncommon to pre-specify two or more subpopulations in Phase III trials and, for this reason, this chapter will focus on the setting with a single pre-defined biomarker.

The key CSE principles and building blocks of the CSE framework in confirmatory subgroup analysis will be reviewed in Section 3.2. Three case studies will be presented to illustrate optimization procedures based on the general CSE approach (see Sections 3.3, 3.4 and 3.5).

R code based on the **Mediana** package introduced in Chapter 1 will be provided throughout this chapter to demonstrate how to perform simulation-based evaluations in the case studies.

3.2 Clinical Scenario Evaluation in confirmatory subgroup analysis

This chapter presents applications of the CSE approach to a general confirmatory subgroup analysis setting. The main elements of this approach were introduced in Chapter 1 and will be utilized here in the context of assessing subgroup effects in Phase III trials. The CSE principles will be applied throughout this chapter to define easy-to-implement clinical optimization algorithms. These algorithms will be presented in Sections 3.3 through 3.5 and will deal with optimal selection of analysis models and their parameters or components, e.g., parameters of multiplicity adjustments and criteria for formulating efficacy claims. The problems considered in the chapter utilize the optimization strategies defined in Chapter 1. This includes direct optimization strategies (including basic and constrained optimization) and tradeoff-based optimization strategies defined in Section 1.3.1 and illustrated in Sections 1.4 and 1.5.

3.2.1 Clinical Scenario Evaluation framework

This section briefly introduces the key components of the CSE framework, i.e., data, analysis and evaluation models, used in clinical trials with pre-defined patient subgroups. As explained in Chapter 1, CSE relies on the following three components:

- Data models define the process of generating trial data.

- Analysis models specify the statistical methods applied to the trial data generated based on the data model.

- Evaluation models determine the measures for evaluating the performance of the analysis strategies defined in the analysis model.

The general data, analysis and evaluation models defined below will serve as "templates" for the models utilized in the case studies presented in Sections 3.3 through 3.5.

Data models

A data model defines the data generation mechanism in a particular clinical trial application. A key feature of multi-population clinical trials is that, in addition to the overall group of patients based on the intent-to-treat population (also known as the population of all comers), several subpopulations are pre-specified based on a set of binary biomarkers.

As an illustration, the most common setting in confirmatory subgroup analysis includes a two-arm clinical trial (treatment versus control) with a single subpopulation. The selected biomarker defines two subsets of the overall trial population, namely, subsets of patients with a biomarker-negative or biomarker-positive status at baseline. This means that the overall population in this clinical trial is partitioned into four groups of patients known as *samples*. The samples are defined as follows:

- Sample 1: Biomarker-negative patients in the control arm.

- Sample 2: Biomarker-positive patients in the control arm.

- Sample 3: Biomarker-negative patients in the treatment arm.

- Sample 4: Biomarker-positive patients in the treatment arm.

The number of patients in each sample is determined by the randomization ratio and prevalence of biomarker positivity in the general population of patients with the condition of interest. A larger number of samples will need to be included in the data model if there are two or more pre-defined subgroups in the trial.

When formulating statistical assumptions in a data model, e.g., expected treatment effects, it is helpful to quantify the *prognostic* and *predictive* properties of the selected biomarker (Mandrekar and Sargent, 2009). To facilitate this process, a comparison of biomarkers with prognostic and predictive properties is provided in Figure 3.1. Using the setting defined above, the figure presents three scenarios with different sets of standardized average effects in the biomarker-negative and biomarker-positive subgroups within each trial arm. The primary endpoint is assumed to be normally distributed and the standardized average effect is defined as the mean effect divided by the common standard deviation, e.g., the mean change in the primary outcome variable from baseline to the last visit normalized by the standard deviation of the change. As a reference, the standardized mean effect of 0.1 corresponds to a weak treatment effect and the effect size 0.5 defines a very strong effect.

In general, a prognostic biomarker can be used to identify patient subgroups with a given prognosis, e.g., poor prognosis, regardless of the treatment assignment. An example of a prognostic biomarker is presented in the top panel of Figure 3.1. Note that no treatment effect is observed within either subset of the overall population. However, the overall effect is greater in the subgroup of biomarker-positive patients compared to the complementary

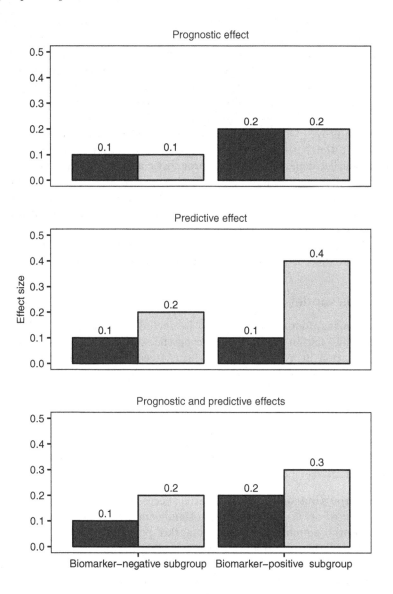

FIGURE 3.1: Treatment effects in subgroups defined by prognostic and predictive biomarkers. Standardized average effects in the control arm (black bars) and treatment arm (gray bars).

subgroup. This indicates that this particular biomarker helps select a subset of the overall population with a more favorable prognosis.

The central panel of the figure provides an example of a biomarker with predictive properties that helps identify treatment responders. Indeed, the treatment is only marginally beneficial in the biomarker-negative subgroup with a rather small difference in the standardized mean effects. The standardized average effect equals 0.1 and 0.2 in the treatment and control arms, respectively. By contrast, the treatment difference is considerably larger in the subgroup of patients with a biomarker-positive status (0.1 in the control arm versus 0.4 in the treatment arm) and thus the selected biomarker helps predict improved treatment effect in a subset of the overall population.

Lastly, the bottom panel of Figure 3.1 corresponds to the case where the biomarker demonstrates both prognostic and predictive properties. Note first that the standardized mean in the control arm is greater among the biomarker-positive patients compared to the complementary subgroup, which demonstrates a prognostic effect. In addition, a differential treatment effect is observed in the biomarker-negative and biomarker-positive subsets with a much larger benefit in the subpopulation of biomarker-positive patients. This differential effect is a sign of a strong predictive biomarker.

Analysis models

The following components need to be included in analysis models utilized in multi-population trials. Considering the setting with a single pre-defined subpopulation in a trial with two arms (treatment and control arms), the primary analysis in the analysis model is based on the following two null hypotheses of no effect:

- Null hypothesis H_0 of no difference between the treatment and control in the overall population.

- Null hypothesis H_+ of no difference between the treatment and control in the biomarker-positive subpopulation.

The trial's outcome will be declared successful if at least one null hypothesis is rejected or, in other words, if a significant treatment effect is established in the overall population and/or biomarker-positive subgroup. It needs to be stressed that there is no formal test for evaluating the treatment effect in the biomarker-negative subgroup but this test can be carried out as part of supportive or secondary efficacy assessments. This hypothesis testing framework is easily extended to settings with two or more subpopulations or trial designs with more than two arms or several endpoints.

The treatment effect is tested within each patient population (overall population and selected subpopulation) using an appropriate statistical test. For example, if the primary endpoint in the trial is continuous and it is appropriate to apply a normal approximation, significance of the treatment difference is typically assessed using analysis of covariance or repeated-measures models with an adjustment for key prognostic variables such as stratification factors and baseline value of the primary endpoint. An important factor that should be considered in the overall population test is the biomarker status (biomarker-positive versus biomarker-negative).

Analysis models arising in confirmatory subgroup analysis also include multiplicity adjustments to account for Type I error rate inflation due to testing several primary null hypotheses and decision rules for interpreting possible outcomes in individual populations. These components of analysis models will be discussed in detail in Sections 3.2.2 and 3.2.3, respectively.

Evaluation models

The last element of CSE specifications is a set of evaluation models. Evaluation models define the measures for assessing the performance of the selected analysis strategies and thus play a central role in formulating success criteria employed in clinical trial optimization procedures. It is critical to choose evaluation models/criteria that are aligned with the clinical objectives of a particular multi-population trial.

Focusing on a two-arm clinical trial with a single subpopulation, let $D(\theta)$ denote the data model, where θ denotes a vector of data model parameters. The analysis model, denoted by $A(\lambda)$, is indexed by a parameter vector λ which serves as the target parameter in the optimization problem. A general evaluation criterion in this problem will be denoted by $\psi(\lambda)$. This criterion also depends on the data model parameters but, as in Chapter 2, this dependence will not be emphasized.

To motivate the discussion of relevant evaluation models in confirmatory subgroup analysis settings, it is instructive to begin with a success criterion based on disjunctive power. The disjunctive power criterion is defined as the probability of establishing a significant effect in at least one trial population, i.e.,

$$\psi_D(\lambda) = P(\text{Reject } H_0 \text{ or Reject } H_+),$$

where the probability is evaluated under the data model $D(\theta)$ and analysis model $A(\lambda)$.

As pointed out in many publications, see, for example, Graf, Posch and Koenig (2015), this criterion is symmetric with respect to the two null hypotheses of interest in the sense that the two hypotheses are treated as if they were interchangeable. Because of this, the criterion based on disjunctive power cannot account for the fact that the consequences of rejecting each individual hypothesis or rejecting two hypotheses simultaneously may substantially differ for the trial's sponsor. In addition, when considering available options for setting up success criteria and associated evaluation models in a clinical trial with two patient populations, it is important to differentiate between statistical outcomes such as rejecting one or more null hypotheses and regulatory outcomes such as a claim of effectiveness in the overall population. As demonstrated below, weighted power criteria based on specific efficacy claims are more relevant in a trial with two or more patient populations since they directly reflect the trial's clinical objectives. These criteria can be set up using basic or partition-based weighted power functions introduced in Chapter 2.

Consider first the simple setting where the trial's sponsor is interested in evaluating the efficacy profile of a new treatment in the overall patient population and, if a significant treatment effect cannot be established in the overall population, the treatment effect will be examined in the subpopulation of biomarker-positive patients (see, for example, Zhao, Dmitrienko and Tamura, 2010). The sponsor could also assess the significance of the treatment effect in the subpopulation after overall efficacy is demonstrated; however, this finding would be of secondary interest in this trial.

As shown in Zhao, Dmitrienko and Tamura (2010), instead of working with the original null hypotheses H_0 and H_+, it is more sensible to partition the outcome that defines success in this trial into the union of two mutually exclusive outcomes:

$$H_0 \cup H_+ = H_0 + \bar{H}_0 \cap H_+,$$

where $\bar{H}_0$ denotes the complement of H_0. The outcomes correspond to the following distinct regulatory claims:

- Reject H_0: This outcome supports a *broad claim* of treatment effectiveness in the overall population of patients.

- Reject H_+ if H_0 is not rejected: This outcome corresponds to a *tailored* or *restricted claim* of treatment effectiveness in the pre-defined subpopulation of patients with a biomarker-positive status.

A clinically meaningful evaluation criterion can then be defined based on partition-based weighted power, i.e.,

$$\psi_{PW}(\boldsymbol{\lambda}) = v_1 P(\text{Broad claim}) + v_2 P(\text{Restricted claim}),$$

Here the non-negative weights v_1 and v_2 reflect the relative importance of the two claims. For example, the weights can be chosen based on the expected market share associated with each efficacy claim. From this perspective, the broad claim is as important or more important than the restricted claim, which implies that v_2 is no greater than v_1. If the weights are selected to add up to 1, this implies that $v_1 \geq 0.5$.

As stated above, the weighted power criterion is an example of partition-based success criteria. Success criteria of this kind are preferred in this setting compared to criteria based on simple weighted power, e.g.,

$$\psi_{SW}(\boldsymbol{\lambda}) = v_0 P(\text{Reject } H_0) + v_+ P(\text{Reject } H_+),$$

where v_0 and v_+ are pre-defined weights that quantify the value of rejecting each null hypothesis. To see this, note that the events corresponding to the rejection of H_0 and H_+ overlap and combining the probabilities of the two events ignores this overlap. This leads to a "biased" success criterion that is often dominated by the probability of rejecting H_+ even if the null hypothesis H_+ is likely to be rejected whenever the overall null hypothesis is rejected.

The setting with two regulatory claims will be discussed in Case studies 3.1 and 3.2. The weighted power criterion will be utilized in problems aimed at selecting optimal multiplicity adjustments and criteria for defining efficacy claims.

An extended framework with three potential efficacy claims was considered in several recent publications, including Millen et al. (2012, 2014). In this case the overall trial's outcome is partitioned based on three mutually exclusive outcomes:

$$H_0 \cup H_+ = H_0 \cap \bar{H}_+ + \bar{H}_0 \cap H_+ + H_0 \cap H_+.$$

The resulting partitioning scheme defines the following three efficacy claims:

- Reject H_0 and fail to reject H_+: This outcome translates to a *broad claim* of treatment effectiveness in the overall population of patients.

- Fail to reject H_0 and reject H_+: This outcome corresponds to a *restricted claim* of treatment effectiveness in the biomarker-positive subpopulation.

- Reject H_0 and reject H_+: This last outcome supports an *enhanced claim* of simultaneous treatment effectiveness in the overall population and pre-defined subpopulation.

A partition-based weighted criterion can be easily defined based on these outcomes:

$$\psi_{PW}(\boldsymbol{\lambda}) = v_1 P(\text{Broad claim}) + v_2 P(\text{Restricted claim}) + v_3 P(\text{Enhanced claim}),$$

where v_1, v_2 and v_3 are non-negative weights that quantify the relative importance of the three claims.

Clinical trials with three regulatory claims will be considered in Case study 3.3. Optimization methods based on the weighted function criterion will be developed to select the most appropriate parameters of the decision-making framework associated with the three efficacy claims.

A variety of other success criteria can be considered in a confirmatory subgroup analysis setting. A general utility-based approach serves as an extension of the weighted power approach described above. Examples of clinical utility functions that can be used to define evaluation models in multi-population clinical trials are given in Zhao, Dmitrienko and Tamura (2010), Graf, Posch and Koenig (2015) and Ondra et al. (2016).

3.2.2 Multiplicity adjustments

A multiplicity adjustment procedure serves as a key component of analysis models used in clinical trials with several null hypotheses of no effect associated with multiple patient populations. Multiplicity is induced in this setting by the evaluation of treatment effects in the overall population and one or more subpopulations. This section provides a brief overview of adjustments applicable to multiplicity problems arising in confirmatory subgroup analysis. Other sources of multiplicity such as multiple dose-control comparisons or multiple endpoints may need to be accounted for in multi-population clinical trials but will not be considered in this section. For more information on approaches to multiplicity adjustment commonly used in clinical trials; see Chapter 2.

The following notation will be used in this section. Let p_0 denote the marginal p-value for testing the null hypothesis of no effect in the overall population (H_0). The marginal p-value associated with the treatment effect test in the pre-defined subpopulation (H_1) is denoted by p_1. The overall Type I error rate (familywise error rate) is denoted by α, e.g., one-sided $\alpha = 0.025$.

Nonparametric procedures

A class of nonparametric multiple testing procedures includes the Bonferroni, Holm and more flexible chain procedures. These procedures impose no assumptions on the joint distribution of the test statistic in a multiplicity problem arising in a multi-population trial. Basic α-splitting methods that rely on the Bonferroni adjustment are quite common in multi-population trials; see, for example, the SATURN trial (Cappuzzo et al., 2010). Consider a multiplicity problem with two null hypotheses (H_0 and H_1) and let w_0 and w_1 denote positive weights with $w_0 + w_1 = 1$ that reflect the relative importance of establishing a significant effect in the overall population and selected subpopulation, respectively. The Bonferroni procedure rejects the null hypothesis H_0 if $p_0 \leq w_0\alpha$ and, similarly, the null hypothesis H_1 if $p_1 \leq w_1\alpha$.

It was explained in Chapter 2 that, despite its popularity in clinical trial applications, a Bonferroni-based approach to controlling the overall Type I error rate is the most conservative approach and multiple more powerful alternatives exist. This includes, for example, the Holm procedure that utilizes the following testing algorithm. First, let $p_{(0)} < p_{(1)}$ denote the ordered p-values for the two null hypotheses of interest, e.g., $p_{(0)} = p_1$ and $p_{(1)} = p_0$ if $p_1 < p_0$. The ordered hypothesis weights are denoted by $w_{(0)}$ and $w_{(1)}$. The Holm procedure rejects the null hypothesis associated with the smaller p-value if $p_{(0)} \leq \alpha w_{(0)}$. If this condition is not satisfied, none of the two hypotheses is rejected. However, if the first ordered null hypothesis is rejected, the other hypothesis is tested at the full α level. In other words, this null hypothesis is rejected by the procedure if $p_{(1)} \leq \alpha(w_{(0)} + w_{(1)}) = \alpha$. The Holm procedure is known to be uniformly more powerful than the Bonferroni procedure in the sense that the former always rejects the hypotheses rejected by the latter and, in addition, can reject other hypotheses.

Semiparametric procedures

Powerful alternatives to the Bonferroni procedure can be found in the class of semiparametric procedures. The Hochberg and Hommel procedures serve as examples of a semiparametric approach to performing a multiplicity adjustment in a clinical trial with two patient populations.

To define the decision rules used in the Hochberg procedure, consider the setting with a single subpopulation and, as above, let $p_{(0)} < p_{(1)}$ denote the ordered p-values for the null hypotheses H_0 and H_1. The Hochberg procedure begins with the larger p-value and rejects both hypotheses if $p_{(1)} \leq \alpha(w_{(0)} + w_{(1)}) = \alpha$. If this condition is not satisfied, the smaller p-value is examined and the corresponding hypothesis is rejected if $p_{(0)} \leq \alpha w_{(0)}$. While the Hochberg procedure is generally less powerful than the Hommel procedure, the two procedures are equivalent to each other in this simple multiplicity with two hypotheses. Further, the Hochberg procedure is uniformly more powerful than the Holm procedure defined above.

As shown in Chapter 2, the Hochberg and Hommel procedures control the overall Type I error rate in this multiplicity problem since the test statistics used for testing the null hypotheses in the two patient populations are positively correlated. The positive correlation is a direct consequence of the fact that the subpopulation is nested within the overall patient population.

Parametric procedures

Parametric procedures provide an improvement over nonparametric procedures by accounting for the joint distribution of the test statistics in a multiplicity problem. For example, if the endpoint in a two-arm trial with a single subpopulation is normally distributed and the fraction of biomarker-positive patients (r) is known before the trial's start or can be controlled using an oversampling strategy (Zhao, Dmitrienko and Tamura, 2010), the two test statistics follow a bivariate distribution with the correlation coefficient given by $\sqrt{r}$. Using this information, it is easy to construct parametric multiplicity adjustments that provide a uniform power improvement over the Bonferroni and Holm procedures. Parametric versions of the Bonferroni and Holm procedures, known as the single-step and step-down Dunnett procedures, are easily defined as explained in Chapter 2. There are several other parametric procedures that can be used in clinical trials with a pre-specified subpopulation, including parametric versions of flexible chain procedures (Millen and Dmitrienko, 2011) and feedback procedure (Zhao, Dmitrienko and Tamura, 2010).

Most of the multiple testing procedures introduced in this section are easily extended to address multiplicity in clinical trials with an arbitrary number of pre-defined patient subgroups. For example, Millen and Dmitrienko (2011) presented chain-based nonparametric and parametric procedures for a clinical trial in patients with schizophrenia that included two pre-specified subgroups. Exceptions include the feedback procedure that was originally defined only for the case of two populations (overall patient population and a single subpopulation) and no extensions to a general setting with several subpopulations have been proposed in the literature.

To facilitate a comparison of the three approaches to defining multiplicity adjustments in multi-population trials, recall from Chapter 2 (see Section 2.2.2) that semiparametric procedures provide a practical compromise between nonparametric and fully parametric procedures. Considering a confirmatory subgroup analysis setting discussed above, note that nonparametric procedures make no assumptions about the joint distribution of the test statistics for assessing the treatment effect in the individual patient populations (e.g., the test statistics for testing the null hypotheses H_0 and H_1) and are less powerful semiparametric and parametric procedures. On the other hand, parametric procedures can be utilized only when the correlation between the test statistics in the two patient populations is known in advance. Since this correlation coefficient is a function of the relative size of the biomarker-positive subgroup in a trial, parametric procedures are applicable only when the fraction of biomarker-positive patients is explicitly controlled, which is quite uncommon in practice.

3.2.3   Decision-making framework

While multiplicity considerations play an important role in confirmatory subgroup analysis in Phase III clinical trials, there are several approaches that are specific to the evaluation of treatment effects in patient subgroups. This includes a general decision-making framework in multi-population clinical trials that relies on the influence and interaction conditions introduced in this section. These conditions were developed as tools for guiding the process of formulating specific regulatory claims for tailored therapies. It is helpful to note that, while multiplicity adjustments are introduced to protect the "statistical error rate," i.e., Type I error rate, the framework based on the two conditions focuses on controlling the "decision-making error rates" (these error rates are known as the influence and interaction error rates and will be defined later in this chapter).

The decision-making framework facilitates interpretation of subgroup analysis results in cases when several regulatory claims can be pursued based on statistically significant findings in the overall patient population as well as pre-defined subpopulations. Operational rules for interpreting possible outcomes in multi-population trials were discussed in Millen et al. (2012, 2014), Rothmann et al. (2012) and Wang and Hung (2014).

Consider a multi-population trial with a single subpopulation of interest based on a pre-specified binary biomarker. This subpopulation includes patients with a biomarker-positive status who are expected to benefit from the experimental treatment. As in Section 3.2.1, let H_0 and H_+ denote the null hypotheses of no effect in the overall trial population and biomarker-positive subpopulation, respectively. The following is a list of four possible outcomes in this trial (a similar classification of trial outcomes can be defined in clinical trials with two or more subpopulations):

- Outcome A: Statistically significant treatment effect is established in the overall population only (H_0 is rejected but H_+ is not rejected).

- Outcome B: Statistically significant treatment effect is demonstrated in the biomarker-positive subpopulation only (H_+ is rejected but H_0 is not rejected).

- Outcome C: Statistically significant treatment effect is shown in the overall population as well as the biomarker-positive subpopulation (H_0 and H_+ are both rejected).

- Outcome D: There is no evidence of a beneficial effect in either patient population (neither null hypothesis is rejected).

Three different regulatory claims can be formulated based on these outcomes. Beginning with Outcome A, a beneficial treatment effect is established in the overall population but there is insufficient evidence to conclude efficacy in the subpopulation. In this case it is natural to pursue the *broad claim* of treatment effectiveness in the overall population. On the other hand, if the treatment is effective in the subpopulation only (Outcome B), the *restricted claim* needs to be considered. The third option is related to Outcome C when a statistically significant treatment effect is demonstrated simultaneously in both populations. As shown below, this outcome is distinct from the first two outcomes and may lead to several different efficacy claims, including the claims of broad and restricted effects as well as the *enhanced claim* based on the broad indication in the overall population and improved treatment effect in the biomarker-positive subpopulation. The underlying decision-making algorithm relies on additional considerations that are relevant in a regulatory environment. Finally, no efficacy claims can be made if the treatment difference is not statistically significant in either population (Outcome D).

Clinical trials with two potential claims

Consider a decision-making framework in the setting where the trial's sponsor is only interested in pursuing the broad and restricted claims (this setting will be considered in Case studies 3.1 and 3.2). It is instructive to first examine a naive rule for formulating an efficacy claim that relies only on statistical arguments, e.g., based only on rejection rules for the two null hypotheses of interest. This rule states that, if both null hypotheses H_0 and H_+ are rejected (Outcome C), the trial's sponsor can pursue the broad claim.

To see why a modified rule is required, note that establishing a statistically significant treatment effect in the overall population does not automatically support a claim of broad effectiveness in this population just like it ordinarily would in a trial with a single patient population. The treatment may appear to

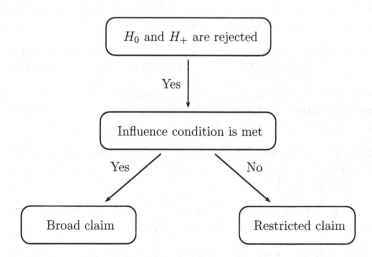

FIGURE 3.2: Recommended decision rules used in a multi-population clinical trial with two potential claims when the treatment effect is significant in the overall population and selected subpopulation.

yield a favorable result in the overall population if the treatment difference in the biomarker-positive subgroup is highly significant but the treatment has no effect in the complementary subgroup of biomarker-negative patients. Using the CRYSTAL trial (Van Cutsem et al., 2009) as an example, the hazard ratio in the biomarker-negative subgroup was very close to 1 and a positive overall effect was clearly driven by a strong treatment effect among patients with a biomarker-positive status (wild-type KRAS subgroup). It would be incorrect to conclude a broad treatment effect in this case and an additional restriction needs to be imposed to construct a clinically meaningful set of rules.

Millen et al. (2012, 2014) proposed to introduce a restriction based on the *influence condition*. The influence condition helps support a streamlined decision-making process that avoids incorrect conclusions in clinical trials with two potential claims. Under the influence condition, the efficacy label will be restricted to the selected subpopulation if there is minimal treatment in the biomarker-negative subgroup or no effect at all. For example, the claim of a broad treatment effect will be replaced with the restricted claim if the estimated effect size in the biomarker-negative subgroup is below a pre-defined threshold. The use of the influence condition in a clinical trial designed to pursue the broad and restricted efficacy claims will be illustrated in Case study 3.2. This case study will discuss the problem of choosing an appropriate value of the threshold to be used in the influence condition.

The recommended criteria based on the influence condition are defined in Figure 3.2. As shown in the figure, the broad claim should be considered if a statistically significant effect is detected in the overall population and, in addition, the influence condition is met. If this condition is not satisfied, it will be most appropriate to recommend the use of the new treatment only in the population of biomarker-positive patients.

Clinical trials with three potential claims

Additional restrictions based on the influence condition as well as the interaction condition are required in a more general setting with three potential efficacy claims (broad, restricted and enhanced claims) to prevent illogical conclusions. This setting will be discussed in Case study 3.3.

Beginning with a basic decision rule for formulating efficacy claims based on statistical considerations, the trial's sponsor can consider pursuing the enhanced claim of a beneficial effect in the overall population as well as the selected subpopulation (combination of the broad and restricted claims) if the two null hypotheses of interest (H_0 and H_+) are simultaneously rejected (Outcome C). It is immediately clear that this rule does not account for the influence condition and, as a consequence, may lead to erroneous conclusions discussed above. Another potential problem with this naive rule is that the enhanced claim can be recommended even if the treatment effect is homogeneous across the biomarker-positive and biomarker-negative subsets. This may happen if the biomarker that was believed to have predictive properties turned out to be non-informative.

To address the limitations of the basic decision rule, the *interaction condition* needs to be applied in conjunction with the influence condition as shown in Figure 3.3. This figure defines the recommended set of decision rules for trials with three potential claims. The influence and interaction conditions are applied sequentially. The latter assesses the degree of treatment-by-biomarker interaction or strength of a differential effect in the biomarker-positive and biomarker-negative subgroups. The condition is satisfied if there is a clinically important interaction that supports the conclusion that the treatment provides a substantial additional benefit in patients with a biomarker-positive status compared to patients in the overall population. The interaction condition can be assessed using any treatment-by-biomarker interaction test. For example, it will be shown in Case study 3.3 that this condition can be defined using a simple test based on the ratio of the observed effect sizes in the biomarker-positive and biomarker-negative subgroups (i.e., the interaction condition is satisfied if this ratio is greater than a pre-defined threshold).

Figure 3.3 shows that the enhanced claim can be made only if the interaction condition is satisfied. If no differential effect is observed and thus the interaction condition is not met, the biomarker is not useful in terms of predicting patients who experience enhanced benefit. In this case the best course of action is to focus on treatment effectiveness in the overall population of patients and pursue the broad claim.

As mentioned above, decision rules in multi-population clinical trials based on the influence and interaction conditions will be illustrated in the context of

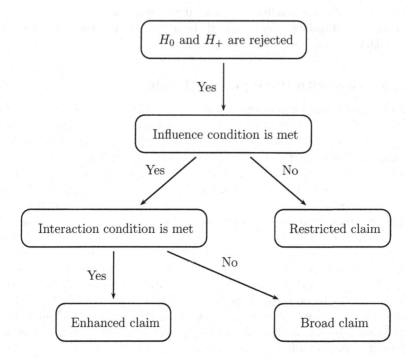

FIGURE 3.3: Recommended decision rules used in a multi-population clinical trial with three potential claims when the treatment effect is significant in the overall population and selected subpopulation.

clinical trial optimization in Case studies 3.2 and 3.3. The specific objectives will include selecting optimal values of the thresholds used in the influence and interaction conditions.

3.3 Case study 3.1: Optimal selection of a multiplicity adjustment

This section discusses optimal selection of multiplicity adjustments and their parameters in a multi-population clinical trial based on an example introduced in Millen, Dmitrienko and Song (2014). Optimization in this context relies on a direct optimization strategy. This case study builds upon the general framework defined in Chapter 1 (see Section 1.4). This framework will be augmented by a thorough review of applicable analysis models (multiplicity adjustments), relevant evaluation criteria and sensitivity assessments.

3.3.1 Clinical trial

A confirmatory Phase III clinical trial in patients with mild or moderate asthma will be used as the main example in this case study. This two-arm trial is aimed at evaluating the efficacy and safety of a single dose of a novel anti-inflammatory therapy compared to placebo. A balanced design with a 1:1 randomization will be considered. A pre-specified biomarker (periostin) will be used in the trial to classify patients into biomarker-positive and biomarker-negative subgroups. This biomarker is believed to be predictive of treatment response and patients with higher biomarker levels (biomarker-positive subgroup) are expected to experience a greater treatment benefit. The complementary subgroup will include biomarker-negative patients. The primary analysis is based on the change from baseline to a 12-week endpoint in the forced expiratory volume in 1 second (FEV1). A larger value of this clinical endpoint indicates a beneficial effect.

Data model

The data model in this case study includes the following components. A balanced design is considered with the total sample size denoted by n. A subset of patients in the overall population, namely, patients with an elevated baseline periostin level, is classified as biomarker-positive. The prevalence of biomarker-positive patients in the general population is denoted by r. The prevalence is expected to be close to $r = 0.4$ but this rate was computed from several heterogeneous historical sources and thus it may be unreliable.

The primary endpoint is normally distributed with the mean μ and standard deviation σ. The available historical data support an assumption of a common standard deviation in the two trial arms and subpopulations of biomarker-negative and biomarker-positive patients. This common standard deviation is given by $\sigma = 0.45$ liters. Since the baseline periostin level is expected to predict treatment response in this clinical trial, the mean value of the primary endpoint is assumed to vary across the trial arms and subpopulations, i.e., across the four samples (independent groups of patients) defined in Section 3.2.1. There is limited information on the prognostic ability of the selected biomarker and, as a result, a common mean is assumed in the biomarker-negative and biomarker-positive subgroups within the placebo arm. In other words, the mean effects are set to the following values:

- Biomarker-negative patients in the placebo arm: Mean effect $\mu_{0-} = 0.12$ liters.

- Biomarker-positive patients in the placebo arm: Mean effect $\mu_{0+} = 0.12$ liters.

Assumptions about the mean values of the primary endpoint in the biomarker-negative and biomarker-positive subgroups within the treatment arm, denoted by μ_{1-} and μ_{1+}, are presented below.

TABLE 3.1: Parameters of the outcome distribution in the four samples in Case study 3.1.

Sample	Trial arm	Subpopulation	Mean	Standard deviation
Sample 1	Placebo	Biomarker-negative	$\mu_{0-} = 0.12$	$\sigma = 0.45$
Sample 2	Placebo	Biomarker-positive	$\mu_{0+} = 0.12$	$\sigma = 0.45$
Sample 3	Treatment	Biomarker-negative	$\mu_{1-} = 0.21$	$\sigma = 0.45$
Sample 4	Treatment	Biomarker-positive	$\mu_{1+} = 0.345$	$\sigma = 0.45$

A differential treatment effect is assumed in the trial in the sense that patients with a negative status are likely to experience standard treatment benefit whereas a much larger treatment difference is anticipated in the target subpopulation of biomarker-positive patents. Let

$$\theta_- = \frac{\mu_{1-} - \mu_{0-}}{\sigma} \text{ and } \theta_+ = \frac{\mu_{1+} - \mu_{0+}}{\sigma}$$

denote the standardized mean treatment differences (effect sizes) in the biomarker-negative and biomarker-positive subpopulations, respectively. The following set of effect sizes will be used in this case study:

- Biomarker-negative subpopulation: $\theta_- = 0.2$.

- Biomarker-positive subpopulation: $\theta_+ = 0.5$.

Note that the assumed effect size in the subset of biomarker-negative patients (θ_-) is viewed as the lowest clinically relevant effect and the treatment difference in the biomarker-positive subgroup represents a very strong beneficial effect.

The resulting set of the outcome distribution parameters, i.e., means and standard deviations, in the four samples is shown in Table 3.1. The associated data model will be referred to as the main data model. This model will be denoted by $D(\theta)$, where $\theta = (\theta_-, \theta_+)$. Two alternative data models will be introduced in Section 3.3.4 as part of qualitative sensitivity assessment.

Analysis model

To define the analysis model, the treatment effect test will be carried out in the overall population and within the selected subpopulation based on the simple two-sample t test. More advanced tests based on analysis of covariance models can be considered to account for important baseline factors, for example, it is recommended that the overall population test should be stratified by the biomarker status. For simplicity, a non-stratified t test will be considered in this case study.

The two primary hypotheses to be tested in the trial are defined as in Section 3.2.1:

- Null hypothesis H_0 of no treatment effect in the overall population.

- Null hypothesis H_+ of no treatment effect in the biomarker-positive subpopulation.

Since there are two opportunities to claim success in this confirmatory Phase III trial, a multiplicity adjustment is required to control the overall Type I error rate at the nominal level of $\alpha = 0.025$ (one-sided). Several candidate multiplicity adjustment methods defined in Section 3.2.2 can be considered in this two-population setting. The most basic and conservative approach to multiplicity adjustment relies on the Bonferroni procedure. The Holm procedure is uniformly more powerful than the Bonferroni and is guaranteed to reject as many or possibly more null hypotheses compared to the Bonferroni. In fact, the Holm procedure was applied in a similar two-population clinical trial in Chapter 1 (see Section 1.4). However, this procedure is inferior in terms of power to the Hochberg procedure. Recall from Section 3.2.2 that the Holm procedure belongs to the class of nonparametric procedures and thus it makes no assumptions about the joint distribution of the test statistics associated with the null hypotheses H_0 and H_+. The Holm is expected to be less powerful than a semiparametric procedure such as the Hochberg procedure that takes advantage of a positive correlation between the hypothesis test statistics. For the reasons presented above, the following two multiple testing procedures will be studied in this case study:

- Bonferroni procedure.

- Hochberg procedure.

The Bonferroni procedure will be used mainly as a reference procedure for assessing the performance of the more powerful Hochberg procedure.

Both multiple testing procedures support an option to assign unequal weights to the null hypotheses H_0 and H_+ to help account for the fact that they are not equally important in this setting. The weights assigned to H_0 and H_+ are defined as follows:

$$w_0 = w, \ w_+ = 1 - w, \ \text{where} \ 0 \leq w \leq 1.$$

The resulting analysis model will be denoted by $A(w)$.

The weight allocation, determined by the w parameter, helps achieve a desirable balance between the two components of the primary analysis in this clinical trial, i.e., between the goals of establishing a significant treatment effect in the overall population and biomarker-positive subset. This parameter will serve as the target parameter in this optimization problem. The testing algorithms used by the weighted Bonferroni and Hochberg procedures are defined in Section 3.2.2. It is important to note that, in the context of the Hochberg procedure, w defines the initial weight assigned to the overall population test. Due to a stepwise testing algorithm used by this procedure, the weight of this test may change depending on the ordering of the test-specific p-values.

Evaluation model

The first step in applying the Clinical Scenario Evaluation framework to this case study involves evaluating the performance of the selected multiplicity adjustment procedures with respect to several sets of statistical assumptions, i.e., several relevant data models. In addition, an optimal analysis model can be identified based on an appropriate success criterion. Optimization will be aimed at selecting the most powerful multiplicity adjustment indexed by the w parameter, i.e., the weight assigned to the overall population test. This parameter will serve as the target parameter in the optimization problem and, once an optimal value of w has been found, an optimal analysis model will be uniquely identified. A direct optimization strategy will be applied to determine optimal values of this parameter, along with optimal intervals, based on a simple grid-search algorithm.

An optimization algorithm can be constructed using the criteria introduced in Section 3.2.1. An evaluation criterion based on disjunctive power can be employed as a good starting point. This criterion function is given by

$$\psi_D(w) = P(\text{Reject } H_0 \text{ or } H_+).$$

Note that this probability is evaluated using the data model $D(\boldsymbol{\theta})$ and analysis model $A(w)$.

As stated in Section 3.2.1, the use of disjunctive power is likely to result in unbalanced conclusions since the relative size of the biomarker-positive subgroup is not accounted for. A utility-based approach based on weighted power provides a viable alternative to disjunctive power. To define a weighted power function (clinical utility function) for this setting, the overall outcome of interest, i.e., establishing a significant treatment effect in either of the two patient populations, is naturally partitioned into two mutually exclusive outcomes that correspond to the following claims:

- Broad claim of treatment effectiveness in the overall population (reject H_0).

- Restricted claim of treatment effectiveness in the biomarker-positive subpopulation only (reject H_+ after failing to reject H_0).

The marginal probabilities of the two claims as a function of the target parameter w are denoted by $\psi_1(w)$ and $\psi_2(w)$, i.e.,

$$\begin{aligned}
\psi_1(w) &= P(\text{Reject } H_0), \\
\psi_2(w) &= P(\text{Fail to reject } H_0 \text{ and Reject } H_+).
\end{aligned}$$

The partition-based weighted power function is defined as a weighted sum of the two marginal power functions:

$$\psi_{PW}(w) = v_1\psi_1(w) + v_2\psi_2(w),$$

where v_1 and v_2 are positive values that define the importance of each outcome or, in other words, the "gain" or market value associated with the broad and restricted claims. The optimization criterion based on this weighted power criterion is more relevant compared to the disjunctive power criterion in this case study since it is generally more desirable to establish a therapeutic benefit in a larger population of patients. As a result, the gain due to a significant effect in the overall population is greater than the gain in the subpopulation and the outcomes associated with the two claims are no longer interchangeable as assumed in the disjunctive power criterion.

It needs to be clarified that the decision rules used in formulating the broad and restricted claims presented above rely solely on statistical considerations and, as explained in Section 3.2.3, additional important considerations need to be taken into account in multi-population clinical trials. These considerations are related to evaluating the influence of a subgroup on the overall population and, in other settings, assessing the interaction effect between a subgroup of interest and its complement. More complex decision rules that incorporate the influence and interaction conditions introduced in Section 3.2.3 will be discussed in Case studies 3.2 and 3.3.

A straightforward approach to quantifying the gains associated with the two claims is to choose the importance parameters that are proportional to the sizes of the two patient populations. If r is the true prevalence of biomarker-positive patients in the asthma clinical trial, the parameters can be found from

$$\frac{v_1}{v_2} = \frac{1}{r}.$$

Since v_1 and v_2 are typically normalized by imposing the restriction that they must add up to 1, the resulting values of the importance parameters are given by

$$v_1 = \frac{1}{1+r}, \quad v_2 = \frac{r}{1+r}.$$

For example, with $r = 0.4$, $v_1 = 0.71$ and $v_2 = 0.29$, which means that establishing a treatment benefit in the overall population is viewed to be 2.5 times more important than demonstrating a significant effect in the subpopulation (this quantity is equal to $1/r$).

To help compare the optimization criteria based on disjunctive and weighted power, it is easy to verify that disjunctive power is simply equal to the sum of the probabilities of broad and restricted claims, i.e.,

$$
\begin{aligned}
\psi_D(w) &= P(\text{Reject } H_0) + P(\text{Fail to reject } H_0 \text{ and Reject } H_+) \\
&= v_1 \psi_1(w) + v_2 \psi_2(w),
\end{aligned}
$$

where $v_1 = v_2 = 1$. It immediately follows from this formula that disjunctive power treats the events associated with the two claims as equally weighted even though the first one (broad claim) is generally more important to the trial's sponsor. A utility-based approach that relies on weighted power provides the means for accounting for unequal expected "gains" associated with the broad and restricted claims. Optimization algorithms based on disjunctive and weighted power will be compared in Sections 3.3.2 and 3.3.3.

3.3.2   Direct optimization based on disjunctive power

To facilitate the comparison between the two evaluation criteria defined above, an optimization algorithm aimed at determining optimal values of the target parameter w (initial weight of the overall population test in the Bonferroni and Hochberg procedures) was first applied using disjunctive power. The target parameter was assumed to range between 0 and 1. As a starting value, the sample size was chosen to guarantee sufficiently high power of the overall population test before a multiplicity adjustment. With the total sample size of 310 patients, the probability of demonstrating a significant treatment effect in the overall population was 80.2% and the probability of a significant effect in the subpopulation was 78.9%. It would have been more natural to perform a sample size calculation in this trial based on an appropriate multiplicity adjustment. However, since the weighting scheme in the Bonferroni or Hochberg procedures was undefined, an unadjusted analysis was utilized as a reasonable proxy. The sample size calculation will be re-run later in this section based on an optimal value of the w parameter.

Multiplicity adjustments based the Bonferroni and Hochberg procedures were applied to control the overall Type I error rate at a one-sided $\alpha = 0.025$. Figure 3.4 displays disjunctive power for the two procedures as a function of the target parameter w. The figure identifies the optimal value of w (denoted by w^*) that results in maximum disjunctive power as well as the 99% optimal interval for each multiple testing procedure. A 99% optimal interval defines a range of nearly optimal values of the target parameter (it includes all values of w for which the criterion function is no more than 1% lower than its maximum value).

It is easy to see from Figure 3.4 that the optimal value of the target parameter w was virtually the same for the two procedures. Table 3.2 provides a summary of the optimal values of w and 99% optimal intervals based on the Bonferroni and Hochberg procedures. It follows from this table that the overall population and biomarker-positive subpopulation should be approximately equally weighted to maximize the probability of success based on disjunctive power. The only tangible difference between the two multiplicity adjustments is that the 99% optimal interval for w computed from the Hochberg procedure was slightly tighter compared to the Bonferroni.

When comparing the performance of the two multiple testing procedures in this case study, it is important to remember that the Hochberg procedure is uniformly more powerful than the Bonferroni procedure (see Section 3.2.2). For this reason, the Hochberg procedure should be preferred to the Bonferroni procedure. However, the burden of multiplicity is rather insignificant in this

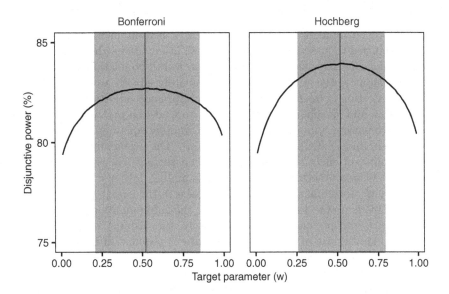

FIGURE 3.4: Disjunctive power for the Bonferroni and Hochberg procedures as a function of the target parameter in Case study 3.1. The vertical lines represent the optimal values of the target parameter and the gray rectangles show the 99% optimal intervals.

TABLE 3.2: Optimal values of the target parameter (w) and optimal intervals based on disjunctive power in Case study 3.1.

Procedure	Optimal value	99% optimal interval
Bonferroni	0.52	$(0.21, 0.85)$
Hochberg	0.52	$(0.26, 0.79)$

simple setting with two null hypotheses and even a basic multiplicity adjustment such as the Bonferroni procedure does a reasonably good job in this case study. For example, it follows from Figure 3.4 that the Hochberg procedure with an optimal value of w provided only one percentage point gain in disjunctive power over the optimal Bonferroni procedure (82.7% versus 84.0%). It is also helpful to examine the marginal power functions for the two population tests after the Bonferroni and Hochberg adjustments. Based on the optimal value of w, the probability of establishing a significant effect in the overall population (i.e., the probability of rejecting H_0) under the Hochberg adjustment was 77.3%, which was substantially higher than the probability of rejecting H_0 under the Bonferroni adjustment (71.6%).

3.3.3   Direct optimization based on weighted power

The optimization algorithm presented above relied on disjunctive power and, as a result, led to a skewed conclusion. Recall that, under the optimal weighting scheme, the treatment effect tests in the overall population and biomarker-positive subpopulation should be approximately equally weighted. This is a simple reflection of the fact that, before a multiplicity adjustment based on the Bonferroni and Hochberg procedures was applied, the probabilities of success in the two patient populations were approximately equal (80.2% in the overall population and 78.9% in the subpopulation). The probability of demonstrating a significant effect in the subset of biomarker-positive patients was indeed high but, from a practical perspective, this finding does not look as attractive as a numerically similar probability of success in the overall population of patients. This is due to the simple fact that the subpopulation is much smaller than the overall population. Unfortunately, the disjunctive power criterion cannot take the size of the underlying patient population into account and, as a consequence, optimization criteria based on disjunctive power often lead to "lopsided" results similar to the one discussed above.

Weighted power represents a meaningful alternative to disjunctive power in this setting since it explicitly accounts for the importance of the two outcomes associated with the broad and restricted claims. The importance parameters used in the definition of partition-based weighted power, i.e., v_1 and v_2, can reflect the relative sizes of the two populations. As shown in Section 3.3.1, if the prevalence of patients with a biomarker-positive status in the general population is assumed to be $r = 0.4$, it is natural to define the weighted power criterion as follows

$$\psi_W(w) = 0.71\psi_1(w) + 0.29\psi_2(w).$$

Using the total sample size of 310 patients, Figure 3.5 displays the selected weighted power function for the Bonferroni- and Hochberg-based multiplicity adjustments as a function of the target parameter w. As in Figure 3.4, the vertical line in this figure identifies the optimal value of w and the 99% optimal interval is represented by the gray rectangle.

Figure 3.5 reveals that the weighted criterion was maximized at a much higher value of the target parameter w compared to the criterion based on disjunctive power. Table 3.3 shows that, after the relative size of the subpopulation was incorporated into the criterion, the optimal weight of the overall population test was shifted toward 1 for both multiplicity adjustments. This clearly indicates that the overall population test plays a key role in maximizing the probability of success based on the weighted power approach.

It is interesting to compare the 99% optimal intervals shown in Table 3.3 and the optimal value of w based on disjunctive power displayed in Table 3.2. Considering the Hochberg procedure, note that, with the disjunctive power criterion, the optimal values of w was quite low, namely, w^* was equal to 0.52. By contrast, the optimal interval based on weighted power was $[0.51, 1]$.

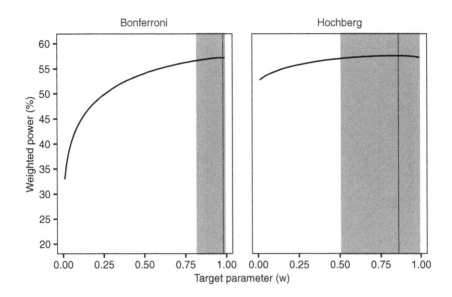

FIGURE 3.5: Weighted power for the Bonferroni and Hochberg procedures as a function of the target parameter in Case study 3.1. The vertical line represents the optimal value of the target parameter and the gray rectangles define the 99% optimal intervals.

TABLE 3.3: Optimal values of the target parameter (w) and optimal intervals based on weighted power in Case study 3.1.

Procedure	Optimal value	99% optimal interval
Bonferroni	0.98	$(0.82, 0.99)$
Hochberg	0.86	$(0.51, 0.99)$

The two criteria used in this case study approached the problem of optimal selection of w from two different perspectives and, as a result, the optimal interval computed from one criterion barely overlapped with the optimal value of the target parameter derived from the other criterion.

Figure 3.5 also illustrates an important property of the Hochberg procedure. It can be seen that the weighted criterion based on this multiplicity adjustment was quite flat over the target parameter's range compared to that of the Bonferroni procedure. The maximum value of weighted power based on the Hochberg procedure was 57.6% and the lowest value achieved at $w = 0$ was 52.3%. To understand why the weighted power function was virtually independent of the target parameter when the Hochberg procedure was considered, it is helpful to examine the marginal probabilities of broad and re-

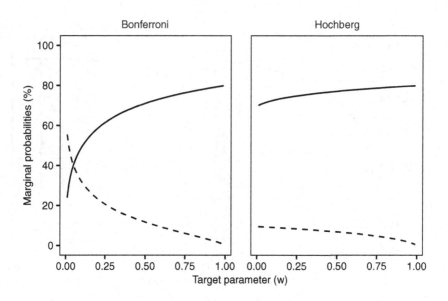

FIGURE 3.6: Marginal probabilities of the broad claim (solid curve) and restricted claim (dashed curve) for the Bonferroni and Hochberg procedures as a function of the target parameter in Case study 3.1.

stricted claims. The marginal power functions for the Hochberg procedure as well as the Bonferroni procedure are displayed in Figure 3.6.

It follows from the left-hand panel of Figure 3.6 that the marginal probabilities of the two claims after the Bonferroni-based multiplicity adjustment are directly driven by the selected value of the w parameter. The right-hand panel of Figure 3.6 displays the marginal probabilities of the two claims of interest for the Hochberg procedure and reveals a completely different pattern. The probability of establishing a significant overall effect was quite high over the entire range of w values. The lowest value of this probability achieved at $w = 0$ was 69.4%. The probability of demonstrating a significant effect in the biomarker-positive subpopulation if no treatment benefit is detected in the overall population was also generally flat as a function of the target parameter. This probability ranged between 0% and 9.4%.

It was pointed out in Section 3.3.1 that, when efficient stepwise procedures are applied, including the Hochberg, the initial hypothesis weights are modified after each rejection. As a result, the marginal power functions of efficient multiple testing procedures are much less sensitive to the initial weights. The initial hypothesis weights are preserved only when a basic procedure such as the Bonferroni is applied.

3.3.4 Qualitative sensitivity assessment

This section and the next section discuss an important component of any clinical trial optimization exercise, namely, sensitivity assessments aimed at "stress-testing" an optimal analysis model based on the optimal multiplicity adjustment. Sensitivity assessments facilitate the process of building robust analysis models that can help mitigate risks in settings with a substantial uncertainty about the true effects of experimental treatments. In this particular setting, sensitivity analysis techniques will be employed to assess the sensitivity of the optimal target parameter with respect to deviations from the main data model assumed in Section 3.3.1. A simple qualitative approach to performing sensitivity analyses in a trial with two pre-defined patient populations is presented in this section. A quantitative approach to sensitivity assessments that relies on a bootstrap algorithm is introduced in Section 3.3.5.

For the sake of simplicity, the discussion of optimal selection of the target parameter focused up to this point on a single data model. Specifically, the optimization algorithms were applied in Sections 3.3.2 and 3.3.3 based on only one set of effect sizes in the biomarker-negative and biomarker-positive subgroups denoted by θ_- and θ_+, i.e.,

$$\theta_- = 0.2, \ \theta_+ = 0.5.$$

When applying clinical trial optimization approaches to multi-population settings, it is important to remember that assumptions around the true treatment differences in the biomarker-positive subset and its complement are typically derived from fairly small data sets collected at early stages of the development program. These assumptions may turn out to be overly optimistic or, on the other hand, the selected treatment difference may underestimate the true magnitude of the beneficial effect. It is recommended to consider a sensitivity assessment to gauge the impact of the hypothesized effect sizes on the conclusions such as the choice of an optimal analysis model. Sensitivity assessments of this kind often focus on the assumed value for θ_+ since this parameter plays a more important role in planning multi-population trials compared to the effect size in the biomarker-negative subpopulation. The effect size in the biomarker-negative subgroup (θ_-) is typically fixed at the assumed value, i.e., $\theta_- = 0.2$ in this example.

Given the uncertainty around the assumed effect size in the biomarker-positive subpopulation, it is natural to consider a range of data models, e.g.,

- Scenario 1 (main data model): $\theta_- = 0.2$ and $\theta_+ = 0.5$.

- Scenario 2 (pessimistic data model): $\theta_- = 0.2$ and $\theta_+ = 0.45$.

- Scenario 3 (optimistic data model): $\theta_- = 0.2$ and $\theta_+ = 0.55$.

Scenario 1 represents the main data model in this case study while Scenarios 2 and 3 introduce some variability in the value of θ_+ to support a qualitative or

TABLE 3.4: Parameters of the outcome distribution in the four samples under the main, pessimistic and optimistic data models in Case study 3.1.

Sample	Trial arm	Subpopulation	Mean	Standard deviation
		Scenario 1 (main)		
Sample 1	Placebo	Biomarker-negative	$\mu_{0-} = 0.12$	$\sigma = 0.45$
Sample 2	Placebo	Biomarker-positive	$\mu_{0+} = 0.12$	$\sigma = 0.45$
Sample 3	Treatment	Biomarker-negative	$\mu_{1-} = 0.21$	$\sigma = 0.45$
Sample 4	Treatment	Biomarker-positive	$\mu_{1+} = 0.345$	$\sigma = 0.45$
		Scenario 2 (pessimistic)		
Sample 1	Placebo	Biomarker-negative	$\mu_{0-} = 0.12$	$\sigma = 0.45$
Sample 2	Placebo	Biomarker-positive	$\mu_{0+} = 0.12$	$\sigma = 0.45$
Sample 3	Treatment	Biomarker-negative	$\mu_{1-} = 0.21$	$\sigma = 0.45$
Sample 4	Treatment	Biomarker-positive	$\mu_{1+} = 0.3225$	$\sigma = 0.45$
		Scenario 3 (optimistic)		
Sample 1	Placebo	Biomarker-negative	$\mu_{0-} = 0.12$	$\sigma = 0.45$
Sample 2	Placebo	Biomarker-positive	$\mu_{0+} = 0.12$	$\sigma = 0.45$
Sample 3	Treatment	Biomarker-negative	$\mu_{1-} = 0.21$	$\sigma = 0.45$
Sample 4	Treatment	Biomarker-positive	$\mu_{1+} = 0.3675$	$\sigma = 0.45$

pivoting-based sensitivity assessment. The outcome distribution parameters corresponding to the three data models are listed in Table 3.4.

The trial's sponsor can conduct a qualitative sensitivity assessment by applying the optimization algorithm to the corresponding data models to compute optimal values of the target parameter for each alternative model. This approach was applied to Scenarios 2 and 3 using the partition-based weighted criterion defined earlier in this section with $n = 310$ patients. Table 3.5 lists the optimal values of w and associated 99% optimal intervals for all three scenarios. The overall conclusions regarding the set of optimal weights were quite consistent across the three data models. Since the true value of θ_+ is unknown, it is reasonable to consider a joint optimal interval for the optimal target parameter which is defined as the intersection of the scenario-specific optimal intervals. It follows from Table 3.5 that the joint 99% optimal interval is given by $[0.64, 0.99]$. The midpoint of this interval could be used as the optimal value of the target parameter, i.e., w can be set to 0.8. The analysis model with the Hochberg procedure based on the corresponding weighting scheme, i.e., $w_0 = w = 0.8$ and $w_+ = 1 - w = 0.2$, is expected to exhibit optimal performance under any of the three data models.

Now that an optimal analysis model has been built, the preliminary sample size calculations need to be re-visited. Recall that the trial's sample size of 310 patients was selected as an initial value that would be used to help ascertain an optimal weight allocation scheme in the multiplicity adjustment procedure. Since the initial weight of the overall population test in this scheme is now set to an optimal value ($w = 0.8$), the optimal analysis model based on the

TABLE 3.5: Optimal values of the target parameter and optimal intervals based on weighted power under the plausible, pessimistic and optimistic data models in Case study 3.1.

Scenario	Optimal value	99% optimal interval
Scenario 1 (main)	0.86	$(0.51, 1.00)$
Scenario 2 (pessimistic)	0.87	$(0.64, 1.00)$
Scenario 3 (optimistic)	0.70	$(0.36, 0.99)$

corresponding Hochberg procedure can be utilized to run the final sample size calculation in the asthma clinical trial.

In general, sample size calculations are performed to achieve a desirable level of the chosen evaluation criterion. The main challenge of using criteria based on clinical utility functions or weighted power is that the associated criteria may not have a straightforward probabilistic interpretation. To illustrate this point, the highest value of the weighted power function for the Hochberg procedure under the main data model (Scenario 1) was 57.7% (see Figure 3.5). Due to lack of probabilistic interpretation, it is not immediately clear if this level is sufficiently high.

To overcome this problem, the following rule of thumb can be applied to run a sample size calculation based on weighted power. Let $\psi_1(n)$ and $\psi_2(n)$ denote the marginal probabilities of broad and restricted claims as a function of the total number of patients in the trial (n) and let $\psi_{PW}(n|v_1, v_2)$ denote the partition-based weighted power function, i.e.,

$$\psi_{PW}(n|v_1, v_2) = v_1\psi_1(n) + v_2\psi_2(n),$$

where the importance parameters v_1 and v_2 are non-negative and add up to 1. Finally, let β denote the pre-defined Type II error rate, e.g., $\beta = 0.2$ corresponds to 80% power.

Consider first an extreme case corresponding to sample size calculations based on the overall population test. If the primary analysis in the asthma clinical trial was formulated in terms of the overall population test and the treatment effect test in the subpopulation of biomarker-positive patients was considered a secondary test, the total number of patients would be computed from

$$\psi_1(n) = 1 - \beta,$$

where $1 - \beta$ defines the target level for this power function. This equation can be re-written in terms of weighted power:

$$\psi_{PW}(n|1, 0) = 1 - \beta$$

since the weighted power function with $v_1 = 1$ and $v_2 = 0$ is equal to $\psi_1(n)$.

Further, as explained at the end of Section 3.3.1, the disjunctive power function, denoted by $\psi_D(n)$, is a special case of the weighed power function with the weights set to $v_1 = 0.5$ and $v_2 = 0.5$, i.e.,

$$\frac{\psi_D(n)}{2} = \frac{\psi_1(n)}{2} + \frac{\psi_2(n)}{2} = \psi_{PW}(n|0.5, 0.5).$$

Therefore, if a sample size calculation was based on disjunctive power, the number of patients in the trial would be found from $\psi_D(n) = 1 - \beta$ or, equivalently, from

$$\psi_{PW}(n|0.5, 0.5) = \frac{1 - \beta}{2}.$$

This means that, in this case, the desirable level of weighted power is $(1 - \beta)/2$. Using a linear interpolation, it is natural to set the desirable level for $\psi_{PW}(n|v_1, v_2)$ to $v_1(1 - \beta)$, where $0.5 \le v_1 \le 1$. Recall from Section 3.2.1 that the broad claim is always as important or more important than the restricted claim and thus $v_1 \ge 0.5$.

Returning to the weighted power function considered in this case study with $r = 0.4$, i.e.,

$$\psi_{PW}(n) = \frac{1}{1+r}\psi_1(n) + \frac{r}{1+r}\psi_2(n),$$

the desirable level for weighted power is

$$\frac{1 - \beta}{1 + r}$$

and thus the total number of patients in the trial should be computed from

$$\psi_{PW}(n) = \frac{1 - \beta}{1 + r} = 0.571.$$

Using a simulation-based approach, the weighted power function was evaluated based on the optimal Hochberg procedure with the target parameter $w = 0.8$ for a range of sample sizes. The calculations were performed under the main data model (Scenario 1) with $\theta_- = 0.2$ and $\theta_+ = 0.5$. The results are presented in Figure 3.7. The figure shows that the weighted power function was equal to the desirable value of 57.1% with $n = 304$. This implies that, with the optimal analysis model, the total sample size in the asthma clinical trial can be set to 304 patients, which provides a small improvement compared to the original sample size of 310 patients.

It is also helpful to compute the marginal probabilities of the broad and restricted claims over the selected range of sample sizes. The two marginal power functions are plotted in Figure 3.8. This figure demonstrates that, with 304 patients, the marginal probability of the broad claim in the overall population was close to 80% (it was equal to 78.3%) whereas the probability of making an effectiveness claim in the subpopulation was very low.

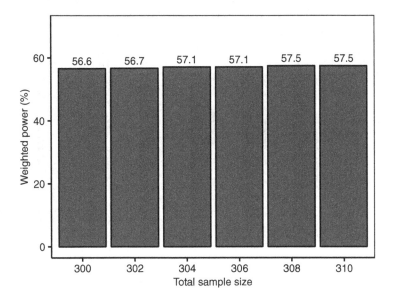

FIGURE 3.7: Weighted power of the optimal Hochberg procedure as a function of the sample size in Case study 3.1.

3.3.5 Quantitative sensitivity assessment

The qualitative sensitivity analyses presented in Section 3.3.4 focused on a single data model parameter, i.e., the effect size in the biomarker-positive subpopulation (θ_+). Another parameter that needs to be included in the sensitivity assessment is the prevalence of biomarker-positive patients in the general population (r). It is often challenging to obtain an accurate estimate of this prevalence rate and it is important to quantify the influence of the hypothesized value of r on power calculations performed in this trial. A quantitative approach to sensitivity assessment in this optimization problem is presented in this section. This approach is aimed at a simultaneous evaluation of the impact of the two key data model parameters, i.e., the treatment effect in the biomarker-positive subpopulation and prevalence of biomarker-positive patients, on the performance of the optimal analysis model in the asthma clinical trial using bootstrap-based perturbations (see Chapter 1 for more information about perturbation-based sensitivity assessments).

As before, the prevalence of biomarker-positive patients in the asthma clinical trial was assumed to be $r = 0.4$. Further, when dealing with the treatment effect, it is convenient to switch from the effect size scale to the mean treatment difference scale and work with the mean parameters, i.e.,

$$\mu_{0-}, \ \mu_{0+}, \ \mu_{1-} \ \text{and} \ \mu_{1+}.$$

Using the main data model based on Scenario 1 defined in Section 3.3.4, the

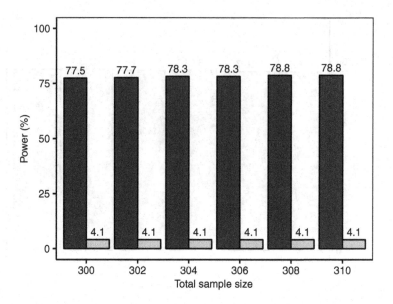

FIGURE 3.8: Marginal probabilities of the broad claim (black bars) and restricted claim (gray bars) for the optimal Hochberg procedure as a function of the sample size in Case study 3.1.

mean effects in the biomarker-positive subgroup and its complement within the placebo arm were fixed at $\mu_{0-} = \mu_{0+} = 0.12$. The mean value of the primary endpoint in the biomarker-negative subgroup within the treatment arm was set to

$$\mu_{1-} = \mu_{0-} + \theta_{-}\sigma = 0.21,$$

where the effect size θ_{-} was equal to 0.2 and the standard deviation of the primary endpoint was $\sigma = 0.45$. To simplify notation, the mean effect in the biomarker-positive subgroup within the treatment arm was denoted by μ and was set to the value consistent with Scenario 1, i.e.,

$$\mu = \mu_{0+} + \theta_{+}\sigma = 0.345$$

since the effect size θ_{+} was equal to 0.5.

Perturbation-based sensitivity assessments for the selected parameters (μ and r) were performed using the parametric bootstrap algorithm defined in Chapter 1 (see Section 1.3.3). Based on this algorithm, multiple *bootstrap data models* were generated using pre-specified distributions for the two parameters of interest. This algorithm included the following two components:

- Beginning with the mean effect in the biomarker-positive subgroup within the treatment arm, create a set of "true" mean values for each bootstrap data model by sampling from the normal distribution centered at μ:

$$\mu_i' \sim N(\mu, \tau^2), \ i = 1, \ldots, k,$$

where τ is the standard deviation of the bootstrap distribution and k is a pre-specified number of bootstrap data models.

- Considering the prevalence rate of biomarker-positive patients, generate a sample of "true" rates for each bootstrap data model from the beta distribution centered at r:

$$r_i' \sim \mathrm{Beta}(\alpha, \beta), \ i = 1, \dots, k,$$

where the parameters of the beta distribution are selected to ensure that the mean is equal to r, i.e., $\alpha/(\alpha + \beta) = r$.

When performing sensitivity assessments for multiple parameters, it is convenient to consider a common uncertainty parameter, denoted by c, that controls the amount of variability around the hypothesized values of μ and r in the bootstrap data models. This parameter can be defined in terms of the common coefficient of variation. In this case, the standard deviation of the bootstrap distribution for the mean effect in the biomarker-positive subgroup within the treatment arm will be given by $\tau = c\mu$ and the parameters of the beta distribution for the prevalence of biomarker-positive patients will be given by

$$\alpha = \frac{1 - r}{c^2} - r, \ \beta = \frac{\alpha(1 - r)}{r}.$$

The assumption of a common coefficient of variation simplifies the presentation of the results; however, alternative approaches may need to be investigated. For example, since $\tau = c\mu$, a larger value of the mean effect implies higher variability and thus a larger standard deviation will be expected in the biomarker-positive subgroup compared to the biomarker-negative subgroup. If this is not a realistic assumption, an alternative approach with a constant standard deviation across the two subgroups needs to be considered. The alternative approach was explored in Chapter 2 (see Case study 2.2).

The marginal probabilities of broad and restricted claims after the Hochberg-based multiplicity adjustment, i.e., $\psi_1(w)$ and $\psi_2(w)$, were computed for each bootstrap data model based on μ_i' and r_i', $i = 1, \dots, k$. It is generally sufficient to generate a relatively small number of bootstrap data models and k was set to 1,000 in this example. The target parameter w was set to 0.8 and the common uncertainty parameter c ranged between 0.1 and 0.4. Simulations were performed using the total sample size of 304 patients to compute the weighted criterion from each bootstrap data model. The criterion used in this quantitative sensitivity assessment was defined earlier in this section, i.e.,

$$\psi_{PW}(w) = 0.71\psi_1(w) + 0.29\psi_2(w).$$

The distribution of weighted power for the selected uncertainty parameters are displayed in Figure 3.9. This figure is similar to Figure 2.7 in Chapter 2 in that it also uses violin plots to display the empirical probability density functions of the weighted criterion computed from the bootstrap data models.

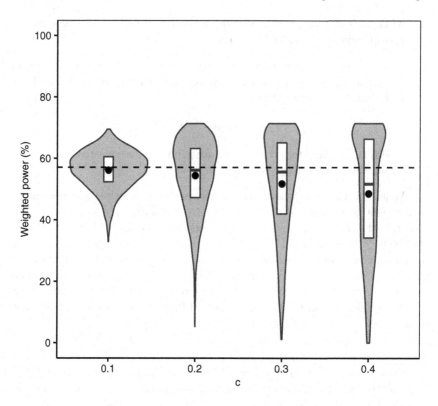

FIGURE 3.9: Distribution of weighted power for several values of the uncertainty parameter (c) in Case study 3.1. The horizontal dashed line identifies weighted power under the original data model (57.1%). The dot indicates the mean and the boxplot identifies the lower and upper quartiles as well as the median.

The figure includes standard box plots to show the lower quartile, median and upper quartile of each distribution for selected values of the uncertainty parameter c. It follows from Figure 3.9 that, with an increasing amount of variability around the assumed values of μ and r, the spread of bootstrap-based weighted power increased as well. The weighted power under the original assumptions, which corresponds to the case where the uncertainty parameter c is set to 0, is represented by a horizontal line. With $c = 0.1$, the weighted power values computed from the bootstrap data models were fairly consistent and clustered around the horizontal line. However, with a larger amount of uncertainty, the distribution became increasingly more skewed with a longer left tail. The largest selected value of the uncertainty parameter ($c = 0.4$) resulted in a heavy-tailed distribution with a high fraction of bootstrap data models where weighted power was quite low.

TABLE 3.6: Descriptive statistics of weighted power as a function of the uncertainty parameter (c) in the quantitative sensitivity assessment performed in Case study 3.1.

Uncertainty parameter	Lower quartile (%)	Median (%)	Mean (%)	Upper quartile (%)
$c = 0.1$	52.4	56.7	56.2	60.5
$c = 0.2$	47.3	56.2	54.4	63.3
$c = 0.3$	42.1	55.7	51.8	65.2
$c = 0.4$	34.2	51.7	48.6	66.4

Despite the obvious changes in the shape of the distributions displayed in Figure 3.9, a visual inspection reveals an important fact that the fraction of bootstrap data models where the weighted power was reduced was roughly equal to the fraction of samples where the probability was improved. To provide a more quantitative assessment of the effect of increasing uncertainty around the hypothesized effect sizes on the expected weighted power, Table 3.6 displays standard descriptive statistics for this quantity estimated from the bootstrap data models.

It can be seen from the table that, due to a longer and heavier tail, the first quartile and mean were shifted towards 0 as the uncertainty parameter increased. The median weighted power was virtually unaffected by changes in the uncertainty parameter and was, in fact, generally close to weighted power evaluated under the original assumptions (i.e., 57.1%). This shows that, despite increasing variability in the underlying parameters, the distribution of bootstrap-based weighted power was not shifted towards lower levels. To be on a safe side, the trial's sponsor may consider increasing the sample size to ensure that the median weighted power is brought back to the desirable level of 57.1% when there is much uncertainty about the assumed values of the μ and r parameters, i.e., if $c = 0.3$ or $c = 0.4$.

To summarize, the results of the quantitative sensitivity assessment demonstrate that an increasing amount of uncertainty around the two key parameters in the main data model (effect size in the biomarker-positive subpopulation and prevalence of biomarker-positive patients) clearly affected the expected range of the selected performance measure (partition-based weighted power) in this clinical trial example. However, the empirical distribution of weighted power computed from a large number of bootstrap data models was centered around a value that was close to the original level of weighted power. This provides an additional level of confidence in the power calculation based on the original data model and implies that, when the two parameters are misspecified, a lower level of weighted power is as likely as a higher level.

3.3.6 Software implementation

Key elements of the simulation-based optimization algorithm presented in this case study can be easily implemented using the **Mediana** package. As explained in Chapter 1, this package was designed to support the general Clinical Scenario Evaluation principles and enables the user to directly define data, analysis and evaluation models for a very broad class of trial settings. The data, analysis and evaluation models for this particular clinical trial example will be specified below.

Data model

A data model specifies a scheme for generating individual patients' data in the set of pre-defined samples, i.e., non-overlapping homogeneous groups of patients, in a clinical trial. In this case study, the overall population of patients is naturally split into four samples that are defined as follows:

- Sample 1 (`Placebo Bio-Neg`) includes biomarker-negative patients in the placebo arm.

- Sample 2 (`Placebo Bio-Pos`) includes biomarker-positive patients in the placebo arm.

- Sample 3 (`Treatment Bio-Neg`) includes biomarker-negative patients in the treatment arm.

- Sample 4 (`Treatment Bio-Pos`) includes biomarker-positive patients in the treatment arm.

Using this definition of samples, the trial's sponsor can model the fact that the treatment's effect is most pronounced in patients with a biomarker-positive status.

For each sample in the data model, the parameters of the outcome distribution (i.e., mean and common standard deviation) defined in Table 3.1 are listed in a single set of outcome parameters.

LISTING 3.1: Outcome parameter specifications in the data model used in Case study 3.1

```
# Outcome parameters
outcome.placebo.neg = parameters(mean = 0.12, sd = 0.45)
outcome.placebo.pos = parameters(mean = 0.12, sd = 0.45)
outcome.treatment.neg = parameters(mean = 0.21, sd = 0.45)
outcome.treatment.pos = parameters(mean = 0.345, sd = 0.45)
```

Consider, for the sake of illustration, a data model with a single set of sample-specific patient counts that corresponds to the total sample size of 310 patients. The number of patients in each individual sample is computed based on the expected prevalence of biomarker-positive patients (40% of patients in the population of interest are expected to have a biomarker-positive status).

LISTING 3.2: Sample size specifications in the data model used in Case study 3.1

```
# Sample size parameters
prevalence.pos = 0.4
sample.size.total = 310

sample.size.placebo.neg = (1-prevalence.pos) / 2 * sample.
    size.total
sample.size.placebo.pos = prevalence.pos / 2 * sample.size.
    total
sample.size.treatment.neg = (1-prevalence.pos) / 2 * sample
    .size.total
sample.size.treatment.pos = prevalence.pos / 2 * sample.
    size.total
```

Finally, the data model can be set up by initializing the `DataModel` object and adding each component to it. The outcome distribution is defined using the `OutcomeDist` object with the `NormalDist` distribution. The data model is shown in Listing 3.3.

LISTING 3.3: Data model in Case study 3.1

```
# Data model
subgroup.cs1.data.model =
  DataModel() +
  OutcomeDist(outcome.dist = "NormalDist") +
  Sample(id = "Placebo Bio-Neg",
         sample.size = sample.size.placebo.neg,
         outcome.par = parameters(outcome.placebo.neg)) +
  Sample(id = "Placebo Bio-Pos",
         sample.size = sample.size.placebo.pos,
         outcome.par = parameters(outcome.placebo.pos)) +
  Sample(id = "Treatment Bio-Neg",
         sample.size = sample.size.treatment.neg,
         outcome.par = parameters(outcome.treatment.neg)) +
  Sample(id = "Treatment Bio-Pos",
         sample.size = sample.size.treatment.pos,
         outcome.par = parameters(outcome.treatment.pos))
```

Analysis model

The analysis model, shown below in Listing 3.4, defines the two individual tests that will be carried out to compare the treatment to placebo in the overall population (OP test) and in the subset of biomarker-positive patients (Bio-Pos test). Each comparison will be carried out based on a one-sided two-sample t-test (TTest method defined in each Test object). A key feature of the analysis strategy in this case study is that the samples defined in the data model are different from the samples used in the analysis of the primary endpoint. As shown in Listing 3.1, four samples were included in the data model. However, from the analysis perspective, the sponsor is interested in examining the treatment effect within two samples, namely, the placebo and treatment samples within the overall population and within the biomarker-positive subpopulation. As shown below, to perform a comparison in the overall population (OP test), the t-test needs to be applied to the following analysis samples:

- Placebo arm is defined by merging the samples Placebo Bio-Neg and Placebo Bio-Pos.

- Treatment arm is defined by merging the samples Treatment Bio-Neg and Treatment Bio-Pos.

Further, the treatment effect test in the subpopulation of biomarker-positive patients (Bio-Pos test) is carried out based on these analysis samples:

- Placebo arm is defined directly based on the sample Placebo Bio-Pos.

- Treatment arm is defined directly based on the sample Treatment Bio-Pos.

In addition, the weighted Bonferroni and Hochberg procedures are requested using the MultAdjProc objects. For the purpose of illustration, the initial weight of the overall population test has been set to 0.8 and thus the weight of the subpopulation test equals 0.2.

LISTING 3.4: Analysis model in Case study 3.1

```
# Analysis model
subgroup.cs1.analysis.model =
  AnalysisModel() +
  Test(id = "OP test",
       samples = samples(c("Placebo Bio-Neg",
                           "Placebo Bio-Pos"),
                         c("Treatment Bio-Neg",
                           "Treatment Bio-Pos")),
       method = "TTest") +
  Test(id = "Bio-Pos test",
       samples = samples("Placebo Bio-Pos",
                         "Treatment Bio-Pos"),
```

```
       method = "TTest") +
 MultAdjProc(proc = "BonferroniAdj",
             par = parameters(weight = c(0.8, 0.2))) +
 MultAdjProc(proc = "HochbergAdj",
             par = parameters(weight = c(0.8, 0.2)))
```

Evaluation model

The evaluation model specifies clinically relevant criteria for assessing the performance of the selected test and multiplicity adjustment defined in the analysis model. As a starting point, it is of interest to compute the probability of achieving a significant outcome in each individual test, e.g., the probability of a significant difference between the treatment and placebo in the overall population and subpopulation of biomarker-positive patents. This is accomplished by requesting a `Criterion` object with the `MarginalPower` method. The method is applied to the two tests defined in the analysis model, i.e., to OP test and Bio-Pos test.

Further, considering more advanced evaluation criteria presented in Section 3.2.1, the first criterion is based on disjunctive power which corresponds to the probability of demonstrating a statistically significant treatment effect in at least one population. This criterion is defined using the `DisjunctivePower` method.

The second evaluation criterion corresponds to weighted power based on combining the probabilities of broad and restricted claims. This criterion is not included in the **Mediana** package but can be implemented as a custom criterion. The user can define this criterion by creating a custom function as described below. The function's first argument (`test.result`) is a matrix of *p*-values corresponding to the test ID defined in the `tests` argument of the `Criterion` object and produced by the `Test` objects defined in the analysis model. Similarly, the second argument (`statistic.result`) is a matrix of results corresponding to the statistic ID defined in the `statistics` argument of the `Criterion` objects produced by the `Statistic` objects defined in the analysis model. In this example, the criteria will only use the `test.result` argument, which will contain the *p*-values produced by the tests associated with the two treatment-placebo comparisons in each population. The last argument (`parameter`) contains the optional parameter(s) defined by the user in the `Criterion` object. In this example, the par argument contains the overall alpha level (`alpha`) as well as the importance values assigned to the broad and restricted claims (v1 and v2).

The `subgroup.cs1.WeightedPower` function, defined in Listing 3.5, computes the probability of broad and restricted claims and then a weighted sum of the two probabilities is calculated. The order in which the tests are included in the evaluation model is important as the first one must correspond to the test in the overall population.

LISTING 3.5: Custom function for computing weighted power in Case study 3.1

```
# Custom evaluation criterion based on weighted power
subgroup.cs1.WeightedPower = function(test.result,
    statistic.result, parameter)  {

  alpha = parameter$alpha
  v1 = parameter$v1
  v2 = parameter$v2

  # Broad claim: Significant OP test
  broad.claim = (test.result[,1] <= alpha)

  # Restricted claim: Significant Bio-Pos test and non-
    significant OP test
  restricted.claim = ((test.result[,1] > alpha) & (test.
    result[,2] <= alpha))

  power = v1 * mean(broad.claim) + v2 * mean(restricted.
    claim)

  return(power)
}
```

A similar approach can be applied to create a custom function for computing the marginal probability of a restricted claim. This function is defined in Listing 3.6.

LISTING 3.6: Custom function for computing the marginal probability of a restricted claim in Case study 3.1

```
# Custom evaluation criterion based on the probability of a
    restricted claim
subgroup.cs1.RestrictedClaimPower = function(test.result,
    statistic.result, parameter)  {

  alpha = parameter$alpha

  # Restricted claim: Significant Bio-Pos test and non-
    significant OP test
  restricted.claim = ((test.result[,1] > alpha) & (test.
    result[,2] <= alpha))

  power = mean(restricted.claim)

  return(power)
}
```

The evaluation model based on the two built-in evaluation criteria (marginal power and disjunctive power) as well as two custom evaluation criteria (weighted power and marginal probability of a restricted claim) is defined in Listing 3.7.

LISTING 3.7: Evaluation model in Case study 3.1

```
# Evaluation model
subgroup.cs1.evaluation.model =
  EvaluationModel() +
  Criterion(id = "Marginal power",
            method = "MarginalPower",
            tests = tests("OP test", "Bio-Pos test"),
            labels = c("OP test","Bio-Pos test"),
            par = parameters(alpha = 0.025)) +
  Criterion(id = "Disjunctive power",
            method = "DisjunctivePower",
            tests = tests("OP test", "Bio-Pos test"),
            labels = c("Disjunctive power"),
            par = parameters(alpha = 0.025)) +
  Criterion(id = "Weighted power",
            method = "subgroup.cs1.WeightedPower",
            tests = tests("OP test", "Bio-Pos test"),
            labels = c("Weighted power"),
            par = parameters(alpha = 0.025,
                v1 = 1 / (1 + prevalence.pos),
                v2 = prevalence.pos /
                    (1 + prevalence.pos))) +
  Criterion(id = "Probability of a restricted claim",
            method = "subgroup.cs1.RestrictedClaimPower",
            tests = tests("OP test", "Bio-Pos test"),
            labels = c("Probability of a restricted claim"),
            par = parameters(alpha = 0.025))
```

Simulation results

As explained in Chapter 1, in order to run simulations based on the data, analysis and evaluation models defined above, the user needs to specify parameters of the simulation process, including the number of simulations. The simulation results based on 100,000 simulation runs are summarized in Table 3.7.

The R code presented above is easily modified and extended to perform other simulation-based assessments described in this section.

3.3.7 Conclusions and extensions

A detailed overview of an optimization exercise aimed at identifying an analysis model with an optimal multiplicity adjustment in a multi-population

TABLE 3.7: Summary of simulation results.

Evaluation criterion	Multiplicity adjustment	Value
Marginal power	Bonferroni	OP test: 77.1%
	Bonferroni	Bio-Pos test: 56.7%
	Hochberg	OP test: 78.9%
	Hochberg	Bio-Pos test: 73.4%
Disjunctive power	Bonferroni	82.1%
	Hochberg	83.0%
Weighted power	Bonferroni	56.5%
	Hochberg	57.5%
Probability of a	Bonferroni	5.0%
restricted claim	Hochberg	4.1%

clinical trial was presented in this section. Both qualitative and quantitative sensitivity assessments were conducted to determine if the selected analysis model would perform optimally under multiple sets of treatment effect assumptions, including extreme assumptions. In the context of quantitative assessments, compound criteria introduced in Chapter 1 (see Section 1.3.3) could also be considered. This includes the minimum criterion that focuses on the worst-case scenario across the assumed sets of treatment effects (Scenarios 1, 2 and 3) as well as the average criterion that relies on averaging the criterion functions across the sets.

It is worth noting that, in addition to the problem of optimally selecting a multiplicity adjustment in multi-population clinical trials presented in this section, other optimization problems can be considered as well. As a quick example, optimization algorithms can be applied to clinical trials with over-sampling strategies (Zhao, Dmitrienko and Tamura, 2010) to focus on optimal selection of the enrichment ratio that controls the proportion of biomarker-positive patients enrolled in the trial. The enrichment ratio can be selected to achieve an optimal balance between higher power in the biomarker-positive subgroup (due to a larger sample size) and a longer enrollment period. The goals of improving power in the subgroup and minimizing the length of the enrollment period compete with each other and thus tradeoff-based optimization strategies from Chapter 1 may be applied in this optimization problem.

The case study focused on a simplified decision-making process that accounts only for multiplicity considerations due to the evaluation of treatment effect in several patient populations. As explained in Section 3.2.3, the recommended decision-making process in clinical trials with several patient populations relies on statistical rules based on multiplicity adjustments as well as additional important considerations that are aimed at formulating meaningful regulatory claims in multi-population settings. The additional considerations will be discussed in Case studies 3.2 and 3.3.

3.4 Case study 3.2: Optimal selection of decision rules to support two potential claims

The asthma clinical trial example introduced in Case study 3.1 will be used to illustrate the process of optimally selecting a decision strategy in a clinical trial with two potential regulatory claims, namely, the broad claim of treatment effectiveness in the overall population and restricted claim that pertains to a subpopulation of marker-positive patients. The discussion will focus on optimal selection of decision rules based on the influence condition using several optimization strategies (tradeoff-based optimization versus constrained optimization). The influence condition was introduced in Section 3.2.3 as a tool for facilitating the interpretation of trial outcomes and formulating regulatory claims in a multi-population setting.

This section focuses on the problem of evaluating treatment benefit in the overall population of patients or pre-defined subpopulation. An additional assessment of a simultaneous beneficial effect in the overall population and selected subpopulation is not considered in this section; however, it may be included as a supportive analysis. An extended version of this setting that includes three potential regulatory claims (broad, restricted and enhanced) will be presented in the next section (see Case study 3.3).

3.4.1 Clinical trial

This case study is based on the same asthma clinical trial example that was used in Case study 3.1.

Data, analysis and evaluation models

The data and analysis models used in this case study are identical to those utilized in Case study 3.1. The evaluation model considered in this case study will incorporate a success criterion based on weighted power. This criterion is conceptually similar to the weighted power criterion employed in Case study 3.1; however, the broad and restricted claims will be re-defined to account for important clinical considerations (see Section 3.4.2). The modified success criterion will be used in Section 3.4.3 to develop an optimization strategy in clinical trials that are conducted to support two potential regulatory claims in the overall population and a pre-specified subpopulation.

3.4.2 Influence condition

Case study 3.1 discussed the computation of the probability of broad and restricted claims in the asthma clinical trial example and focused on optimal selection of a multiplicity adjustment strategy. It was concluded that, using an optimal Hochberg-based multiplicity adjustment with the initial weight of the overall population test set to $w = 0.8$, the probability of making a broad claim of treatment effectiveness in the overall patient population was 78.3% with 304 patients. Using the same data and analysis models, the probability of the restricted claim was 4.1%.

Needless to say, statistical methods such as multiplicity adjustments play an important role in multi-population clinical trials. An application of an appropriate multiple testing procedure guarantees control of the overall Type I error rate in the problem of testing two null hypotheses H_0 and H_+ of no treatment effect in the overall population and marker-positive subpopulation, respectively. There are, however, additional important issues that are not addressed by multiplicity adjustments. It was emphasized in Section 3.2.3 that, to formulate meaningful regulatory claims in this trial, the sponsor needs to ensure that a significant difference in the overall population is not caused by a highly beneficial effect in the biomarker-positive subgroup while the treatment is not actually effective in the complementary subgroup

The influence condition presented in Section 3.2.3 serves as a tool for facilitating the decision-making process in clinical trials with two patient populations. The condition states that the broad claim of treatment effectiveness in the overall patient population can be supported only if there is sufficient evidence of a beneficial treatment effect in the biomarker-negative subset and thus a significant treatment effect in the overall population is not directly driven by a strong effect in the biomarker-positive subpopulation. If the influence condition is met, the trial's sponsor can rule out the possibility of incorrectly characterizing the efficacy profile in the overall population.

When the influence condition is taken into account, it is no longer correct to use the simple rules for making the broad and restricted claims used in Case study 3.1, i.e.,

- Broad claim of treatment effectiveness in the overall population is made if H_0 is rejected.

- Restricted claim of treatment effectiveness in the subpopulation is made if H_+ is rejected but H_0 is not rejected.

The modified decision rules are displayed in Figure 3.2 and can be summarized as follows:

- Broad claim is made if (1) H_0 is rejected and H_+ is not rejected or (2) H_0 and H_+ are both rejected and the influence condition is met.

- Restricted claim is made if at least one of the two conditions is met: (1) H_+ is rejected but H_0 is not rejected or (2) H_0 and H_+ are both rejected but the influence condition is not satisfied.

A more straightforward frequentist formulation of the influence condition will be utilized in this case study. The influence condition is said to be met if

$$\widehat{\theta}_- \geq \lambda_1,$$

where $\widehat{\theta}_-$ is the estimated effect size in the biomarker-negative subgroup and λ_1 is a pre-specified non-negative quantity that serves as a threshold for defining a minimal clinically important effect in the biomarker-negative subpopulation. This parameter will be referred to as the *influence threshold*. This inequality shows that a sufficiently large treatment effect is present in the subset of patients with a biomarker-negative status.

As a general comment, it is more relevant to formulate a decision-making framework aimed at specifying relevant efficacy claims using an estimation-based approach, as shown above, rather than pursuing rules that rely on p-values. However, if it is relevant in a particular context, the influence condition can be defined using the treatment effect p-value in the biomarker-negative subgroup, e.g., the condition will be met if this p-value is significant at a predefined level. In addition, a Bayesian formulation of the influence condition can be considered (Millen, Dmitrienko and Song, 2014) and the optimization approaches presented below can also be applied using Bayesian rules.

To illustrate the importance of evaluating the influence of a strong treatment effect in a subgroup on the inferences in the overall patient population, a simulation study was conducted to compute the *influence error rate* in the asthma clinical trial. The influence error rate helps assess the likelihood of committing an influence error in a particular setting. This error rate is defined as the probability of erroneously concluding a positive treatment effect in the overall population or, in other words, the probability of a broad claim when in reality only marker-positive patients benefit from the treatment. To compute the influence error rate, the probability of rejecting the null hypothesis H_0 was evaluated under the main data model introduced in Case study 3.1 but the effect size in the biomarker-negative population was set to 0, i.e.,

$$\theta_- = 0, \ \theta_+ = 0.5.$$

The influence error rate was computed in the setting where the influence condition was not imposed and, in addition, with the condition applied based on the influence threshold $\lambda_1 = 0.1$. This value of the threshold represented the smallest clinically significant effect in this clinical trial example. In other words, the observed effect size of 0.1 or more in the biomarker-negative subpopulation was considered sufficient to justify a broad claim of treatment effectiveness across the entire patient population.

The results of the simulation study are displayed in Figure 3.10. The calculations were performed based on the Hochberg procedure with $w = 0.8$ and the recommended sample size computed in Case study 3.1, i.e., the total sample size of 304 patients. The figure demonstrates that, without applying the influence condition, the probability of incorrectly making a broad efficacy claim in the overall population when in truth the treatment is only beneficial in the biomarker-positive subset can be highly inflated. In this particular case, the influence error rate was almost 40%. This implies a high risk of formulating an incorrect claim and potentially recommending the new treatment to patients with a biomarker-negative status who do not benefit from the treat-

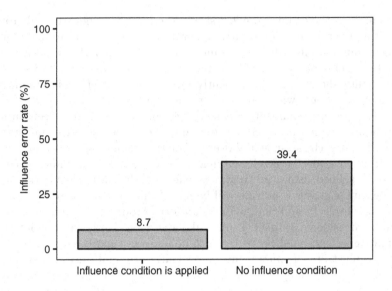

FIGURE 3.10: Influence error rate with and without the influence condition in Case study 3.2. The influence condition is applied with the threshold $\lambda_1 = 0.1$.

ment. With the influence condition based on a clinically relevant threshold, the probability of committing an influence error was considerably lowered and was, in fact, close to 9%. If a larger value of λ_1 was chosen, the influence error rate would be further reduced.

It is instructive to examine the effect of imposing the influence condition on the marginal probabilities of broad and restricted claims in the asthma clinical trial. Figure 3.11 shows the probabilities of making broad and restricted claims using the main data model ($\theta_- = 0.2$ and $\theta_+ = 0.5$). The simulations were performed using the same sample size and multiplicity adjustment procedure as in Figure 3.10.

It follows from Figure 3.11 that a broad claim of a beneficial treatment effect in the overall population was expected to be made much less frequently if the influence error rate was controlled. For example, the probability of a broad claim was reduced from 78.3% to 49.0% after the influence condition was imposed. Further, the probability of making a restricted claim increased from 4.1% to 33.4%. This was due to the fact that outcomes associated with the broad claim in the original setting without influence error rate control were often re-classified and the claim was restricted to the biomarker-positive subset because a strong treatment effect in that subset affected the conclusions in the overall population.

To better understand the role of the influence condition, note that a re-

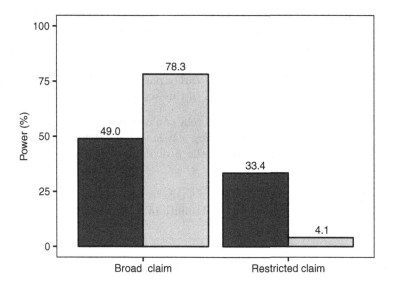

FIGURE 3.11: Marginal probabilities of the broad and restricted claims with the influence condition (black bars) and without the influence condition (gray bars) in Case study 3.2. The influence condition is applied with the threshold $\lambda_1 = 0.1$.

jection of the null hypothesis H_0 is sufficient to support a broad claim if the influence condition is not applied. When the modified decision rules that incorporate the influence condition are considered, additional conditions need to be met to justify a claim of treatment effectiveness in the overall patient population when H_0 and H_+ are both rejected. Specifically, the influence condition must also be satisfied, which lowers the probability of the broad claim. At the same time, if the influence condition is not met, there is a possibility of supporting a restricted claim. This leads to an increased probability of making a restricted claim. To summarize, the influence threshold directly affects the balance between the probabilities of the broad and restricted claims in multi-population clinical trials. Optimal selection of this important parameter will be discussed in the next section.

3.4.3 Optimal selection of the influence threshold

It was shown in Section 3.4.2 that the choice of the influence threshold λ_1 has a significant impact on the overall conclusions in a clinical trial with a pre-specified subpopulation. This parameter can be selected based on clinical or statistical considerations. Clinical judgment was used to determine the value of the influence threshold in Section 3.4.2. Statistical approaches to selecting the threshold and associated optimization algorithms are presented below.

An optimization problem will be set up to help determine the most appropriate value or range of values of the threshold in the influence condition. The threshold will be treated as the target parameter. Optimization strategies based on two criteria are discussed in this section:

- The first optimization criterion relies on a tradeoff-based optimization approach and is aimed at achieving a balance between the competing goals of simultaneously maximizing the probabilities of making broad and restricted claims.

- The second criterion is based on a constrained optimization approach and focuses on maximizing the probability of a broad claim while controlling the influence error rate.

Tradeoff-based optimization algorithm

Since the choice of the target parameter λ_1 clearly affects a balance between the probabilities of broad and restricted claims in this clinical trial example, it appears natural to think of a tradeoff-based criterion for determining an optimal value of λ_1 derived from the two marginal probabilities. The corresponding performance functions are defined as follows:

$$\psi_1(\lambda_1) = P(\text{Broad claim}|\lambda_1), \quad \psi_2(\lambda_1) = P(\text{Restricted claim}|\lambda_1).$$

Note that both probabilities are evaluated under the main data model using the modified decision rules for defining the broad and restricted claims that incorporate the influence condition (see Section 3.4.2). The threshold in the influence condition is set to λ_1. Multiplicity adjustment is carried out using the Hochberg procedure with $w = 0.8$ and the total sample size is set to $n = 304$ patients.

As an illustration, the performance functions $\psi_1(\lambda_1)$ and $\psi_2(\lambda_1)$ are plotted in Figure 3.12 as a function of λ_1 with $0 \leq \lambda_1 \leq 0.3$. This figure demonstrates that the goal of maximizing the probability of a broad claim indeed conflicts with the goal of maximizing the probability of a restricted claim. When the target parameter λ_1 was set to 0, the first probability approached 80% whereas the second probability was very close to 0. The two probabilities were equal to each other when λ_1 was about 0.24 and the probability of making a restricted claim was greater than the other probability when the target parameter exceeded 0.24. This means that an additive tradeoff-based criterion can be introduced in this problem with the criterion function defined as a weighted sum of the two performance functions:

$$\psi_{AT}(\lambda_1) = v_1\psi_1(\lambda_1) + v_2\psi_2(\lambda_1).$$

Here v_1 and v_2 define the relative importance of the two competing goals. An

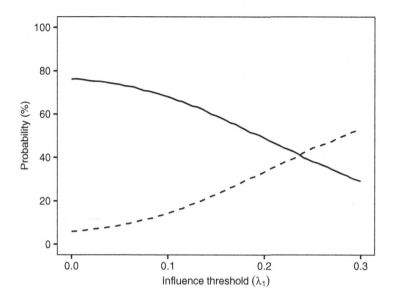

FIGURE 3.12: Marginal probability of the broad claim (solid curve) and restricted claim (dashed curve) as a function of the target parameter (influence threshold) in Case study 3.2.

optimal value of the target parameter λ_1, as well as a set of nearly optimal values, can be found by maximizing this criterion function.

Figure 3.12 also illustrates an important feature of this optimization problem. A visual inspection of the two curves in this figure suggests that the two performance functions add up to a constant value, which indicates that they are approximately linearly related. This means that trial's sponsor faces a collinearity problem discussed in Chapter 1 (see Section 1.3.1). Due to collinearity, the criterion function $\psi_{AT}(\lambda_1)$ is no longer concave and optimization based on this function leads to a trivial solution. If the weight assigned to $\psi_1(\lambda_1)$ is greater than the weight assigned to $\psi_2(\lambda_1)$, i.e., $v_1 > v_2$, the criterion function will be a monotonically increasing function of λ_1. This immediately implies that the optimization criterion will be maximized at the upper end of the selected range, i.e., at $\lambda_1 = 0.3$. On the other hand, if a greater weight is assigned to $\psi_2(\lambda_1)$, the optimization criterion will be dominated by this performance function and the minimum value of target parameter will be optimal, i.e., the optimization criterion will be maximized at $\lambda_1 = 0$. As a result, an additive tradeoff-based optimization criterion based on the probabilities of broad and restricted claims is not relevant in this setting.

Constrained optimization algorithm

It was shown in the preceding section that a tradeoff-based optimization strategy based on the probabilities of broad and restricted claims produces trivial solutions due to collinearity and thus it is not useful in practice. Another downside of the optimization algorithm based on balancing the probabilities of broad and restricted claims is that it does not explicitly incorporate influence error rate control. Even if the corresponding tradeoff-based criterion did lead to non-trivial solutions for the target parameter λ_1, there would be no guarantee that optimal values of λ_1 resulted in a reasonably low influence error rate. A potentially high influence error rate is undesirable from the sponsor's perspective and thus it will be impractical to employ this optimization strategy.

Given the important consideration related to the influence error rate control, it is natural to apply a constrained optimization approach and define an optimization criterion aimed at maximizing an appropriate power function while protecting the probability of an influence error at a desirable level. The partition-based weighted criterion introduced in Case study 3.1, i.e.,

$$\psi_{PW}(\lambda_1) = 0.71 P(\text{Broad claim}|\lambda_1) + 0.29 P(\text{Restricted claim}|\lambda_1),$$

will be used as the key measure of performance. This criterion accounts for the relative importance of claiming treatment effectiveness in the overall population of patients and in the subpopulation of biomarker-positive patients only. As before, the probabilities of the broad and restricted claims are computed based on the decision rules that incorporate the influence condition with the influence threshold set to λ_1.

Considering the following criterion functions:

$$\psi_1(\lambda_1) = \psi_{PW}(\lambda_1), \quad \psi_2(\lambda_1) = P(\text{Influence error}|\lambda_1),$$

the goal is to maximize $\psi_1(\lambda_1)$ over the set of threshold values where $\psi_2(\lambda_1) \leq \gamma$. Here γ is the highest acceptable level of the influence error rate, e.g., $\gamma = 0.1$ or $\gamma = 0.2$.

It needs to be pointed out that the probabilities used in the weighted criterion are evaluated under the main data model with $\theta_- = 0.2$ and $\theta_+ = 0.5$. The second criterion function relies on the probability of a broad claim which is evaluated under the assumption that the treatment provides no benefit in the biomarker-negative subset, e.g., $\theta_- = 0$ and $\theta_+ = 0.5$.

The two functions used in this optimization problem are plotted in Figure 3.13. As shown in the figure, the influence error rate was a monotonically decreasing function of the target parameter λ_1 and it is easy to identify the sets of threshold values corresponding to error rate control at a 10% or 20% level. Specifically, the influence error rate did not exceed 10% ($\gamma = 0.1$) if $\lambda_1 \geq 0.186$ and was not greater than 20% ($\gamma = 0.2$) if $\lambda_1 \geq 0.106$. Given the monotonicity of the first performance function, it is now trivial to find an optimal value of the target parameter. For example, if the acceptable influence

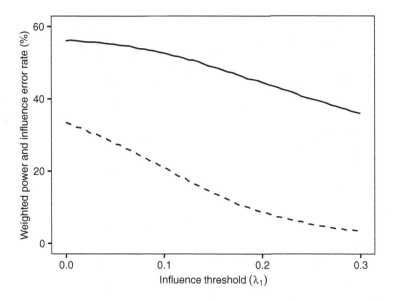

FIGURE 3.13: Partition-based weighted power (solid curve) and influence error rate (dashed curve) as a function of the target parameter (influence threshold) in Case study 3.2.

error rate is set to $\gamma = 0.1$, an optimal threshold is equal to 0.186. This means that, under an optimal decision rule, the broad claim of treatment effectiveness in the overall population should be considered only if the observed effect size in the biomarker-negative subset is no less than 0.186.

As a side note, it follows from Figure 3.13 that imposing a restriction based on the influence error rate results in lower weighted power. With $\gamma = 0.1$, the weighted power was reduced to 45.9% and, if the acceptable influence error rate was set to 20%, the highest level of weighted power was 52.4%. The latter value is lower than the weighted power level computed before the influence condition was applied (i.e., 57.1%) and it would generally be advisable to adjust the sample size to improve the overall probability of success in the first setting.

Continuing with the exploration of optimal values of the target parameter, the shape of the weighted power function influences optimal intervals for this parameter. For example, the optimal value of λ_1 corresponding to the influence error rate of 10% and accompanying 90% optimal interval are shown in Figure 3.14. Note that, due to the requirement to protect the influence error rate, the set of eligible λ_1 values is restricted to the interval $\lambda_1 \geq 0.186$. As a consequence, the optimal interval displayed in Figure 3.14 as well as any other optimal interval considered in this optimization problem are one-sided. It follows from the figure that the 90% optimal interval for the influence threshold

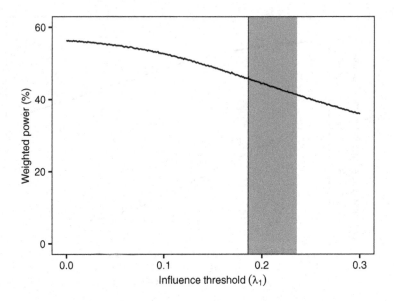

FIGURE 3.14: Weighted power as a function of the target parameter (λ_1) in Case study 3.2. The vertical line represents the optimal value of the target parameter with the influence error rate controlled at 10% and the gray rectangle defines the 90% optimal interval.

TABLE 3.8: Optimal values of the target parameter (influence threshold) and optimal intervals for selected influence error rates (γ) in Case study 3.2.

Acceptable influence error rate	Optimal value	90% optimal interval	95% optimal interval
$\gamma = 0.1$	0.186	$(0.186, 0.235)$	$(0.186, 0.209)$
$\gamma = 0.2$	0.106	$(0.106, 0.170)$	$(0.106, 0.138)$

was quite tight and the optimal intervals based on a 95% or 99% level would be very thin.

Table 3.8 lists the 90% and 95% optimal intervals for the target parameter λ_1 when the influence error rate is set to $\gamma = 0.1$ and $\gamma = 0.2$. The 95% optimal interval was narrow for both values of γ, which indicates that the optimal values of the target parameter were well defined in this clinical trial example. With the influence thresholds set to the optimal values, the probability of broad and restricted claims were, respectively, 52.1% and 30.3% with $\gamma = 0.1$ and 67.3% and 15.1% with $\gamma = 0.2$.

3.4.4 Software implementation

The **Mediana** package can be used to perform simulations in this case study. As mentioned in Section 3.4.1, Case studies 3.1 and 3.2 share the same data and analysis models. The only major difference between the two case studies is that the evaluation model in the latter includes updated definitions of broad and restricted claims that incorporate the influence condition. To evaluate this condition, the effect size in the biomarker-negative subpopulation must be computed, which requires a slight modification of the analysis model.

Analysis model

The computation of the effect size in the biomarker-negative subpopulation is performed by including the `Statistic` object with the `EffectSizeContStat` method in the analysis model. This method computes the effect size for normally distributed endpoints.

LISTING 3.8: Analysis model in Case study 3.2

```
# Analysis model
subgroup.cs2.analysis.model =
  AnalysisModel() +
  Test(id = "OP test",
 samples = samples(c("Placebo Bio-Neg", "Placebo Bio-Pos"),
             c("Treatment Bio-Neg", "Treatment Bio-Pos")),
      method = "TTest") +
  Test(id = "Bio-Pos test",
      samples = samples("Placebo Bio-Pos",
                         "Treatment Bio-Pos"),
      method = "TTest") +
  Statistic(id = "Effect Size in Bio-Neg",
            samples = samples("Placebo Bio-Neg",
                               "Treatment Bio-Neg"),
            method = "EffectSizeContStat") +
  MultAdjProc(proc = "HochbergAdj",
              par = parameters(weight = c(0.8, 0.2)))
```

Evaluation model

A custom function needs to be defined in the evaluation model to implement the criterion based on weighted power using the general approach used in Case study 3.1. The only difference is that, in this case, the `statistic.result` argument of the function will be used to specify the matrix of effect sizes in the biomarker-negative subpopulation. This custom function computes weighted power based on the modified broad and restricted claims with the influence condition.

LISTING 3.9: Custom function for computing weighted power in Case study 3.2

```
# Custom evaluation criterion based on weighted power
subgroup.cs2.WeightedPower = function(test.result,
    statistic.result, parameter)  {

  alpha = parameter$alpha
  v1 = parameter$v1
  v2 = parameter$v2
  influence_threshold = parameter$influence_threshold

  # Broad claim: (1) Reject OP test but not Bio-Pos or (2)
    Reject OP and Bio-Pos test and influence condition is
    met
  broad.claim = ((test.result[,1] <= alpha & test.result
    [,2] > alpha) | (test.result[,1] <= alpha & test.result
    [,2] <= alpha & statistic.result[,1] >= influence_
    threshold))

  # Restricted claim: (1) Reject Bio-Pos test but not OP or
    (2) Reject Bio-Pos and OP test and influence not met
  restricted.claim = ((test.result[,1] > alpha & test.
    result[,2] <= alpha) | (test.result[,1] <= alpha & test
    .result[,2] <= alpha & statistic.result[,1] < influence
    _threshold))

  power = v1 * mean(broad.claim) + v2 * mean(restricted.
    claim)

  return(power)
}
```

Custom functions to compute the probabilities of broad and restricted claims, i.e., **subgroup.cs2.BroadClaimPower** and **subgroup.cs2.Restricted ClaimPower**, can be written in a similar way.

The resulting evaluation model is presented below. For the purpose of illustration, the influence threshold (i.e., **influence_threshold**) is set to 0.186 in the **par** argument of the functions for computing weighted power and probabilities of broad and restricted claims.

LISTING 3.10: Evaluation model in Case study 3.2

```
# Evaluation model
subgroup.cs2.evaluation.model =
  EvaluationModel() +
  Criterion(id = "Marginal power",
            method = "MarginalPower",
            tests = tests("OP test", "Bio-Pos test"),
            labels = c("OP test","Bio-Pos test"),
```

```
             par = parameters(alpha = 0.025)) +
Criterion(id = "Disjunctive power",
           method = "DisjunctivePower",
           tests = tests("OP test", "Bio-Pos test"),
           labels = c("Disjunctive power"),
           par = parameters(alpha = 0.025)) +
Criterion(id = "Weighted power",
      method = "subgroup.cs2.WeightedPower",
      tests = tests("OP test", "Bio-Pos test"),
      statistics = statistics("Effect Size in Bio-Neg"),
      labels = c("Weighted power"),
      par = parameters(alpha = 0.025,
         v1 = 1 / (1 + prevalence.plus),
         v2 = prevalence.plus / (1 + prevalence.plus),
         influence_threshold = 0.186)) +
   Criterion(id = "Probability of a broad claim",
         method = "subgroup.cs2.BroadClaimPower",
         tests = tests("OP test", "Bio-Pos test"),
         statistics = statistics("Effect Size in Bio-Neg"),
         labels = c("Probability of a broad claim"),
         par = parameters(alpha = 0.025,
              influence_threshold = 0.186)) +
   Criterion(id = "Probability of a restricted claim",
         method = "subgroup.cs2.RestrictedClaimPower",
         tests = tests("OP test", "Bio-Pos test"),
         statistics = statistics("Effect Size in Bio-Neg"),
         labels = c("Probability of a restricted claim"),
         par = parameters(alpha = 0.025,
              influence_threshold = 0.186))
```

Simulation results

Based on the R code presented above, 100,000 simulation runs were carried out. The simulation results are summarized in Table 3.9.

TABLE 3.9: Summary of simulation results.

Evaluation criterion	Value
Marginal power	OP test: 78.9%
	Bio-Pos test: 73.4%
Disjunctive power	83.0%
Weighted power	46.0%
Probability of a broad claim	52.0%
Probability of a restricted claim	31.0%

3.4.5 Conclusions and extensions

This section dealt with optimization considerations in a multi-population clinical trial with a single pre-defined subpopulation. An optimization algorithm was constructed to develop an optimal decision-making strategy based on two potential regulatory claims in this multi-population trial (broad and restricted claims).

As in Case study 3.1, the optimization exercise presented in this section can be augmented by performing sensitivity analyses. For example, it is recommended that the trial's sponsor should investigate the effect of misspecifying key data and analysis model parameters on the conclusions related to the choice of the target parameter (threshold used in the influence condition, λ_1). This includes an important analysis model parameter such as the initial weight of the overall population test (w) used in the multiplicity adjustment procedure such as the Hochberg procedure. In general, if the influence threshold is chosen using a constrained optimization approach by controlling the influence error rate, the weights utilized in the multiplicity adjustment procedure have very little impact on an optimal value of λ_1. An additional sensitivity analysis can be performed with respect to supportive parameters of the data model such as the population prevalence of biomarker-positive patients (r). A perturbation-based sensitivity assessment of this kind can be conducted as in Case study 3.1.

3.5 Case study 3.3: Optimal selection of decision rules to support three potential claims

This section will discuss optimality considerations in a multi-population Phase III clinical trial with three potential regulatory claims: broad, restricted and enhanced claims. The decision-making rules will be set up using the influence and interaction conditions defined in Section 3.2.3 and the case study introduced in this section will be used to illustrate the process of optimally selecting a decision strategy for these three claims. A solution to this optimization problem will be found in the class of constrained optimization algorithms with a bivariate grid search.

3.5.1 Clinical trial

The clinical trial example used in this case study is based on the panitumumab trial in a population of patients with metastatic colorectal cancer (Amado et al., 2008). Using the same patient population, consider a Phase III trial for a novel treatment versus control (best supportive care) that utilizes a balanced design with a 1:1 randomization scheme. The treatment is a fully human antibody against the EGFR (epidermal growth factor receptor) and is expected to benefit mostly patients in a pre-specified subset. This subset is defined based on each patient's KRAS (Kirsten rat sarcoma viral oncogene homolog) status and includes patients with wild-type KRAS. These patients will be referred to as biomarker-positive patients and patients with a mutated KRAS status will be referred to as biomarker-negative patients. For simplicity, it will be assumed that the KRAS status can be ascertained in all patients. The treatment effect in this two-arm trial will be evaluated based on progression-free survival (PFS).

Data model

The data model in this clinical trial example is specified using the general approach outlined in Section 3.2.1. As stated above, the clinical trial uses a balanced biomarker-driven design. The fraction of biomarker-positive patients in this patient population is expected to be approximately 55%. It is assumed that the time to disease progression follows an exponential distribution. The hazard rates in each subset and trial arm can be computed from the median PFS times derived from Phase II trial data and relevant clinical trial publications. The statistical assumptions used in this clinical trial are summarized in Table 3.10. As shown in the table, the hazard rate is denoted by η. In addition, δ will denote the treatment difference (hazard ratio) and θ will denote the effect size (log-transformed hazard ratio).

Using the terminology introduced in Section 3.2.1 (see Figure 3.1), the binary classifier based on the KRAS status demonstrates purely predictive effect. Table 3.10 lists the assumed outcome distribution parameters (median PFS times and hazard rates) in the four samples. This table shows that a common median PFS value (or common hazard rate) is assumed in the two subsets within the control arm (Samples 1 and 2) and thus the biomarker exhibits no prognostic effect. Further, due to a strong predictive effect, a much larger treatment benefit is assumed in the subpopulation of biomarker-positive patients (Sample 4) compared to the complementary subpopulation (Sample 3) within the treatment arm. The hazard ratios in the two subpopulations are given by

$$\delta_- = \frac{\eta_{1-}}{\eta_{0-}} = 0.882, \quad \delta_+ = \frac{\eta_{1+}}{\eta_{0+}} = 0.6.$$

These hazard ratios correspond to the following hypothesized effect sizes:

$$\theta_- = -\ln\delta_- = 0.125, \quad \theta_+ = -\ln\delta_+ = 0.511.$$

For simplicity, the data model considered in this case study will not account for potential censoring in the trial, which includes administrative censoring and loss to follow-up. This approach is similar to the one assumed when calculations aimed at computing the target number of events are performed. The optimization algorithm presented below can be easily applied to extended data models that include detailed specifications of important design elements

TABLE 3.10: Parameters of the outcome distribution (median PFS times and hazard rates) in the four samples in Case study 3.3.

Sample	Trial arm	Subpopulation	Median PFS time (months)	Hazard rate
Sample 1	Control	Biomarker-negative	$m_{0-} = 7.5$	$\eta_{0-} = 0.0924$
Sample 2	Control	Biomarker-positive	$m_{0+} = 7.5$	$\eta_{0+} = 0.0924$
Sample 3	Treatment	Biomarker-negative	$m_{1-} = 8.5$	$\eta_{1-} = 0.0815$
Sample 4	Treatment	Biomarker-positive	$m_{1+} = 12.5$	$\eta_{1+} = 0.0555$

such as the enrollment and follow-up periods, assumptions about withdrawal rates, etc. These data models support the calculation of the required number of patients in the trial.

Analysis model

The clinical trial in patients with colorectal cancer is designed to simultaneously evaluate the effect of the new treatment in two pre-defined patient populations (overall population of all-comers and subset of biomarker-positive patients). The associated null hypotheses of no treatment difference are defined in the same way as in the asthma clinical trial example considered in Case studies 3.1 and 3.2, i.e.,

- Null hypothesis H_0 of no effect in the overall patient population.

- Null hypothesis H_+ of no effect in the biomarker-positive subpopulation (wild-type KRAS subset).

The treatment effect on progression-free survival will be assessed in each patient population using the log-rank test. As in Case study 3.1, a stratified version of the log-rank test should be considered in the overall population but, for simplicity, the non-stratified test will be included in this analysis model.

Potential inflation of the overall Type I error rate due to testing the two null hypotheses will be addressed by applying the Hochberg-based multiplicity adjustment (see Section 3.2.2). As in the asthma clinical trial example, the Hochberg procedure will account for unequal importance of the treatment effect tests in the overall population and selected subpopulation by assigning initial weights to the two null hypotheses. The weights of H_0 and H_+ will be set to $w_0 = w$ and $w_+ = 1 - w$, respectively, where w ranges between 0 and 1.

Evaluation model

The analysis model assumed in this case study is conceptually quite similar to the model used in the asthma clinical trial example in the sense that both models are built around two null hypotheses of no treatment effect and associated multiplicity adjustment. There is, however, an important difference when the evaluation models are considered. The key assumption made in Case studies 3.1 and 3.2 was that the sponsor planned to pursue two potential regulatory claims of treatment effectiveness in the overall population and pre-selected subpopulation. In the current setting, another claim, known as the *enhanced claim*, will be added.

The broad and restricted claims need to be modified when the enhanced claim is introduced as a potential option. As shown in Case study 3.1, in the more straightforward setting with two potential claims, the overall outcome of interest (significant treatment effect in at least one of the two patient populations) is partitioned into two mutually exclusive outcomes, i.e.,

$$H_0 \cup H_+ = H_0 + \bar{H}_0 \cap H_+.$$

The two resulting outcomes correspond to the broad claims of treatment effectiveness in the overall population and restricted claim of treatment effectiveness in the biomarker-positive subpopulation, respectively. As explained in Section 3.2.1, when three regulatory claims are considered in a clinical trial, these claims are based on a different partitioning of the overall outcome:

$$H_0 \cup H_+ = H_0 \cap \bar{H}_+ + \bar{H}_0 \cap H_+ + H_0 \cap H_+.$$

This means that the three claims of interest in this case study are defined as follows:

- Broad claim in the overall population (reject H_0 only).

- Restricted claim in the biomarker-positive subpopulation (reject H_+ only).

- Enhanced claim in the overall population and biomarker-positive subpopulation (reject both H_0 and H_+).

It was stressed in Section 3.2.3 that these simple rules do not account for key clinical considerations in a multi-population setting and may lead to spurious conclusions. To address this problem, the influence and interaction conditions need to be introduced.

The influence condition was discussed at length in Case study 3.2 and, as in that case study, a frequentist formulation of the condition will be applied in the oncology trial example. The influence condition will be met if the observed log-hazard ratio in the subpopulation of patients with a biomarker-negative status exceeds a pre-defined influence threshold, i.e.,

$$\widehat{\theta}_- \geq \lambda_1.$$

The interaction condition serves as a tool for assessing the magnitude of the differential treatment effect in the two subsets of the overall population. This condition supports the decision-making process that leads to the enhanced claim by ensuring that the treatment effect in the overall population is positive and, in addition, the treatment provides further benefit in the biomarker-positive subgroup. This interaction condition is satisfied if

$$\frac{\widehat{\theta}_1}{\overline{\theta}_-} \geq \lambda_2$$

provided the influence condition is met and thus $\widehat{\theta}_-$ is known to be non-negative. Here $\lambda_2 \geq 1$ is the pre-defined interaction threshold. As a quick illustration, if the threshold is equal to 1.2, this implies that a 20% improvement is expected on the effect size scale in the biomarker-positive subset compared to the complementary subset (biomarker-negative) to support the conclusion of additional benefit in the former. For example, if the hazard ratio observed in the complementary subgroup is $\widehat{\delta}_- = 0.8$, the hazard ratio in the biomarker-positive subgroup needs to be less than

$$\exp(\lambda_2 \, \widehat{\theta}_-) = \exp(\lambda_2 \ln \widehat{\delta}_-) = \exp(1.2 \times \ln 0.8) = 0.72$$

to satisfy the interaction condition.

To prevent incorrect decisions in a clinical trial with three potential claims, the definitions of the broad, restricted and enhanced claims need to be updated by incorporating the influence and interaction conditions. The modified decision rules were displayed in Figure 3.3 and are defined as follows:

- Broad claim of treatment effectiveness in the overall population is made if (1) H_0 is rejected and H_+ is not rejected or (2) H_0 and H_+ are both rejected, the influence condition is met but the interaction condition is not met.

- Restricted claim of treatment effectiveness in the subpopulation is made if at least one of the two conditions is met: (1) H_0 is not rejected but H_+ is rejected or (2) both null hypotheses are rejected but the influence condition is not satisfied.

- Enhanced claim of treatment effectiveness in the overall population and biomarker-positive subpopulation is made if H_0 and H_+ are both rejected and, in addition, the influence and interaction conditions are both met.

The evaluation model in a trial with the three claims will be defined based on weighted power. Recall that a utility-based approach was recommended in Case study 3.1 to define an optimization criterion in settings with two regulatory claims (broad and restricted claims). This approach relied on computing partition-based weighted power, i.e., a weighted sum of the performance functions associated with the two claims:

$$\psi_1(\boldsymbol{\lambda}) = P(\text{Broad claim}|\boldsymbol{\lambda}), \quad \psi_2(\boldsymbol{\lambda}) = P(\text{Restricted claim}|\boldsymbol{\lambda}),$$

where $\boldsymbol{\lambda} = (\lambda_1, \lambda_2)$.

When another performance function is introduced, i.e.,

$$\psi_3(\boldsymbol{\lambda}) = P(\text{Enhanced claim}|\boldsymbol{\lambda}),$$

it is natural to define a weighted power criterion of the following form:

$$\psi_{PW}(\boldsymbol{\lambda}) = \sum_{i=1}^{3} v_i \psi_i(\boldsymbol{\lambda}).$$

The three importance parameters used in this definition, i.e., v_1, v_2 and v_3, are non-negative values that, as before, quantify the relative importance of the three claims. Since the enhanced claim is the most desirable one, its importance parameter should be greater than the other two parameters, i.e., $v_3 \geq 1/3$. Lastly, the marginal probabilities of the three regulatory claims used in the weighted criterion are computed under the influence and interaction conditions. The conditions are applied with the influence and interaction thresholds set to λ_1 and λ_2, respectively.

The importance parameters in the weighted criterion can be selected using a general idea similar to that used in Case study 3.1 (see Section 3.3.1). Specifically, the parameters are chosen to be proportional to the size of the patient populations associated with each claim. The overall population serves as a reference point and thus the broad claim can be assigned a weight of 1. The second claim is restricted to a subset of the overall population with the relative size of r ($r < 1$) and, consequently, its weight is r. The enhanced claim is associated with establishing a beneficial treatment effect simultaneously in two patient populations. The combined size of the two populations is $1 + r$ and thus the weight of the third claim can be set to $1 + r$. Finally, the weights need to be standardized to ensure that their sum is equal to 1. The resulting importance parameters are given by

$$v_1 = \frac{1}{2(1+r)}, \quad v_2 = \frac{r}{2(1+r)}, \quad v_3 = \frac{1}{2}.$$

Since the population prevalence of biomarker-positive patients is assumed to be $r = 0.55$ in this case study, the partition-based weighted criterion as a function of the two target parameters is defined as follows:

$$\psi_W(\boldsymbol{\lambda}) = 0.32\psi_1(\boldsymbol{\lambda}) + 0.18\psi_2(\boldsymbol{\lambda}) + 0.5\psi_3(\boldsymbol{\lambda}).$$

This definition will be used in Section 3.5.3 to identify decision rules for formulating efficacy claims with optimal values of the thresholds λ_1 and λ_2.

3.5.2 Interaction condition

The interaction condition was defined earlier in this section as a tool for evaluating the differential treatment effect within the trial's population, i.e., the strength of treatment-by-subgroup interaction. It is instructive to examine the impact of this condition on the decision-making process in clinical trials with three potential regulatory claims. The impact can be quantified using the concept of the *interaction error rate*, which is defined similarly to the influence error rate introduced in Section 3.4.2. The interaction error rate is computed based on the probability of erroneously making the enhanced claim in a two-population clinical trial. This error rate is evaluated under the null hypothesis of no differential treatment effect, i.e., the selected biomarker is not predictive of enhanced treatment efficacy and a common treatment difference is assumed in the biomarker-positive and biomarker-negative subpopulations.

To illustrate the evaluation of the interaction error rate, consider the clinical trial in patients with colorectal cancer. The interaction error rate is the probability of making the enhanced claim of simultaneous treatment effectiveness in the overall population and pre-defined subpopulation if the hazard ratio in the biomarker-negative subpopulation (θ_-) is in fact equal to that in the biomarker-positive subpopulation (θ_+) provided a significant treatment effect is established in both patient populations. In other words, a common median PFS needs to be assumed in the two subpopulations. The following hazard ratios were used in the calculations:

$$\delta_- = \frac{0.0555}{0.0924} = 0.6, \ \delta_+ = \frac{0.0555}{0.0924} = 0.6.$$

The calculations incorporated the Hochberg-based multiplicity adjustment with the initial weight of the overall population test set to $w = 0.8$. The influence and interactions thresholds λ_1 and λ_2 were set to 0 and 1, respectively.

To run the calculations, the number of events in the clinical trial was computed based on the weighted power function introduced in Section 3.5.2. Using an extension of the arguments presented in Section 3.3.4, the following rule can be applied to determine the target level for weighted power with three components based on the probabilities of three efficacy claims.

Let $\psi_{PW}(n|v_1, v_2, v_3)$ denote a general weighted criterion, i.e.,

$$\psi_{PW}(n|v_1, v_2, v_3) = v_1\psi_1(n) + v_2\psi_2(n) + v_3\psi_3(n),$$

with $v_i \geq 0$, $i = 1, 2, 3$, and $v_1 + v_2 + v_3 = 1$. Here n denotes the total number of events (disease progressions) in the trial. Let β denote the desirable value of the Type II error rate, e.g., $\beta = 0.2$.

First of all, it is easy to check that

$$H_0 \cap \bar{H}_+ + H_0 \cap H_+ = H_0 \text{ and } \bar{H}_0 \cap H_+ + H_0 \cap H_+ = H_+.$$

This means that the weighted power function with $v_1 = 0.5$, $v_2 = 0$ and $v_3 = 0.5$ is equal to one half of the probability of rejecting the null hypothesis of no effect in the overall population, i.e.,

$$\psi_{PW}(n|0.5, 0, 0.5) = \frac{1}{2}\psi_1(n) + \frac{1}{2}\psi_3(n) = \frac{1}{2}P(\text{Reject } H_0).$$

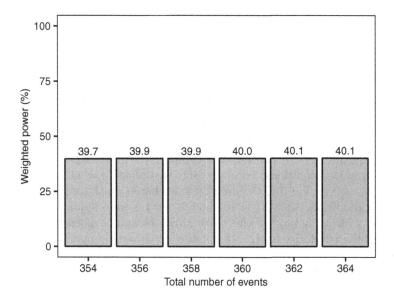

FIGURE 3.15: Weighted power as a function of the total number of events in Case study 3.3. The influence and interaction conditions are applied with $\lambda_1 = 0$ and $\lambda_2 = 1$, respectively.

Since a clinical trial designed to test the treatment effect in the overall population would typically be powered at $1 - \beta$, the target value for weighted power with $v_1 = 0.5$, $v_2 = 0$ and $v_3 = 0.5$ should be $(1 - \beta)/2$.

A similar argument shows that

$$\psi_{PW}(n|0, 0.5, 0.5) = \frac{1}{2}\psi_2(n) + \frac{1}{2}\psi_3(n) = \frac{1}{2}P(\text{Reject } H_+).$$

and thus the target value for weighted power with $v_1 = 0$, $v_2 = 0.5$ and $v_3 = 0.5$ should be set to $(1 - \beta)/2$.

Finally, note that weighted power with $v_1 = v_2 = v_3 = 1/3$ equals one third of disjunctive power (probability of rejecting at least one null hypothesis) and, since sample size or event count calculations based on disjunctive power rely on equating this definition of power to $1 - \beta$, the desirable level for weighted power with $v_1 = v_2 = v_3 = 1/3$ is naturally set to $(1 - \beta)/3$.

Applying a linear interpolation, it is easy to show the target value for $\psi_{PW}(n|v_1, v_2, v_3)$ is simply equal to $v_3(1 - \beta)$. For example, in the oncology clinical trial, the importance of the enhanced claim was set to 0.5 and therefore, the total number of PFS events in this trial can be computed from

$$0.32\psi_1(n) + 0.18\psi_2(n) + 0.5\psi_3(n) = 0.5(1 - \beta) = 0.4.$$

Figure 3.15 depicts the weighted power as a function of the total number of events. It can be seen from this figure that the target level of 40% was achieved with 360 events in this clinical trial. It is important to remember that the resulting number of events is heavily influenced by the chosen values of λ_1 and λ_2 and may be viewed as a preliminary estimate of the final event count. It will be shown in Section 3.5.3 that this event count calculation can be updated as part of the algorithm aimed at selecting optimal values of the influence and interaction thresholds.

Returning to the problem of evaluating the interaction error rate, Figure 3.16 displays the interaction error rate in the following three settings. First, the interaction error rate was computed without imposing the influence or interaction conditions. Secondly, only the influence condition was required with $\lambda_1 = 0.1$. Thirdly, the decision rules based on the influence and interaction conditions with $\lambda_1 = 0.1$ and $\lambda_2 = 1.5$ were applied. As explained above, with $\lambda_2 = 1.5$, the effect size in the biomarker-positive subset should exceed the effect size in the other subset by 50% to support an enhanced efficacy claim. A restriction based on the influence and interaction conditions led to a dramatic drop in the interaction error rate. Figure 3.16 shows that the interaction error rate was extremely high in the first setting (it exceeded 94%). Similarly, when only the influence condition was imposed, the interaction error rate remained very high. This result is not that surprising since, if the influence condition is the only condition required to support an enhanced claim, this decision could be made if both H_0 and H_+ were rejected and the observed effect size in the biomarker-negative subpopulation was greater than the influence threshold. The interaction error rate is evaluated under the null hypothesis of no differential treatment effect, i.e., when the effect size of the biomarker-negative subpopulation (θ_-) is equal to that in the biomarker-positive subpopulation (θ_+). In this case study, θ_+ was set to 0.511 and thus the probability to pass the influence condition would be very high. Finally, the probability of committing an interaction error was lowered to below 20% when the interaction condition was introduced. It is to be expected that increasing the interaction threshold λ_2 will result in a lower interaction error rate. For example, it can be verified by running additional simulations that the interaction error rate approaches 10% if the interaction threshold λ_2 is set to 2. Alternatively, the interaction error rate can be reduced by selecting a greater value of the influence threshold λ_1. As shown in Figure 3.3, it is more difficult to satisfy the influence condition with a larger λ_1. This reduces the probability of reaching the enhanced claim and, as a consequence, the interaction error rate decreases.

To better understand the relationship between the interaction condition and the probabilities of the three potential outcomes in this clinical trial, the marginal probabilities of the broad, restricted and enhanced claims were evaluated with and without the influence and interaction conditions. The calculations were run using the same data and analysis models as above. Figure 3.17 presents the three sets of marginal probabilities and shows that a simultaneous application of the two conditions had a considerable impact on

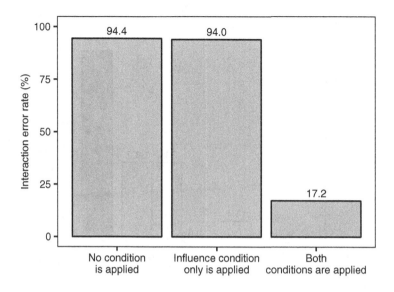

FIGURE 3.16: Interaction error rate with and without the influence and interaction conditions in Case study 3.3. The influence and interaction conditions are applied with $\lambda_1 = 0.1$ and $\lambda_2 = 1.5$, respectively.

the probabilities of making the individual claims. When the influence and interaction considerations were not accounted for in the decision-making process, the probability of the enhanced claim was much higher than the other two probabilities and approached 90%. This was due to the fact the treatment effect was very likely to be significant in the overall as well as biomarker-positive populations. Secondly, when only the influence condition was imposed, this condition affected the balance between the restricted and enhanced claims compared to the naive decision-making approach that relies on neither condition. Note that, in this setting, the influence condition must be satisfied in order to claim the enhanced label. If this condition is not satisfied, the restricted label is claimed. Finally, when a modified decision rule based on the influence and interaction conditions with $\lambda_1 = 0.1$ and $\lambda_2 = 1.5$ was applied, the interaction error rate was reduced, which resulted in lowering the probability of the enhanced claim (this probability dropped from 88.7% when neither condition was applied to 53.0% with the influence condition only and to 43.4% with both conditions imposed). Further, the outcomes where the conclusion of a differential treatment effect in the biomarker-positive and biomarker-negative subsets was reached in error were re-classified.

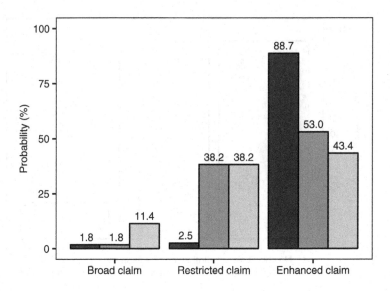

FIGURE 3.17: Marginal probabilities of the broad, restricted and enhanced claims without the influence and interaction conditions (black bars), with the influence condition only (dark gray bars) and with the influence and interaction conditions (light gray bars) in Case study 3.3. The influence and interaction conditions are applied with $\lambda_1 = 0.1$ and $\lambda_2 = 1.5$, respectively.

3.5.3 Optimal selection of the influence and interaction thresholds

It was demonstrated above that imposing an additional restriction (a restriction based on the interaction condition) clearly affects the probabilities of key outcomes in a clinical trial with several patient populations. Additional calculations similar to those presented in Figure 3.16 show that selecting larger values of the influence and interaction thresholds result in a lower probability of the enhanced claim and affect the balance between the probabilities of the broad and restricted claims. Given the important role played by the two thresholds, the sponsor of a multi-population clinical trial would be interested in determining an optimal set of the parameters used in the influence and interaction conditions, i.e., λ_1 and λ_2.

A general clinical trial optimization approach can be employed to develop a "multivariate" algorithm aimed at the selection of an optimal analysis model (i.e., Hochberg-based multiplicity adjustment with an optimal weight parameter) as well as optimal values of the thresholds used in the influence and interaction conditions. For simplicity, a bivariate optimization algorithm for identifying optimal thresholds will be considered in this case study. The w parameter that represents the initial weight of the overall population test in the Hochberg procedure will be fixed at the value selected in Case study 3.1, i.e., $w = 0.8$. The influence and interaction thresholds (λ_1 and λ_2) will serve as the target parameters in this optimization problem.

A natural approach to setting up an evaluation criterion for finding optimal values of the target parameters is to extend the approach that was applied in Case study 3.2 in the context of a clinical trial with two potential efficacy claims. Recall that an optimization algorithm was constructed in that case study to maximize an appropriately defined weighted power function while controlling the influence error rate. Likewise, a weighted power criterion can be utilized in this setting and optimization will be aimed at maximizing weighted power under relevant restrictions on the influence and interaction error rates. The decision rules based on the resulting values of the target parameters will provide a high probability of success in this trial and, at the same time, guarantee acceptable probabilities of incorrectly committing influence or interaction errors.

To implement this approach, the definition of weighted power introduced at the end of Section 3.5.1 will be used, i.e.,

$$\psi_{PW}(\boldsymbol{\lambda}) = 0.32\psi_1(\boldsymbol{\lambda}) + 0.18\psi_2(\boldsymbol{\lambda}) + 0.5\psi_3(\boldsymbol{\lambda}),$$

where, as before, $\boldsymbol{\lambda} = (\lambda_1, \lambda_2)$. This definition relies on the assumption that the prevalence of biomarker-positive patients in the general population of patients with colorectal cancer is $r = 0.55$. A bivariate grid search will be performed to identify optimal values of the target parameters λ_1 and λ_2 that maximize $\psi_{PW}(\boldsymbol{\lambda})$ under the following restrictions:

$$P(\text{Influence error}|\lambda_1) \leq \gamma_1, \ P(\text{Interaction error}|\lambda_1, \lambda_2) \leq \gamma_2,$$

where the acceptable values of the influence and interaction error rates are denoted by γ_1 and γ_2. As a quick note, the probability of an influence error depends only on the first target parameter (λ_1) whereas the probability of an interaction error is influenced by both parameters.

Details of the optimization algorithm are provided below. All calculations were run with the total event count set to 360 events based on the Hochberg procedure with the initial weight of the overall population test set to $w = 0.8$. First of all, Figure 3.18 presents a heat map of weighted power values as a function of the two target parameters. The influence threshold λ_1 ranges between 0 and 0.3 and the interaction threshold λ_2 ranges between 1 and 2. It follows from the figure that weighted power decreased monotonically as either target parameter increased and, if no restrictions based on error rate control were imposed, weighted power would be maximized by simply setting λ_1 to 0 and λ_2 to 1. This maximum value of weighted power would equal 40.0%. Since the restrictions are in fact imposed, it is important to examine the influence and interaction error rates for the same combinations of the target parameters.

Heat maps for the influence and interaction error rates for the same sets

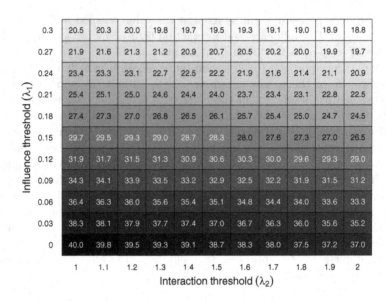

FIGURE 3.18: Weighted power as a function of the influence threshold (λ_1) and interaction threshold (λ_2) in Case study 3.3.

of λ_1 and λ_2 are shown in Figures 3.19 and 3.20. As a quick reminder, the influence error rate was evaluated under the assumption of no beneficial effect in the biomarker-negative subpopulation, i.e., the calculation was performed by forcing the hazard ratio in this subpopulation to be equal to 1:

$$\delta_- = 1, \ \delta_+ = 0.6.$$

The interaction error rate was computed by forcing the hazard ratios to be the same in the two subsets of the overall population:

$$\delta_- = 0.6, \ \delta_+ = 0.6.$$

The influence error rate decreased monotonically with the increasing influence threshold λ_1 in Figure 3.19 (as indicated above, the influence error rate does not depend on the interaction threshold and any changes across the columns of this heat map were due to Monte Carlo error). It is worth noting that the probability of an influence error decreased at a much slower rate in this clinical trial example compared to Case study 3.2 (see Figure 3.13). As a quick comparison, the influence error rate was around 35% with $\lambda_1 = 0$ and quickly dropped to below 10% at $\lambda_1 = 0.1$ in Case study 3.2. The influence error rate is affected by the total sample size in a clinical trial and population prevalence of biomarker-positive patients. For example, this error rate tends to decrease quite rapidly with the increasing threshold if the total number of patients or events is large and population prevalence is low.

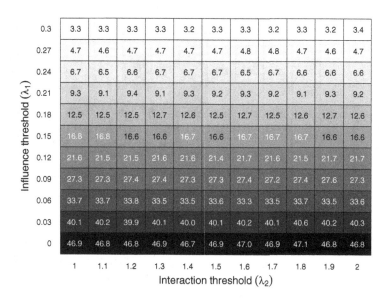

FIGURE 3.19: Influence error rate as a function of the influence threshold (λ_1) and interaction threshold (λ_2) in Case study 3.3.

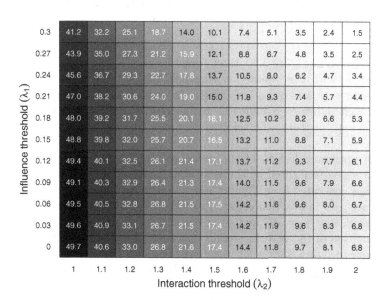

FIGURE 3.20: Interaction error rate as a function of the influence threshold (λ_1) and interaction threshold (λ_2) in Case study 3.3.

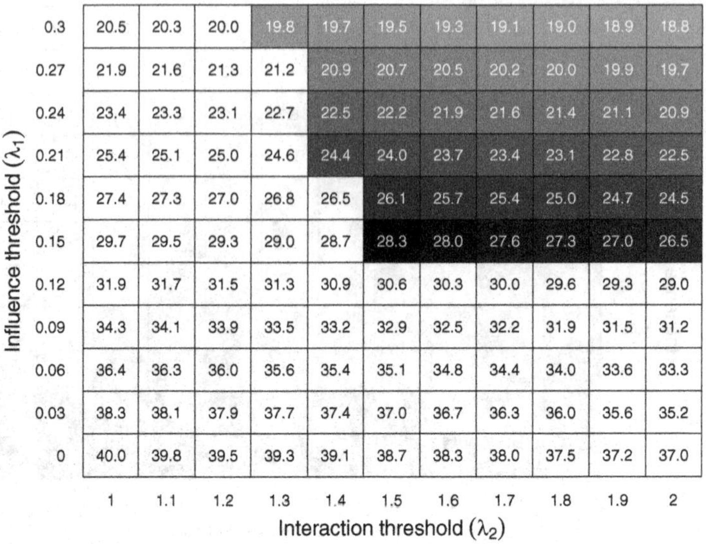

Influence threshold (λ_1)	1	1.1	1.2	1.3	1.4	1.5	1.6	1.7	1.8	1.9	2
0.3	20.5	20.3	20.0	19.8	19.7	19.5	19.3	19.1	19.0	18.9	18.8
0.27	21.9	21.6	21.3	21.2	20.9	20.7	20.5	20.2	20.0	19.9	19.7
0.24	23.4	23.3	23.1	22.7	22.5	22.2	21.9	21.6	21.4	21.1	20.9
0.21	25.4	25.1	25.0	24.6	24.4	24.0	23.7	23.4	23.1	22.8	22.5
0.18	27.4	27.3	27.0	26.8	26.5	26.1	25.7	25.4	25.0	24.7	24.5
0.15	29.7	29.5	29.3	29.0	28.7	28.3	28.0	27.6	27.3	27.0	26.5
0.12	31.9	31.7	31.5	31.3	30.9	30.6	30.3	30.0	29.6	29.3	29.0
0.09	34.3	34.1	33.9	33.5	33.2	32.9	32.5	32.2	31.9	31.5	31.2
0.06	36.4	36.3	36.0	35.6	35.4	35.1	34.8	34.4	34.0	33.6	33.3
0.03	38.3	38.1	37.9	37.7	37.4	37.0	36.7	36.3	36.0	35.6	35.2
0	40.0	39.8	39.5	39.3	39.1	38.7	38.3	38.0	37.5	37.2	37.0

Interaction threshold (λ_2)

FIGURE 3.21: Weighted power as a function of the influence threshold (λ_1) and interaction threshold (λ_2) in Case study 3.3. A dark-colored cell identifies a combination of the thresholds where the influence error rate and interaction error rate are simultaneously controlled at a 20% level.

As shown in Figure 3.20, the interaction error rate was influenced by both λ_1 and λ_2 with the interaction threshold having a more pronounced effect. The error rate was quite high when the interaction threshold was less than 1.5, which indicates a high risk of incorrectly recommending an enhanced claim when, in truth, the selected biomarker is not predictive of treatment response.

An optimal selection of the influence and interaction thresholds in this case study is facilitated by the heat map displayed in Figure 3.21. This heat map was generated from Figures 3.19 and 3.20 by applying restrictions on the influence and interaction error rates. Both error rates were controlled at a 20% level, i.e., $\gamma_1 = 0.2$ and $\gamma_2 = 0.2$. Each cell in the heat map, i.e., each combination of the two thresholds, was colored white if either error rate was not preserved or a dark color was used when both error rates were controlled. The problem of identifying an optimal combination of the two thresholds simplifies to the problem of finding the cell with the highest weighted power in the subset of dark-colored cells in this heat map. The highest weighted power was achieved with

$$\lambda_1 = 0.15, \ \lambda_2 = 1.5.$$

These optimal values maximize the weighted power criterion under clinically

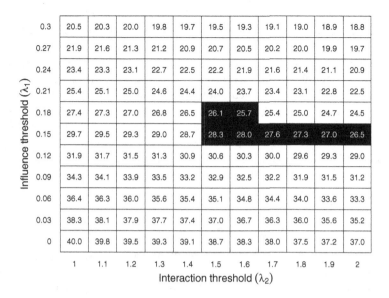

FIGURE 3.22: Weighted power as a function of the influence threshold (λ_1) and interaction threshold (λ_2) in Case study 3.3. The dark-colored cells define a 90% optimal region for the two thresholds.

meaningful restrictions on the probabilities of incorrect decisions in this clinical trial with three potential regulatory claims.

Figure 3.22 displays an approximate 90% optimal region in the optimization problem with $\gamma_1 = 0.2$ and $\gamma_2 = 0.2$. The optimal region is a two-dimensional region which is found based on the same principle as optimal intervals for univariate target parameters considered in Case studies 3.1 and 3.2. Using weighted power associated with the optimal thresholds identified above (i.e., 28.3%), the dark-colored cells in Figure 3.22 were defined as the cells where weighted power was not more than 10% lower than this maximum value on a relative scale. The 90% optimal region consisted of a small cluster of cells in the heat map that resulted in operating characteristics of the decision rules for selecting regulatory claims than were quite similar to those based on the optimal configuration of the two target parameters. The set of nearly optimal values of the influence and interaction thresholds was found approximately in the zone with $0.15 \leq \lambda_1 \leq 0.18$ and $1.5 \leq \lambda_2 \leq 2$.

The optimization algorithm presented above is easily extended to settings where the influence and interaction error rates are controlled at different levels. It can be shown that the optimal combination of the influence and interaction thresholds is quite sensitive to the cap on the influence error rate. For example, if this cap was set to $\gamma_1 = 0.1$ and the interaction error rate was controlled at the same level (i.e., $\gamma_2 = 0.2$), the maximum value of weighted power decreased to 24.4%. By contrast, if the acceptable level of the interaction error rate was lowered to 10% ($\gamma_1 = 0.2$ and $\gamma_2 = 0.1$), the highest value of weighted power changed by only one percentage point (from 28.3% to 27.3%).

A final comment deals with the calculation of the target event count in the oncology clinical trial. Even if the acceptable levels of the influence and interaction error rates are reasonably high, the maximum value of weighted power can end up being quite low. It follows from Figure 3.21 that, with the acceptable levels of the error rates set to $\gamma_1 = 0.2$ and $\gamma_2 = 0.2$, the maximum value of weighted power (28.3%) was way below the target value of 40% computed in Section 3.5.2. To avoid an underpowered trial, the number of events will need to be increased in this case to ensure that weighted power is reasonably close to 40%.

3.5.4   Software implementation

As in Case studies 3.1 and 3.2, the **Mediana** package can be used to perform simulations in the clinical trial considered in this section. The process of defining the data, analysis and evaluation models in this cases study is generally similar to that used in Case study 3.1. It needs to be slightly modified to account for the fact that the trial's primary objective is formulated in terms of analyzing time to disease progression (PFS), which means that the data and analysis models need to be set up based on an exponential distribution and the log-rank test. Moreover, the definitions of broad, restricted and enhanced claims need to be updated to incorporate the influence and interaction conditions.

Data model

The outcome distribution in this case study is exponential and its parameters are defined using the hazard rates presented in Table 3.10.

LISTING 3.11: Outcome parameter specifications in Case study 3.3

```
# Outcome parameters
outcome.placebo.neg = parameters(rate = log(2)/7.5)
outcome.treatment.neg = parameters(rate = log(2)/8.5)
outcome.placebo.pos = parameters(rate = log(2)/7.5)
outcome.treatment.pos = parameters(rate = log(2)/12.5)
```

It is important to note that, if no censoring mechanism is specified in a data model with a time-to-event endpoint, all patients will reach the endpoint of interest (i.e., progression) and thus the number of patients will be equal to the number of events. Using this property, it is sufficient to define the number of patients in each sample, according to the prevalence of biomarker-negative and biomarker-positive patients. The prevalence of biomarker-positive patients in the general population (**prevalence.pos**) is set to 0.55.

LISTING 3.12: Sample sizes specification in Case study 3.3

```
# Sample size parameters
prevalence.pos = 0.55
sample.size.total = 270

sample.size.placebo.neg = round(((1-prevalence.pos) / 2) *
    sample.size.total)
sample.size.placebo.pos = round((prevalence.pos / 2 *
    sample.size.total))
sample.size.treatment.neg = round(((1-prevalence.pos) / 2)
    * sample.size.total)
sample.size.treatment.pos = round((prevalence.pos / 2 *
    sample.size.total))
```

Using these specifications, the data model can be set up as in Case study 3.1 by adding each component to an empty data model. The exponential distribution is defined in the OutcomeDist object.

LISTING 3.13: Data model in Case study 3.3

```
# Data model
subgroup.cs3.data.model =
  DataModel() +
  OutcomeDist(outcome.dist = "ExpoDist") +
  Sample(id = "Placebo Bio-Neg",
         sample.size = sample.size.placebo.neg,
         outcome.par = parameters(outcome.placebo.neg)) +
  Sample(id = "Placebo Bio-Pos",
         sample.size = sample.size.placebo.pos,
         outcome.par = parameters(outcome.placebo.pos)) +
  Sample(id = "Treatment Bio-Neg",
         sample.size = sample.size.treatment.neg,
         outcome.par = parameters(outcome.treatment.neg)) +
  Sample(id = "Treatment Bio-Pos",
         sample.size = sample.size.treatment.pos,
         outcome.par = parameters(outcome.treatment.pos))
```

By default, the outcome type is set to **fixed**, which means that a design with a fixed patient follow-up is assumed even though the primary endpoint in this clinical trial is a time-to-event endpoint. This is due to the fact that, as was explained earlier, no censoring is assumed in this trial and all patients are followed until the event of interest (disease progression) is observed. In the presence of censoring, the outcome type will be set to **event** and the design parameters, e.g., length of the enrollment and follow-up periods, will need to be specified as well.

Analysis model

The analysis model in this clinical trial is very similar to the one defined in Case study 3.2. The only components of the model that need to be modified are the statistical method utilized in the primary analysis (method = "LogrankTest") and method for computing the effect size in the biomarker-negative subpopulation (method = "EffectSizeEventStat"). In addition, the ratio of effect sizes between the biomarker-positive and biomarker-negative subpopulations needs to be computed. This is accomplished by specifying a Statistic object with the RatioEffectSizeEventStat method. This method computes the ratio of effect sizes for exponentially distributed endpoints.

LISTING 3.14: Analysis model in Case study 3.3

```
# Analysis model
subgroup.cs3.analysis.model =
  AnalysisModel() +
  Test(id = "OP test",
       samples = samples(c("Placebo Bio-Neg", "Placebo Bio-
  Pos"),
                              c("Treatment Bio-Neg", "Treatment
  Bio-Pos")),
       method = "LogrankTest") +
  Test(id = "Bio-Pos test",
       samples = samples("Placebo Bio-Pos",
                              "Treatment Bio-Pos"),
       method = "LogrankTest") +
  Statistic(id = "Effect Size in Bio-Neg",
            samples = samples("Placebo Bio-Neg", "Treatment
  Bio-Neg"),
            method = "EffectSizeEventStat") +
  Statistic(id = "Ratio Effect Size Bio-Pos vs Bio-Neg",
            samples = samples("Placebo Bio-Pos",
                                "Treatment Bio-Pos",
                                "Placebo Bio-Neg",
                                "Treatment Bio-Neg"),
            method = "RatioEffectSizeEventStat")    +
  MultAdjProc(proc = "HochbergAdj",
              par = parameters(weight = c(0.8, 0.2)))
```

Evaluation model

As in the evaluation model used in Case study 3.2, custom functions need to be written to support the evaluation of the probabilities of the individual claims and weighted power. Note that the definitions of broad, restricted and enhanced claims need to be updated to account for the interaction condition (see Section 3.5.1). As an illustration, a custom function for computing weighted power (`subgroup.cs3.WeightedPower`) is defined below. Custom functions for evaluating the probabilities of broad, restricted and enhanced claims are set up in a similar way. The `statistic.result` argument in the `subgroup.cs3.WeightedPower` function is a matrix containing the value of the effect size in the biomarker-negative subpopulation and the ratio of effect sizes between the two subpopulations.

LISTING 3.15: Custom function for computing weighted power in Case study 3.3

```
# Custom evaluation criterion based on weighted power
subgroup.cs3.WeightedPower = function(test.result,
    statistic.result, parameter)  {

  alpha = parameter$alpha
  v1 = parameter$v1
  v2 = parameter$v2
  v3 = parameter$v3
  influence_threshold = parameter$influence_threshold
  interaction_threshold = parameter$interaction_threshold

  # Broad claim: (1) Reject OP test but not Bio-Pos or (2)
  #   Reject OP and Bio-Pos test and influence condition is
  #   met but the interaction condition is not met
  broad.claim = ((test.result[,1] <= alpha & test.result
    [,2] > alpha) | (test.result[,1] <= alpha & test.result
    [,2] <= alpha & statistic.result[,1] >= influence_
    threshold & statistic.result[,2] < interaction_
    threshold))

  # Restricted claim: (1) Reject Bio-Pos test but not OP or
  #   (2) Reject Bio-Pos and OP test and influence not met
  restricted.claim = ((test.result[,1] > alpha & test.
    result[,2] <= alpha) | (test.result[,1] <= alpha & test
    .result[,2] <= alpha & statistic.result[,1] < influence
    _threshold))

  # Enhanced claim: (1) Reject Bio-Pos and OP test or
  #   reject both and influence not met
  enhanced.claim = ((test.result[,1] <= alpha & test.result
    [,2] <= alpha & statistic.result[,1] >= influence_
    threshold & statistic.result[,2] >= interaction_
    threshold))

  power = v1 * mean(broad.claim) + v2 * mean(restricted.
    claim) + v3 * mean(enhanced.claim)

  return(power)
}
```

The evaluation model is presented below. The influence threshold (`influence_threshold`) and interaction threshold (`interaction_threshold`) are set to their optimal values, i.e., 0.15 and 1.5, respectively, in the computation of the probabilities of the three claims of interest and weighted power.

LISTING 3.16: Evaluation model in Case study 3.3

```
# Evaluation model
subgroup.cs3.evaluation.model =
  EvaluationModel() +
  Criterion(id = "Marginal power",
            method = "MarginalPower",
            tests = tests("OP test", "Bio-Pos test"),
            labels = c("OP test","Bio-Pos test"),
            par = parameters(alpha = 0.025)) +
  Criterion(id = "Disjunctive power",
            method = "DisjunctivePower",
            tests = tests("OP test", "Bio-Pos test"),
            labels = c("Disjunctive power"),
            par = parameters(alpha = 0.025)) +
  Criterion(id = "Weighted power",
        method = "subgroup.cs3.WeightedPower",
        tests = tests("OP test", "Bio-Pos test"),
        statistics = statistics("Effect Size in Bio-Neg",
                                "Ratio Effect Size Bio-Pos
    vs Bio-Neg"),
        labels = c("Weighted power"),
        par = parameters(alpha = 0.025,
        v1 = 1 / (2 * (1 + prevalence.pos)),
        v2 = prevalence.pos / (2 * (1 + prevalence.pos)),
        v3 = 1/2,
        influence_threshold = 0.15,
        interaction_threshold = 1.5)) +
  Criterion(id = "Probability of a broad claim",
        method = "subgroup.cs3.BroadClaimPower",
        tests = tests("OP test", "Bio-Pos test"),
        statistics = statistics("Effect Size in Bio-Neg",
                                "Ratio Effect Size Bio-Pos
    vs Bio-Neg"),
        labels = c("Probability of a broad claim"),
        par = parameters(alpha = 0.025,
                         influence_threshold = 0.15,
                         interaction_threshold = 1.5)) +
  Criterion(id = "Probability of a restricted claim",
        method = "subgroup.cs3.RestrictedClaimPower",
        tests = tests("OP test", "Bio-Pos test"),
        statistics = statistics("Effect Size in Bio-Neg",
                                "Ratio Effect Size Bio-Pos
    vs Bio-Neg"),
        labels = c("Probability of a restricted claim"),
```

```
      par = parameters(alpha = 0.025,
                       influence_threshold = 0.15,
                       interaction_threshold = 1.5)) +
  Criterion(id = "Probability of an enhanced claim",
      method = "subgroup.cs3.EnhancedClaimPower",
      tests = tests("OP test", "Bio-Pos test"),
      statistics = statistics("Effect Size in Bio-Neg",
                              "Ratio Effect Size Bio-Pos
  vs Bio-Neg"),
      labels = c("Probability of an enhanced claim"),
      par = parameters(alpha = 0.025,
                       influence_threshold = 0.15,
                       interaction_threshold = 1.5))
```

Simulation results

Simulation results based on the R code presented above are summarized in Table 3.11 (the simulations were run with 100,000 replications).

TABLE 3.11: Summary of simulation results.

Evaluation criterion	Value
Marginal power	OP test: 90.4%
	Bio-Pos test: 91.2%
Disjunctive power	92.8%
Weighted power	28.3%
Probability of a broad claim	11.6%
Probability of a restricted claim	49.7%
Probability of an enhanced claim	31.6%

3.5.5 Conclusions and extensions

This section focused on the problem of optimal selection of the parameters of the decision rules (influence and interaction thresholds) used in multi-population clinical trials. A constrained algorithm was developed to identify optimal values of the target parameters that resulted in highest weighted power under clinically relevant constraints on the influence and interaction error rates.

The clinical trial example considered in the case study utilized a time-to-event endpoint and power evaluations were performed without accounting for potential censoring due to loss to follow-up or administrative reasons. This setting is commonly used when the required number of events is computed in oncology trials or other trials with time-to-event outcomes. The next step typically involves calculating the number of patients to be enrolled in the trial when the trial design parameters such as the lengths of the enrollment and follow-up periods are specified. The general approach to optimal selection of the influence and interaction thresholds or other analysis model parameters in this setting will be analogous to the approach presented above.

The optimization problem considered in this case study can be extended by introducing other relevant target parameters. As in other case studies, examples include important analysis model parameters such as the initial weights assigned to the null hypothesis of interest in the multiplicity adjustment. It was assumed in Section 3.5.3 that the weights were fixed (i.e., the weight assigned to the null hypothesis of no treatment effect in the overall population was 80% and the remaining weight was assigned to the null hypothesis of no effect in the pre-specified subpopulation). However, it is reasonable to consider selecting an optimal value of this parameter based on the hypothesized hazard rates.

Further, it is recommended to perform comprehensive sensitivity analyses to assess the robustness of the conclusions with respect to the assumed hazard ratios in the patient populations. Using a quantitative approach similar to that presented in Case study 3.1 (see Section 3.3.5), gamma priors can be assigned to the hazard rates specified in Table 3.10 and a permutation-based algorithm can be applied to evaluate the impact of parameter misspecification on the key operating characteristics such as weighted power. The algorithm can be run using several values of the uncertainty parameter that correspond to increasing variances of the gamma distributions.

4

Decision Making in Clinical Development

Kaushik Patra

Alexion

Ming-Dauh Wang

Eli Lilly and Company

Jianliang Zhang

MedImmune

Aaron Dane

AstraZeneca

Paul Metcalfe

AstraZeneca

Paul Frewer

AstraZeneca

Erik Pulkstenis

MedImmune

4.1 Introduction

Decision making is a critical part of drug development involving information, risk awareness/tolerance, quantification of evidence, and uncertainty. The impact of decisions made is significant. For example, stopping development of a compound due to futility; advancing or not-advancing a compound to the next stage of development; or weighing Phase II data and deciding whether to launch a large and long Phase III program to support a regulatory approval all have significant implications. There is a need to improve productivity by stopping the development of inferior treatments as early as possible, and by accelerating the development of effective treatments (Arrowsmith et al., 2013; Paul et al., 2010). The drug development landscape is replete with examples of failures that may be examined retrospectively via "post-mortem," and second-guessed as to whether the decision making at earlier stages of development was sufficiently robust. In some cases, promising Phase II data are not repeated in Phase III (Brutti et al., 2008; Kirby et al., 2012). In addition, the number of decisions to be made along the way adds to the potential risk. What is the right dose? Should a program be stopped or accelerated? Is there a patient population to develop an enrichment strategy around? As a result, drug developers have increasingly desired quantitative methods to accurately assess all available data and to quantify risk or provide operating characteristics for important decisions. Two closely related concepts are the Go/No-Go (GNG) paradigm where criteria are set to move from Phase II clinical trial data to Phase III studies (Chuang-Stein et al., 2011; Kola et al., 2004; Sabin et al., 2014) and probability of success (POS) calculations that endeavor to quantify how likely future data are to deliver success (Chuang-Stein et al., 2006; O'Hagan et al., 2005). Even the concept of success itself may be defined differently depending on the situation. One sponsor may define success as two statistically significant Phase III trials (technical success), while other sponsors may desire to further quantify the likelihood of meeting a desired target product profile, realizing that statistical success and market acceptance are increasingly becoming two distinct objectives.

Very often Phase II trials are designed to achieve some level of (possibly reduced) statistical significance on a regulatory (or other surrogate) endpoint, or to estimate it with a desired level of precision. An alternative approach may be to design Phase II trials with the goal of enabling sufficiently robust decision making based on operating characteristics of the trial with respect to GNG criteria and associated POS calculations. The Clinical Scenario Evaluation approach (CSE), Benda et al. (2010), is well suited to compare competing trial designs and decision-making criteria, or to assess operating characteristics of various scenarios against sets of assumptions. Key components of the CSE framework are defined in Chapter 1 and this chapter will approach the topics of GNG decision making and POS evaluation from a general CSE perspective. Several proof-of-concept or Phase II trials will be used to illustrate the concepts.

Key CSE considerations in the context of GNG decision making and determination of probability of success will be defined in Section 4.2. A number of case studies will be presented to illustrate the optimization procedures based on the general CSE approach.

4.2 Clinical Scenario Evaluation in Go/No-Go decision making and determination of probability of success

This chapter presents applications of the CSE approach to a general setting for GNG decision making and determination of probability of success in the early phase of clinical development. Main elements of Clinical Scenario Evaluation were introduced in Chapter 1 and will be utilized here in the context of assessing GNG decisions and probability of success. The CSE approach will be applied throughout this chapter to provide a foundation for a number of clinical trial scenarios. These algorithms will deal with optimal selection of analysis models and their parameters or components such as the sample size or probabilistic thresholds related to GNG decisions and probability of success.

4.2.1 Clinical Scenario Evaluation approach

This section introduces the key components of the CSE approach, i.e., data, analysis and evaluation models, used during early phase of clinical development in the context of GNG decision and probability of success evaluation. As explained in Chapter 1, CSE relies on the following three components:

- Data models define the process of generating trial data.

- Analysis models specify the statistical methods applied to the trial data generated based on the data model.

- Evaluation models determine the measures for evaluating the performance of the analysis strategies defined in the analysis model.

The general data, analysis and evaluation models defined below will serve as templates for the models utilized in the case studies presented in Sections 4.4 through 4.8.

Data models

A data model defines the data generation mechanism in a particular clinical trial application. The anchor of any clinical development program is the *target product profile* (TPP) which defines the desired efficacy and safety criteria for a compound. Chuang-Stein et al. (2011) and Lalonde et al. (2007) described the concept of a *lower reference value* (LRV) and a *target value* (TV) that define the TPP. The LRV represents a modest level of efficacy (dignity line), or the lowest level of efficacy that would be of interest (downside). The TV is the target base case efficacy that the sponsor would like to achieve in order to establish the compound as a preferred option or strong competitor relative to the existing standard of care. Setting the TV and LRV typically involves a combination of the synthesis of available evidence in the literature, evaluation of regulatory precedent or feedback (if applicable), and clinical judgment often elicited from external experts.

Consider a clinical trial that is conducted to test the effect of an experimental drug (Treatment 1) on an endpoint of interest in comparison with another treatment (Treatment 2), with the measurement of the endpoint denoted by X_i for Treatment i, $i = 1, 2$. Suppose that n_i patients are enrolled to receive Treatment i, and that will result in the data $X_i = \{X_{i1}, \cdots, X_{in_i}\}, i = 1, 2$, at the end of the trial. For ease of presentation, denote $\mathbf{X} = \{X_i, i = 1, 2\}$, $\boldsymbol{\theta} = \{\theta_i, i = 1, 2\}$, and $\mathbf{n} = \{n_i, i = 1, 2\}$. When considering plausible data models for a Phase II trial, the data may be generated based on the assumption that the treatment effect profile is equivalent to TV. However, the LRV may not be exactly equivalent to the null hypothesis. In some cases LRV may be set to a null value where any improvement over the standard of care would be considered meaningful. In other cases, one may consider LRV as the smallest meaningful difference worth detecting.

Analysis models

The analysis models for the GNG evaluation or POS calculation may depend on the analysis models specified only to test the null hypotheses (such as calculation of p-values based on a frequentist method) or to calculate the metrics related to posterior distribution of a parameter of interest based on Bayesian formulation.

To define a general analysis model, the distribution of X_i is assumed to be defined by the parameter $\boldsymbol{\theta}$. Suppose that the trial is designed to test the null hypothesis

$$H_0: \ M(\boldsymbol{\theta}) \in R$$

against the alternative

$$H_a: \ M(\boldsymbol{\theta}) \in R^c,$$

where M is a metric that measures the distance between θ_1 and θ_2, R is a subspace in the Euclidean space, and R^c is the complement.

Let $T(\mathbf{X})$ denote the statistic for testing H_0 against H_a at the end of the trial at a given one-sided Type I error rate α ($\alpha = 0.025$). Usually fixed values of $\boldsymbol{\theta}$ under H_0 and H_a are assumed for sample size calculations without consideration of their variability. For example, the difference $\Delta = \theta_1 - \theta_2$ (assumed univariate) is often of interest, and $H_0: \Delta = \Delta_0$ is tested against $H_a: \Delta = \Delta_a$. A conventional method of sample size determination would be to calculate the number of patients in the trial that gives at least a probability of $1 - \beta$ (or power) for exhibiting $T(X) > t_\alpha$ under the alternative hypothesis, where t_α is the $100(1 - \alpha)$ percentile of T under the null hypothesis. The value of Δ_0 is typically set as zero, and the value of Δ_a is commonly chosen as representative of the clinically or commercially desired target, such as LRV (denoted as Δ_{LRV}) or TV (denoted as Δ_{TV}) specified in the TPP. The power is highly dependent on the assumed fixed value of Δ_a.

As a quick example, if $\mathbf{X} = \{X_i, i = 1, 2\}$ denotes a set of binary responses (0 or 1) where "1" indicates a clinical response and $\Delta = \theta_1 - \theta_2$ indicates the treatment effect to be tested (θ_1 and θ_2 being the population response rates for Treatments 1 and 2, respectively), the analysis model can be specified by a chi-squared test or a confidence interval. If the objective is to make a GNG decision, a frequentist confidence interval approach (Frewer et al., 2016; Lalonde et al., 2007) can be implemented or a general Bayesian framework employing a credible interval approach can be proposed. We will elaborate on these analysis models in subsequent sections.

Evaluation models

The last element of CSE specifications is a set of evaluation models. Evaluation models define the measures for assessing the performance of the selected analysis strategies and thus play a central role in formulating selection criteria. It was emphasized in Chapter 1 that it is critical to choose evaluation models/criteria that are aligned with the objectives of an optimal decision related to investment in clinical development.

For GNG and POS, evaluation models will be closely related to operating characteristics around correct decision making as well as associated uncertainty. Relevant evaluation criteria are discussed below.

4.2.2 Go/No-Go decision criteria

Depending on the approach adopted by a sponsor, the GNG decision can be based on a simple statistical significance (p-value) criterion or by approximating the probabilities of Go and No-Go decisions based on TPP-provided thresholds and acceptable risks; see Lalonde et al. (2007). In any GNG decision, the following two types of risk are important to consider:

- False No-Go risk: Risk associated with a No-Go decision when the target case profile is true.

- False Go risk: Risk associated with a Go decision when the minimal case profile is the true.

Let τ_{TV} and τ_{LRV} denote the acceptable maximal values associated with the above risks, respectively. These values can be application-specific and depend on the risk tolerance level. The trial's sponsor could pre-specify $\tau_{TV} = 10\%$ and $\tau_{LRV} = 20\%$. These choices will imply that the risk of terminating a commercially competitive compound with $\Delta \geq \Delta_{TV}$ should not exceed 10% while there should be at most 20% risk of progressing a compound that has suboptimal efficacy, i.e., $\Delta \leq \Delta_{TV}$.

A dual criterion to formulate a Go/Indeterminate/No-Go decision structure is set up as follows

- Go decision if $\text{PCT}_{20} > \text{LRV}$ and $\text{PCT}_{90} > \text{TV}$.

- Indeterminate decision if $\text{PCT}_{20} \leq \text{LRV}$ and $\text{PCT}_{90} > \text{TV}$.

- No-Go decision if $\text{PCT}_{90} \leq \text{TV}$.

Here PCT_x denotes the xth percentile of the distribution of the treatment effect Δ. Frewer et al. (2016) investigated this approach further with emphasis on evaluation of different scenarios leading to indeterminate outcomes.

In this chapter, we examine an alternative analysis model proposed by Pulkstenis et al. (2017) under a Bayesian extension of these decision criteria that supports GNG decisions related to a product-specific TPP (Case study 4.1). Bayesian methods allow probabilistic statements regarding the hypothesized treatment effects (product case profiles) pre-specified in a TPP. The posterior distribution readily provides an answer to the question: How likely is the product to achieve the TPP given the current data/knowledge?

As the GNG decision is made based on observed results at the end of the trial, the evaluation of evidence supporting efficacy can naturally be made using the posterior distribution $\pi(\Delta|\mathbf{x})$ of Δ given the data ($\mathbf{x}$) [Bayes' theorem]. Table 4.1 provides the link between TPP case profiles and the associated posterior probabilities to be used to issue the GNG decision. In this table, $F_\Delta(\cdot \mid \mathbf{x})$ denotes the cumulative distribution function of the posterior distribution of Δ. Although the segments $\{\mathbf{M}, \mathbf{L}, \mathbf{T}\}$ of the parameter space are mutually exclusive, one may combine $\mathbf{L}$ and $\mathbf{T}$ together to form a domain for a Go decision.

Let τ_{TV} and τ_{LRV} denote the risk thresholds corresponding to false No-Go and false Go decisions. Let us also assume that $\tau_{TV} = 10\%$ and $\tau_{LRV} = 20\%$. These choices in a Bayesian setting will imply that the maximum acceptable risk of that ($\Delta \in T$) in the presence of a No-Go decision should not exceed 10% while there should be at most 20% risk of ($\Delta \in M$) in the presence of a Go decision. Based on these considerations, Table 4.2 provides a set of rules for the Go, Indeterminate and No-Go decisions derived from the posterior probabilities (Criteria 1 and 2). The rules are illustrated in Figure 4.1.

A No-Go decision is reached if the posterior distribution-based evidence suggests that the probability associated with the target case profile is less than or equal to τ_{TV}. A Go decision is reached if the posterior probability of the minimal TPP profile is at most τ_{LRV} and the probability of the target profile is at least τ_{TV}. Remaining combinations will lead to an Indeterminate decision. These decisions can also be made based on an asymmetric $100 \times (1 - \tau_{TV} - \tau_{LRV})\%$ Bayesian credible interval $(\hat{\Delta}_{LRV}, \hat{\Delta}_{TV})$ as shown in Figure 4.2. The lower and upper tail probabilities are set to τ_{LRV} and τ_{TV} respectively, i.e.,

$$\int_{\Delta < \hat{\Delta}_{TV}} \pi(\Delta|\mathbf{x})\, d\Delta = 1 - \tau_{TV}, \quad \int_{\Delta < \hat{\Delta}_{LRV}} \pi(\Delta|\mathbf{x})\, d\Delta = 1 - \tau_{LRV}. \quad (4.1)$$

TABLE 4.1: Posterior probabilities associated with three TPP case profiles.

Minimal (**M**: $\Delta \le \Delta_{\mathrm{LRV}}$)	$P_\Delta(\mathbf{M} \mid \mathrm{x}) = \int_{\Delta \in \mathbf{M}} \pi(\Delta \mid \mathbf{x}) d\Delta = F_\Delta(\Delta_{\mathrm{LRV}} \mid \mathbf{x})$
Lower (**L**: $\Delta_{\mathrm{LRV}} < \Delta < \Delta_{\mathrm{TV}}$)	$P_\Delta(\mathbf{L} \mid \mathrm{x}) = \int_{\Delta \in \mathbf{L}} \pi(\Delta \mid \mathbf{x}) d\Delta$ $= F_\Delta(\Delta_{\mathrm{TV}} \mid \mathbf{x}) - F_\Delta(\Delta_{\mathrm{LRV}} \mid \mathbf{x})$
Target (**T**: $\Delta \ge \Delta_{\mathrm{TV}}$)	$P_\Delta(\mathbf{T} \mid \mathrm{x}) = \int_{\Delta \in \mathbf{T}} \pi(\Delta \mid \mathbf{x}) d\Delta = 1 - F_\Delta(\Delta_{\mathrm{TV}} \mid \mathbf{x})$

TABLE 4.2: Bayesian dual decision rules for the GNG framework.

Decision	Posterior probability-based criteria	Credible interval-based criteria
Go	Criterion 1: $P_\Delta(\mathbf{T} \mid \mathrm{x}) > \tau_{TV}$ Criterion 2: $P_\Delta(\mathbf{M} \mid \mathrm{x}) < \tau_{LRV}$	$\hat{\Delta}_{TV} > \Delta_{TV}$ and $\hat{\Delta}_{LRV} > \Delta_{LRV}$
Indeterminate	Criterion 1: $P_\Delta(\mathbf{T} \mid \mathrm{x}) > \tau_{TV}$ Criterion 2: $P_\Delta(\mathbf{M} \mid \mathrm{x}) > \tau_{LRV}$	$\hat{\Delta}_{TV} > \Delta_{TV}$ and $\hat{\Delta}_{LRV} < \Delta_{LRV}$
No-Go	Criterion 1: $P_\Delta(\mathbf{T} \mid \mathrm{x}) \le \tau_{TV}$ Criterion 2: NA	$\hat{\Delta}_{TV} < \Delta_{TV}$

Note that the posterior probability-based criteria and credible interval-based criteria can be used interchangeably. In summary, when the credible interval includes Δ_{TV}, but not Δ_{LRV}, a Go decision is prescribed; if the credible interval does not include Δ_{TV}, a No-Go decision is issued and, finally, an Indeterminate decision is adopted if the credible interval includes both Δ_{LRV} and Δ_{TV}.

The proposed framework is anchored with probability thresholds to make decisions rather than the magnitude of point estimates subjectively determined to be "good enough." This allows the trial's sponsor to know what levels of efficacy are likely to trigger different decisions and also to incorporate historical information through an informative prior, if existing clinical data are available. The concept of posterior probability can be used at any stage of the clinical development starting from pre-POC studies; for example, the biomarker data generated from Phase I studies may inform further clinical development in this quantitative setting.

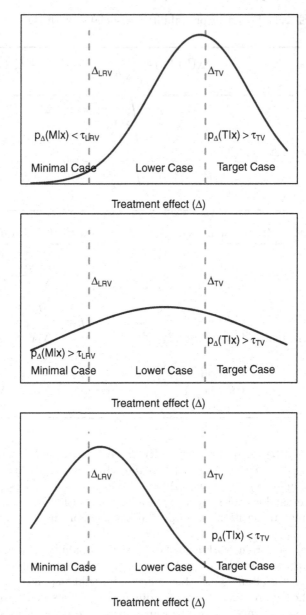

FIGURE 4.1: Visualization of posterior distributions associated with a Go decision (top panel), Indeterminate decision (center panel) and No-Go decision (bottom panel).

4.2.3   Probability of success

The common and long-standing approach to sample size determination for a clinical trial is based on assuming fixed values of unknown parameters to strike

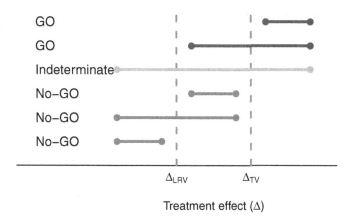

FIGURE 4.2: Visualization of GNG decisions based on credible intervals.

a balance between acceptable study power and Type I error rate. However, ignorance of the uncertainty around the parameters often leads to an underestimated sample size or an overoptimistic estimate of the chances of success, which in turn accounts for more frequent than expected trial failure. As a remedy to this problem, the approach termed *Probability of Success* (POS) has been promoted for more accurate estimation of the probability of a trial in achieving trial significance (Chuang-Stein et al., 2006; O'Hagan et al., 2005; Wang et al., 2013; Wang, 2015) but can also be extended to the probability of achieving a target level of efficacy. POS relaxes the fixed-value basis and assumes that the treatment effect parameters come from random distributions instead, which would then require more intense computation, often by simulation.

The POS approach will be reviewed in the generally more understood frequentist perspective, as well as from the Bayesian viewpoint. In application of POS, distributions of the parameters of interest are typically elicited from data collected in earlier trials of the same study treatment or published results of similar treatments. Often unnoticed, these sources of prior information for designing a new trial biasedly represent only positive outcomes of all conducted trials, which would result in an undersized trial if used without adjustment. This critical issue will be discussed and appropriate adjustment methods will be developed; see Case studies 4.4 and 4.5 for more information.

Mixed Bayesian-frequentist approach

Instead of focusing on a fixed value of the treatment effect θ in a clinical trial, a distribution which reflects up-to-date knowledge of this parameter is assumed.

Statistical power averaged over the distribution of θ is more representative of what the trial can achieve in terms of POS. Using more general notation, let the prior distribution of θ be denoted as $\pi(\theta)$. At the time of designing a trial, the data $\mathbf{X}$ is yet unobserved, which is predicted given the prior $\pi(\theta)$ and the assumed density $f(\mathbf{x}|\theta)$. That is, the predictive density of θ is given by

$$\tilde{f}(\mathbf{x}) = \int f(\mathbf{x}|\theta)\pi(\theta)\, d\theta.$$

Then the POS is defined as

$$\text{POS} = \int \mathbf{I}\{T_0(\mathbf{x}) > t_\alpha \mid \mathbf{x}\}\tilde{f}(\mathbf{x})\, d\mathbf{x},$$

where T_0 is the test statistics under H_0, and $\mathbf{I}$ is the indicator function that returns 0 or 1 given the input. The predictive density function $\tilde{f}$ is typically not easy to derive and it is recommended to re-write the POS as follows

$$\text{POS} = \int \left(\int \mathbf{I}\{T_0(\mathbf{x}) > t_\alpha \mid \mathbf{x}\}f(\mathbf{x}|\theta)\, d\mathbf{x} \right) \pi(\theta)\, d\theta,$$

which is more conducive to simulation-based calculations.

By considering uncertainty of assumptions, the POS is typically lower than the power that would result from a conventional power calculation for a given sample size. This is because power drops as the assumed treatment effect decreases more than the gain in power seen with a larger treatment effect. It indicates that the conventional sample size determination tends to over-estimate the probability of a trial being successful, and the POS approach would better reflect the ability of a trial to achieve the intended objective.

Other criteria can be added to define "success" in a clinical trial. For example, in the case of frequentist hypothesis testing based on $\Delta = \theta_1 - \theta_2$, it could be critical to not only obtain a significant p-value for the test but also observe an estimate of Δ that is above a meaningful threshold, say, $\delta \geq 0$ (Chuang-Stein et al., 2011; O'Hagan et al., 2005). This threshold resembles the target value (TV) defined earlier in this chapter. If Δ is estimated by the observed mean difference $\bar{x}_1 - \bar{x}_2$, the POS would be calculated by

$$\text{POS} = \int \left(\int \mathbf{I}\{T_0(\mathbf{x}) > t_\alpha \text{ and } \bar{x}_1 - \bar{x}_2 > \delta \mid \mathbf{x}\}f(\mathbf{x}|\theta)\, d\mathbf{x} \right) \pi(\theta)\, d\theta.$$

Showing a significant test on Δ is a requirement for regulatory approval, whereas exhibiting a large clinically meaningful treatment difference is a key consideration for the trial sponsor and, increasingly, for health reimbursement authorities around the world.

It is worth noting that the POS concept has been proposed and applied to conducting interim assessments in an ongoing trial (Dmitrienko and Wang, 2006; Spiegelhalter et al. 2004; Wang, 2007). It was termed the *predictive power approach* and positioned as an alternative to the *conditional power approach* (Lan et al., 1982). Applications of this methodology to clinical trial design could be seen as a special case of its use in interim assessments, as no interim data are available for update and the prediction of the required sample size is based purely on pre-study prior knowledge. This mixed Bayesian-frequentist approach is more appropriate for confirmatory clinical trials because frequentist analysis for the primary endpoint is usually required.

Fully Bayesian approach

Though a frequentist test and the associated treatment effect p-value are still generally required for judging the success of a clinical trial intended for regulatory approval, p-values are often not conducive to decision making (Wasserstein and Lazar, 2016). An alternative approach (fully Bayesian approach) relies on a Bayesian analysis at the end of the trial that would provide a statement about the treatment effect θ in terms of its distribution. This approach provides useful information for the subsequent clinical trials.

Using the notation introduced above, this posterior probability is $P(\theta \in H_a|\mathbf{X})$, which is the updated probability of the alternative hypothesis at the end of the trial and would indicate success of the trial if it is greater than a pre-specified threshold $\eta > 0$. Upon observing $\mathbf{X} = \mathbf{x}$ at the end of the trial, $P(\theta \in H_a|\mathbf{X})$ is realized as

$$P(\theta \in H_a|\mathbf{x}) = \int \mathbf{I}\{\theta \in H_a\}g(\theta|\mathbf{x})d\theta,$$

where $g(\theta|\mathbf{x}) = f(\mathbf{x}|\theta)\pi^\star(\theta)$ if another prior $\pi^\star(\theta)$ is used for the final analysis. Then sample size determination is made by the calculation of POS expressed by POS $= \int \mathbf{I}\{P(\theta \in H_a|\mathbf{x}) > \eta\}\tilde{f}(\mathbf{x})d\mathbf{x}$. To facilitate simulation-based calculations, the POS can be expressed as

$$\text{POS} = \int \left(\int \mathbf{I}\{P(\theta \in H_a|\mathbf{x}) > \eta\}f(\mathbf{x}|\theta)d\mathbf{x} \right) \pi(\theta) \, d\theta.$$

Note that the prior $\pi(\theta)$ used at the trial's design stage is called the *design prior* and the prior $\pi^\star(\theta)$ assigned for final analysis is termed the *analysis prior* (Brutti et al., 2008). Different opinions are held for whether the two priors should be assumed different.

Regarding the selection of the value of η, Dmitrienko and Wang (2006) suggested that "η is mathematically related to the frequentist significance level and, for this reason, is often set to a value between 0.9 and 0.975." This recommendation is reasonable for confirmatory trials but seems too stringent in early-phase exploratory trials. In the latter case, a value between 0.6 and 0.8 would facilitate more practical decision making in early-phase development. Also, returning to the fact that POS tends to be lower than frequentist power, the statement holds true if the analysis prior is non-informative. However, the use of more informative and optimistic analysis priors could increase the value of POS compared to frequentist power.

Simulation-based POS calculations

Although analytical formulas may be derived for simple cases, POS is generally approximated by simulation. Let n denote the total sample size in a clinical trial. Beginning with the mixed Bayesian-frequentist approach, POS is estimated using the following algorithm:

1. Simulate a value of θ from $\pi(\theta)$.
2. Given the value of θ, simulate n observations from $f(x|\theta)$.
3. Given the observations, declare success if $T_0(\mathbf{x}) > t_\alpha$.
4. Repeat the above steps a large number of times. The proportion of successes is an estimate of POS.

For the fully Bayesian approach, the following algorithm is used:

1. Simulate a value θ from the design prior $\pi(\theta)$.
2. Given the value of θ, simulate n observations from $f(x|\theta)$.
3. Given the observations and the analysis prior $\pi^\star(\theta)$, calculate the posterior probability $P(\theta \in H_a|\mathbf{x})$ and declare values greater than η as a success.
4. Repeat the above steps a large number of times. The proportion of successes is an estimate of POS.

The number of simulations needed in Step 4 of the simulation-based algorithms would generally depend on the complexity of sampling from the distribution of the test statistic $T_0(\mathbf{x})$ in the mixed Bayesian-frequentist approach or computing $P(\theta \in H_a|\mathbf{x})$ in the fully Bayesian approach. In particular, Markov Chain Monte Carlo (MCMC) is often applied in the latter case and convergence checks are required to ensure a reliable calculation of POS.

4.2.4 Probability of success applications

Overall, an appropriately defined probability of success can help provide a realistic assessment of whether a clinical trial is likely to meet its stated goals. Although POS is not intended to replace the well-established concept of statistical power, it can be used alongside standard power calculations to provide additional information critical for informed decision making and risk assessment throughout a drug development program.

Comparison of POS and Go/No-Go approaches

Treating the treatment effect assumptions at the start and analysis at the end as the two bookends of designing a trial, the approaches introduced earlier in this section (POS-based and Go/No-Go approaches) can be summarized as follows:

- The frequentist Go/No-Go approach is non-Bayesian on both design and analysis ends.

- The Bayesian version of Go/No-Go is Bayesian on the analysis end.

- The mixed Bayesian-frequentist POS is Bayesian on the design end.

- The fully Bayesian version of POS is Bayesian on both ends.

The appropriateness and selection of one approach over another would depend on the phase of the trial and sponsor's preferences. One general comment is that Bayesian methods applied on the design end, as represented by the POS approaches, would better reflect what a trial can really achieve. Bayesian analysis at the end, as adopted by the Bayesian Go/No-Go and fully Bayesian approaches, tends to facilitate post-trial decision making.

Software implementation

Conceptually, computing a POS value for a single trial or even entire Phase III program is fairly simple. First, an appropriate Bayesian model is fitted to existing data in a trial. It is important to check the model and ensure that it fits the data adequately. The model is used to simulate clinical trials or Phase III programs. For each of those simulations, a success is defined using appropriate criteria and the average over the simulation runs is used to compute an overall POS. Informative prior data or shrinkage models can be applied, perhaps as a meta-regression, and, in principle, simulations can be performed down to the individual patient level, handling multiple testing and a Phase III program consisting of multiple trials in detail. In essence, this algorithm is really just a Monte-Carlo evaluation of the underlying integrals that define the POS and it is difficult to see how any standard tools can be produced beyond those that are used for general-purpose modeling and simulation. However, the full problem is not necessarily that which needs to be solved. While it may be conceptually attractive and sometimes necessary to fit the POS problem into a general-purpose modeling and simulation framework, much of the time the full power of this approach is not needed and simpler tools can be used. For example, the **assurance** R package available at

```
https://github.com/scientific-computing-solutions/assurance/
```

can be used. This package provides simple code for POS calculations in a variety of scenarios covering broadly used clinical trial endpoints. The package was internally fully documented and an example of its use is provided below.

Consider a Phase II trial with a time-to-event endpoint and suppose that the hazard ratio of 0.7 was observed in this trial, with 20 events on one arm and 25 events on the other. The trial's sponsor in interested in computing the assurance (POS) of a later trial that will be analyzed after 248 events have been observed. To perform this calculation, as shown in Listing 4.1, the `assurance` needs to be loaded and then the Phase II trial data and the structure of the Phase III trial need to be defined. Note that, in this particular case, it is possible to compute POS directly without using simulations.

LISTING 4.1: Basic POS calculations using the Assurance package

```
library("assurance")
hrData = new.survival(0.7, x1=20, x2=25)
later = new.twoArm(size=study.size(total.size=248),
    significance=0.05)
assurance(hrData, later, 100000)
## [1] 0.62993
assurance(hrData, later)
## [1] 0.6295942
```

Now, standard R tools can be used to explore the Phase III trial. Suppose, for instance, that the definition of success in this trial relies on both statistical significance and specific clinical criteria, as discussed previously. The code in Listing 4.2 explores both the effect of the size of the Phase III trial and the magnitude of the treatment effect required on the overall POS.

LISTING 4.2: Advanced POS calculations using the Assurance package

```
library("assurance")
hrData = new.survival(0.7, x1=20, x2=25)
sizes = seq(100, 1000, by=10)
hurdles = c(0.6, 0.7, 0.8, 0.9)
pos =
  vapply(hurdles,
    function(hurdle) {
      vapply(sizes,
        function(size) {
            later = new.twoArm(size=study.size(size),
                               significance=0.05,
                               hurdle=log(hurdle))
            assurance(hrData, later)
        }, 0)
    },
  sizes)
```

More complex scenarios and other endpoints may be examined using this package. Further details are provided in the package's documentation.

4.3   Motivating example

This section introduced a proof-of-concept (POC) trial and illustrates the operating characteristics (evaluation model) of an analysis model based on

TABLE 4.3: Response rates under three data models in the SLE trial.

Data model	Response rate in the placebo arm	Response rate in the treatment arm	Sample size per arm
Data model 1	$\theta_1 = 0.2$	$\theta_2 = 0.3$	$n = 231$
Data model 2	$\theta_1 = 0.2$	$\theta_2 = 0.35$	$n = 109$
Data model 3	$\theta_1 = 0.2$	$\theta_2 = 0.4$	$n = 64$

a traditional hypothesis testing approach in a GNG setting. The discussion will be followed by evaluation of the general Bayesian framework defined in Section 4.2.

4.3.1 Clinical trial

A proof-of-concept trial in patients with systemic lupus erythematous (SLE) will be used as a motivating example. The primary endpoint in this trial is a binary response variable called SLEDAI Responder Index-4 (SRI-4). It is defined as an improvement in the SLE Disease Activity Index by 4 or more points, no new organ involvement with at least moderately active disease on the British Isles Lupus Assessment Group instrument and no disease worsening in the Physicians Global Assessment. This clinical trial is designed as a randomized two-arm trial (experimental treatment versus placebo) with a balanced design.

Suppose that the TPP specifies the LRV and TV for the treatment effect, i.e., the difference between the response rates in the two arms, as $\Delta_{LRV} = 10\%$ and $\Delta_{TV} = 20\%$. Positive values of the treatment effect indicate a beneficial treatment effect. The trial may be powered at an alternative treatment effect of Δ_{LRV} or Δ_{TV} or any other intermediate value. The choice of this value will impact the trial's minimum statistically significant treatment effect that may or may not support a range of hypothesized efficacy relative to the TPP.

Let θ_1 and θ_2 denote the underlying response rates in the treatment and placebo arms, respectively, and $\Delta = \theta_1 - \theta_2$ denote the unknown treatment effect. Suppose that the trial's sponsor is interested in considering three treatment effect scenarios. These scenarios are listed in Table 4.3 and define three data models that will be explored throughout this chapter. The scenario-specific sample sizes (n) shown in the table were computed using a standard formula, i.e.,

$$n = \frac{\left(z_{1-\alpha/2}\sqrt{\bar{\theta}(1-\bar{\theta})} + z_{1-\beta}\sqrt{\theta_1(1-\theta_1) + \theta_2(1-\theta_2)}\right)^2}{(\theta_2 - \theta_1)^2},$$

where $z_{1-\alpha/2}$ and $z_{1-\beta}$ are the standardized normal quantiles, $\bar{\theta} = \frac{1}{2}(\theta_1 + \theta_2)$. The calculations assumed 80% power ($\beta = 0.20$) and a two-sided $\alpha = 0.10$.

The treatment effect test will be carried out based on the simple Pearson chi-squared test. Asymptotic confidence intervals for the difference in response rates will be calculated. With the set-up described above, the GNG decision-making paradigm will be evaluated using the standard frequentist criterion that relies on statistical significance. The frequentist decision rule is defined as follows:

- Go if the observed p-value is statistically significant and observed treatment effect is positive.

- No-Go otherwise.

Under this rule, only two decisions are possible (Go and No-Go) and no Indeterminate decision is encountered. Note that the probability of a Go decision is equal to statistical power at the underlying alternative hypothesis and equal to the one-sided Type I error rate if the treatment difference is set to zero.

Table 4.4 provides the observed treatment effects and associated p-values when marginal statistical significance is observed in each of the three data models. The corresponding treatment effect scenarios would lead to a Go decision for the next trial under the frequentist decision rule. In addition, the following considerations emerge:

1. The observed treatment effect may or may not satisfy the TPP case profiles when the treatment difference is statistically significant.

2. The probability of a Go decision can be quite high even if the observed treatment effect falls into the suboptimal efficacy zone $(\Delta \leq \Delta_{LRV})$.

3. For scenarios where the observed treatment effect falls into the acceptable efficacy zone $(\Delta > \Delta_{LRV})$, the strength of the evidence is often not quantified.

Not all data models would be aligned with the TPP case profiles as pointed out in the first point above. With the increasing sample size in the trial under the three data models, the likelihood of achieving the lower end of TPP, i.e., $\Delta_{LRV} = 10\%$, diminished as the magnitude of the observed treatment effect decreased (from 14.1% to 6.5%). The corresponding 90% asymptotic confidence intervals supported the same conclusions. Under Data model 1, the confidence interval (0.1%, 12.9%) almost completely excluded the TPP. Further, Under Data model 3, although the confidence interval (1.3%, 26.9%) included the TPP, it came with considerable uncertainty because of its width.

To illustrate the second point, Table 4.5 lists the probabilities (operating characteristics) associated with GNG decisions based on the frequentist decision rule as a function of the true treatment difference Δ_T. Note that the probability of an Indeterminate decision was zero as this decision was not feasible. Each data model had a high likelihood $(1-\alpha/2)$ of issuing a No-Go for zero treatment effect. However, across the minimal case profile of the TPP $(\Delta = 10\%)$, the false Go rates increased to between 38% and 80% with the performance worsening with increased sample size. This behavior of the

TABLE 4.4: Summary of minimally significant effects under the three data models.

Data model	Observed response (responders/sample size)		Minimally significant effect (p-value)	90% confidence interval
	Placebo	Treatment		
Data model 1	19.9% (46/231)	26.4% (61/231)	6.5% (0.097)	(0.1%,12.9%)
Data model 2	20.2% (22/109)	30.3% (33/109)	10.1% (0.084)	(0.5%,19.7%)
Data model 3	20.3% (13/64)	34.4% (22/64)	14.1% (0.071)	(1.3%,26.9%)

TABLE 4.5: Operating characteristics of the frequentist decision criterion under the three data models.

Δ_T	Data model 1	Data model 2	Data model 3
	P(Go)		
0%	5%	5%	5%
10%	80%	53%	38%
15%	98%	81%	62%
20%	100%	95%	81%
	P(Indeterminate)		
0%	0%	0%	0%
10%	0%	0%	0%
15%	0%	0%	0%
20%	0%	0%	0%
	P(No-Go)		
0%	95%	95%	95%
10%	20%	47%	62%
15%	2%	19%	38%
20%	0%	5%	19%

frequentist decision rule is understandable since hypothesis testing is formulated for establishing evidence against the null hypothesis and not necessarily evidence in support of the TPP.

While one can readily compute the strength of evidence in support of the TPP based on the observed treatment effect, in practice this is often not done as part of the decision-making process. Hence the actual level of evidence is often unknown and in many cases would not be acceptable upon careful inspection and evaluation in light of the TPP.

In this example, with minimal statistically significant treatment effects, one can use the methods described in Section 4.2.2 to compute the probability of the various TPP case profiles as shown in Table 4.6. It is easy to see that, under Data models 1 and 2, the target case profile was effectively ruled out (it

TABLE 4.6: Strength of evidence for the TPP case profiles when marginal statistical significance is observed under the three data models.

Data model	Posterior probability			
	$P_\Delta(\mathbf{M}\vert x)$	$P_\Delta(\mathbf{L}\vert x)$	$P_\Delta(\mathbf{T}\vert x)$	$P_\Delta(\mathbf{L}\cup\mathbf{T}\vert x)$
Data model 1	0.82	0.18	0.00	0.18
Data model 2	0.50	0.46	0.04	0.50
Data model 3	0.32	0.48	0.20	0.68

was less than 5% likely) and that the minimal case profile was in fact 50-80% likely. These data patterns would actually result in a No-Go decision if the rules defined in Table 4.2 were applied while the design based on Data model 3 would yield an Indeterminate decision.

This illustration highlights the importance of proper selection of the decision rule and that using frequentist rules based on statistical significance does have a corresponding set of value judgments relative to the TPP but they are simply unknown. Careful inspection reveals, in this case, that these decision rules are not satisfactory and would be inconsistent with how one would value efficacy relative to an informed TPP.

4.3.2   Software implementation

R code for evaluating operating characteristics of the frequentist decision rule shown in Table 4.5 is presented in Listing 4.3.

LISTING 4.3: Operating characteristics of the frequentist decision rule

```
OpCharFreq = function(n,true.t=0.2,pbo.rate=0.2,alpha=0.10)
  {
  # n = Sample size per arm
  # true.t = True treatment difference
  # pbo.rate = True placebo response rate
  # alpha = Significance level (two-sided)

  mi=0:n; ri=mi/n; n1=n+1
  rdiff=array(outer(ri,t(ri),"-"),c(n1,n1))
  sei=sqrt((array(outer(mi*(n-mi),t(mi*(n-mi)),"+"),c(n1,n1
    ))+1)/n^3)
  sign=rdiff/sei>qnorm(1-alpha/2)
  probi=array(outer(dbinom(mi,n,pbo.rate+true.t),t(dbinom(
    mi,n,pbo.rate)),"*"),c(n1,n1))
  pr.go=sum(probi[sign])
  list(Pr.GO=pr.go,Pr.NoGO=1-pr.go)
  }
```

The following function call computes the operating characteristics of the frequentist decision rule under Data model 1 when the true treatment difference (Δ_T) is set to 20%.

```
OpCharFreq(n=231,true.t=0.2)
```

4.4 Case study 4.1: Bayesian Go/No-Go decision criteria

After examining the key properties of the frequentist decision rule that relies on statistical significance in light of informing a TPP in a clinical trial, this section evaluates operating characteristics of the Bayesian GNG decision-making paradigm described in Section 4.2.2.

4.4.1 Clinical trial

Data model

The data model to be used in this case study is the same as described in Section 4.3.1.

Analysis model

Consider the clinical trial example introduced in Section 4.3 and let $\pi(\theta_2)$ and $\pi(\theta_1)$ denote two independent prior distributions for the response rates. The posterior distribution of the proportions is given by

$$\pi(\theta_2, \theta_1 | \mathbf{x}) \propto L(\mathbf{x} | \theta_2, \theta_1) \pi(\theta_2) \pi(\theta_1),$$

where $L(\mathbf{x} | \theta_2, \theta_1)$ denotes the likelihood function. The posterior distribution of the treatment effect, $\pi(\Delta | \mathbf{x})$, can be derived from $\pi(\theta_2, \theta_1 | \mathbf{x})$. Let $x_2 \sim Bin(n, \theta_2)$ and $x_1 \sim Bin(n, \theta_1)$ denote the number of SRI-4 responders in the placebo and treatment arms, respectively. Assume that both $\pi(\theta_2)$ and $\pi(\theta_1)$ represent non-informative priors, i.e., uniform distributions. Then the posterior distributions of θ_2 and θ_1 will be $Beta(\alpha_2, \beta_2)$ and $Beta(\alpha_1, \beta_1)$, respectively, where $\alpha_i = x_i + 1$ and $\beta_i = n - x_i + 1$, $i = 1, 2$. Consequently, the prior and posterior distributions of Δ can be generated by calculating the difference between θ_2 and θ_1 generated from their respective prior and posterior distributions. Sverdlov et al. (2014) provided exact Bayesian posterior inferences for the difference in response rates as well as R code to facilitate computations. The cumulative distribution function for Δ corresponding to the posterior distribution $\pi(\Delta | x)$ is given by:

$$F_\Delta(t) = \begin{cases} \int_{-t}^1 F_{\theta_1}(t+\mu) f_{\theta_2}(\mu) d\mu, & 1 \le t \le 0, \\ \int_0^{1-t} F_{\theta_1}(t+\mu) f_{\theta_2}(\mu) d\mu + \int_{1-t}^1 f_{\theta_2}(\mu) d\mu, & 0 \le t \le 1. \end{cases}$$

Using this posterior, the probabilities associated with the TPP case profiles can be computed (Table 4.1) and the decision rules for GNG (Table 4.2) can be applied.

Evaluation model

Let us now examine the operating characteristics of the proposed Bayesian GNG criteria described in Section 4.2.2 for various underlying values of Δ denoted by Δ_T) and the analysis model described previously. The posterior distribution of Δ will be simulated and the decision probabilities will be quantified based on the simulation steps described below. The simulations can be performed in two ways: using exact computation of the posterior distribution (Sverdlov et al., 2014) or a simulation-based approach which may be required in cases where exact computations on the posterior do not exist or are overly complicated.

The following algorithm is used to perform an exact computation of the posterior distribution:

1. Simulate the number of responders, $x_2 \sim Bin(n, \theta_2)$ and $x_1 \sim Bin(n, \theta_1)$, where $\theta_1 = \theta_2 + \Delta_T$, in the placebo and treatment arms, respectively.

2. Calculate $\alpha_i = x_i + 1$ and $\beta_i = n - x_i + 1$, $i = 1, 2$.

3. Calculate $P(\mathbf{T} \mid x_1, x_2)$ and $P(\mathbf{M} \mid x_1, x_2)$ based on the exact posterior distribution of $\Delta = \theta_1 - \theta_2$.

4. Issue a decision of Go, Indeterminate, or No-Go based on the rules as described in Table 4.2.

5. Repeat the above steps for a specified number of iterations, e.g., 10,000,

6. Calculate the proportion of cases with each decision.

Alternatively, the following simulation-based algorithm can be applied:

1. Simulate the number of responders, $x_2 \sim Bin(n, \theta_2)$ and $x_1 \sim Bin(n, \theta_1)$, where $\theta_1 = \theta_2 + \Delta_T$, in the placebo and treatment arms, respectively.

2. Calculate $\alpha_i = x_i + 1$ and $\beta_i = n - x_i + 1$, $i = 1, 2$.

3. Simulate M (say, 1,000) pairs of response rates, θ_i, from $Beta(\alpha_i, \beta_i)$, $i = 1, 2$, and calculate $\Delta = \theta_1 - \theta_2$ for each simulated pair.

4. Calculate empirical quantiles $\hat{\Delta}_{LRV}$ and $\hat{\Delta}_{TV}$ and form the $100 \times (1 - \tau_{TV} - \tau_{LRV})\%$ credible interval.

5. Issue a decision of Go, Indeterminate, or No-Go based on the rules as described in Table 4.2.

6. Repeat the above steps for a specified number of iterations, e.g., 10,000.

7. Calculate the proportion of cases with each decision.

Table 4.7 provides the decision probabilities under the full simulation approach under the three data models defined in Section 4.3 for several values of the true treatment difference Δ_T. As shown in this table, all three data models provided a sufficiently high level of the probability of a Go decision when the true treatment effect met the target profile ($\Delta_T = \Delta_{TV} = 0.2$) and a high level of the probability of a No-Go decision when there was no treatment effect. In addition, the latter probability remained relatively low at 11% when $\Delta_T = \Delta_{TV} = 0.2$. It is immediately apparent that even across underlying values that span the TPP, a variety of decisions may ultimately result. The probability of an Indeterminate decision was zero under Data model 1 for all cases described in Table 4.7 leading to clarity in the decision-making process. This clarity comes at the expense of a very large trial which may be deemed undesirable (recall that the sample size per arm was 231 in Data model 1). A practical tradeoff may be to accept some level of a non-zero probability of an Indeterminate decision. Under Data model 3, this probability ranged from 24% to 30% across the TPP which may be viewed as acceptable or not depending on desired precision. Note that Data model 2 cut the Indeterminate zone approximately in half relative to Data model 3. This reflects the inherent uncertainty present in mid-stage trials, where the sponsor needs to decide on whether or not to advance the compound based on limited information. However, this uncertainty can be calibrated by the user via sample size and controlled at the design stage.

As a result, the Phase II trial may be designed to produce acceptable operating characteristics in light of acceptable error rates and level of uncertainty. Data model 2 may be an optimal choice among the three because it leads to a relatively low probability of an Indeterminate decision. Figure 4.3 provides a visual representation of the decision probabilities under this data model.

4.4.2 General sensitivity assessments

It is also helpful to evaluate how sensitive the operating characteristics of Bayesian decision criteria are relative to the values in the TPP. While it would not be advisable to alter a TPP in order to improve operating characteristics, one can learn how the TPP itself impacts operating characteristics, which in turn gives insight into how challenging the drug development process may be with respect to decision making. For example, if Δ_{LRV} is set to 0.12 and

TABLE 4.7: Operating characteristics of the
Bayesian decision criterion under the three data
models.

Δ_T	Data model 1	Data model 2	Data model 3
		P(Go)	
0%	0%	0%	1%
10%	11%	19%	20%
15%	51%	49%	42%
20%	89%	79%	65%
		P(Indeterminate)	
0%	0%	1%	4%
10%	0%	12%	27%
15%	0%	16%	30%
20%	0%	10%	24%
		P(No-Go)	
0%	100%	99%	95%
10%	90%	69%	54%
15%	49%	34%	28%
20%	11%	11%	11%

TABLE 4.8: Operating characteristics of the
Bayesian decision criterion under the three data
models using an alternate TPP with $\Delta_{LRV} = 0.12$ and
$\Delta_{TV} = 0.20$.

Δ_T	Data model 1	Data model 2	Data model 3
		P(Go)	
10%	9%	11%	12%
15%	45%	36%	29%
20%	85%	68%	53%
		P(Indeterminate)	
10%	2%	20%	34%
15%	6%	29%	43%
20%	4%	22%	36%
		P(No-Go)	
10%	90%	69%	54%
15%	49%	34%	28%
20%	11%	11%	11%

the original value of Δ_{TV} is kept, i.e., $\Delta_{TV} = 0.20$, Table 4.8 provides the
estimated decision probabilities using this alternate TPP.

It can be seen from Table 4.8 that the probability of an Indeterminate
decision increased dramatically and the probability of a Go decision decreased
compared to the TPP based on the original values of Δ_{LRV} and Δ_{TV}. This is
intuitive as decision-making uncertainty increases if the TPP case profiles are

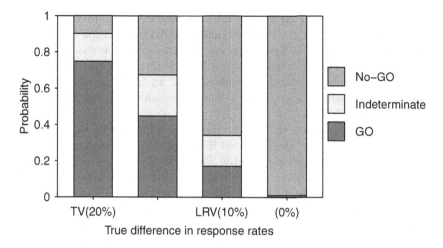

FIGURE 4.3: Decision probabilities of the Bayesian decision criterion under Data model 2.

not well distinguished as measured by the distance between Δ_{LRV} and Δ_{TV}. Figure 4.4 displays the decision probabilities under this alternate TPP.

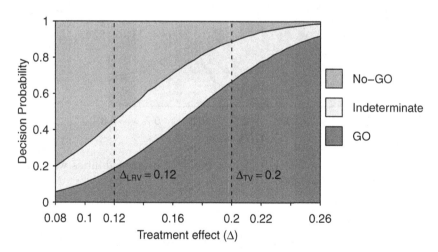

FIGURE 4.4: Decision probabilities of the Bayesian decision criterion under Data model 2 using an alternate TPP with $\Delta_{LRV} = 0.12$ and $\Delta_{TV} = 0.20$.

Further, Figure 4.5 provides a visual summary of the impact of considering different TPPs under Data model 2, where the TPPs differ in terms of the relative distance between Δ_{LRV} and Δ_{TV} (measured by the ratio Δ_{LRV}/Δ_{TV}) for the fixed $\Delta_{TV} = 0.2$. The probability of a No-Go decision did not change as it only depended on Δ_{TV}; however, the tradeoff between the probability of a Go decision and probability of an indeterminate decision was a function of the ratio Δ_{LRV}/Δ_{TV}. The probability of an Indeterminate decision approached zero when $\Delta_{LRV}/\Delta_{TV} = 0.36$ or became unacceptably large when $\Delta_{LRV}/\Delta_{TV} = 0.8$.

This example shows that, while there are a number of ways to design a proof-of-concept study, the proposed Bayesian GNG decision criteria directly inform a reasonably well constructed TPP. The allowable size of the Indeterminate zone is an important determination that should reflect the risk the trial's sponsor is willing to take regarding generation of data that are inconclusive at the end. This must be weighed against the trial's cost and how quickly data may be available for decision making. An early decision that carries more uncertainty may be superior to waiting for complete clarity that removes the uncertainty risk, but at the opportunity cost of time spent.

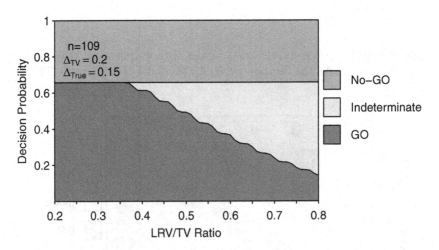

FIGURE 4.5: Impact of Δ_{LRV} on the decision probabilities when Δ_{TV} is fixed under Data model 2.

4.4.3 Bayesian Go/No-Go evaluation using informative priors

The Bayesian framework of GNG evaluation provides ability to improve decision making by incorporating relevant prior information, if available. For instance, if promising results are available from a "small" historical SLE trial similar to one described in Section 4.3, the GNG decision can be enhanced by

TABLE 4.9: Operating characteristics of the Bayesian decision criterion with non-informative priors and informative priors under the three data models. NI denotes non-informative priors for both response rates.

Δ_T	Data model 1				Data model 2				Data model 3			
					Prior distribution/historical treatment effect							
	NI	10%	15%	20%	NI	10%	15%	20%	NI	10%	15%	20%
	P(Go)				$n_h = 20$							
0%	0%	0%	0%	0%	0%	0%	0%	1%	1%	1%	2%	3%
10%	11%	8%	10%	12%	19%	19%	23%	28%	20%	17%	23%	29%
15%	51%	46%	51%	55%	49%	48%	54%	60%	41%	37%	45%	52%
20%	89%	87%	89%	91%	78%	75%	82%	85%	65%	61%	68%	75%
					$n_h = 40$							
0%	0%	0%	0%	0%	0%	0%	1%	2%	1%	1%	2%	5%
10%	11%	6%	9%	13%	19%	16%	25%	35%	20%	15%	26%	41%
15%	51%	40%	48%	57%	49%	44%	56%	67%	41%	35%	51%	66%
20%	89%	83%	88%	92%	78%	74%	83%	90%	65%	60%	74%	85%
	P(No-Go)				$n_h = 20$							
0%	100%	100%	100%	100%	99%	100%	99%	99%	95%	96%	94%	91%
10%	89%	92%	90%	88%	69%	74%	69%	63%	54%	60%	52%	43%
15%	49%	54%	49%	45%	35%	41%	35%	29%	27%	34%	27%	21%
20%	11%	13%	11%	9%	11%	14%	11%	8%	12%	15%	10%	7%
					$n_h = 40$							
0%	100%	100%	100%	100%	99%	100%	99%	98%	95%	98%	94%	87%
10%	89%	94%	91%	87%	69%	81%	70%	59%	54%	69%	52%	36%
15%	49%	60%	52%	43%	35%	49%	37%	25%	27%	42%	27%	15%
20%	11%	17%	12%	8%	11%	19%	11%	6%	12%	20%	11%	5%

constructing an informative prior distribution based on the historical results as opposed to using a non-informative prior.

To illustrate this point, consider a two-arm historical SLE trial with $n_h = 20$ patients per arm that resulted in the observed treatment difference of 20% (the placebo and experimental treatment response rates were $\theta_{2h} = 0.2$ and $\theta_{1h} = 0.4$, respectively). This treatment effect was consistent with $\Delta_{TV} = 0.2$. For simplicity, assume that this historical treatment effect is fully relevant to the current trial in the sense that the results can be used to construct a prior distribution without any down weighting.

Given this background information, the prior distribution, $\pi(\theta_2)$, defined in Section 4.4.1 can be constructed as Beta(α_{2h}, β_{2h}) where $\alpha_{2h} = n_h \theta_{2h} = 4$ and $\beta_{2h} = n_h(1 - \theta_{2h}) = 16$. Similarly, the prior $\pi(\theta_1)$ can be constructed as Beta(8,12). The GNG evaluation in this set-up can be carried out by following similar simulation steps as described in Section 4.4.1. The operating characteristics of the resulting Bayesian decision criterion under the three data models are summarized in Table 4.9.

It follows from the table that, for example, when $\Delta_T = 20\%$ and a clinical trial with $n = 64$ patients per arm is considered, the probability of a Go decision improved to the level of 75% and 85% for $n_h = 20$ and 40, respectively. In comparison, the probability of a Go decision was 65% corresponding to the non-informative Beta(1, 1) prior as shown in Table 4.7. These decision probabilities are listed in Table 4.9 under the column labelled "20%" and row labelled "20%." Similarly, the probability of a No-Go decision decreased to 7% and 5% in comparison to 11%. On the other hand, if the historical trial showed a marginal treatment effect consistent with $\Delta_{LRV} = 0.1$, the probability of a Go decision decreased to 61% and 60% compared to 65%. These numerical comparisons show a clear advantage of incorporating informative priors into the decision-making process. The relative advantage of using an informative prior diminishes, however, when the trial sample size increases as in the case of Data model 3 with $n = 231$ per arm. In summary, in comparison to a non-informative prior, when the treatment effect under an informative prior is consistent with Δ_{LRV}, the probability of a Go decision tended to be lower and the probability of a No-Go decision tended to be higher. However, when the informative prior is consistent with Δ_{TV}, the probability of a Go decision is generally higher, whereas the probability of a No-Go decision tends to be lower.

4.4.4 Sample size considerations

Sample size is computed in clinical trials by evaluating appropriate operating characteristics. In this particular setting, sample size calculations can be performed based on the goal of reducing the probability of an Indeterminate decision to an acceptable level. The trial's sponsor may use a graphical tool or an analytical formula proposed below to decide on the final sample size based on risk tolerance and desired operating characteristics. To describe the sample size calculations, consider a situation where the sponsor selected a less discriminating TPP, i.e., $\Delta_{LRV} = 0.12$ and $\Delta_{TV} = 0.20$. Also assume that Data model 3 with 64 patients per arm was initially considered. The computation of posterior probabilities will be identical to those described in Section 4.4.1.

Figure 4.6 presents the simulated decision probabilities for a range of sample sizes with $\Delta_T = 15\%$. It can be seen from this figure that the probability of a Go decision increased with the sample size and exceeded the probability of an Indeterminate decision quite rapidly. In this setting, this crossover happened at approximately $n = 92$ patients per arm which required an additional 28 subjects per arm compared to Data model 3. This type of visual presentation can be a useful tool to decide on the sample size increase in a trial that would benefit the decision-making process. While unlimited resources are prohibitive in Phase II trials, the sponsor may consider increasing the sample size up to the point when the probability of a Go decision exceeds that of an Indeterminate decision or to the point when the probability of an Indeterminate decision is sufficiently small.

Alternatively, the sample size in a trial can be determined through an iterative algorithm to achieve an acceptable magnitude of the probability of an Indeterminate decision. Specifically, assuming an asymptotic normality of the response rates in the proof-of-concept trial, set the probability of an Indeterminate decision to 30%, i.e., $\tau_I = 0.3$, given the true treatment difference Δ_T.

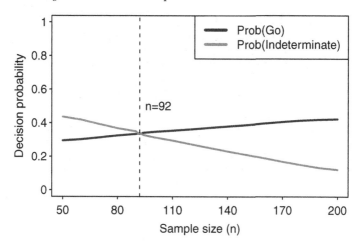

FIGURE 4.6: Probability of Go and Indeterminate decisions as a function of the sample size.

The sample size is computed iteratively as follows:

$$n_i = \frac{2\left[\Phi^{-1}(c)\sqrt{\hat{\sigma}^2_{TV}} + z_{\tau_{LRV}}\sqrt{\hat{\sigma}^2_{LRV}}\right]^2}{(\Delta_T - \Delta_{LRV})^2},$$

where

$$c = \Phi\left((\Delta_{TV}-\Delta_T)\sqrt{\frac{n_{i-1}}{2\hat{\sigma}^2_{TV}}} + z_{\tau_{TV}}\right) + \tau_I.$$

Further,

$$\hat{\sigma}^2_{LRV} = \bar{\theta}_{LRV}(1 - \bar{\theta}_{LRV}) \text{ with } \bar{\theta}_{LRV} = \theta_0 + \frac{\Delta_{LRV}}{2},$$

$$\hat{\sigma}^2_{TV} = \bar{\theta}_{TV}(1 - \bar{\theta}_{TV}) \text{ with } \bar{\theta}_{TV} = \theta_0 + \frac{\Delta_{TV}}{2}$$

and z_u is the normal quantile corresponding to u.

To illustrate, consider the selected TPP, i.e., $\Delta_{LRV} = 0.12$ and $\Delta_{TV} = 0.20$, and let $\tau_{TV} = 10\%$ and $\tau_{LRV} = 20\%$. Under the true treatment difference given by

$$\Delta_T = \frac{\Delta_{TV} + \Delta_{LRV}}{2} = 0.16,$$

the sample size of $n = 110$ per arm will be required to ensure the probability of an Indeterminate decision to 30%. To illustrate the relationship between P(Indeterminate) and corresponding sample size requirements, Table 4.10 provides a summary of sample size calculations assuming that this probability ranges between 0% and 40% with the true effects $\Delta_T = 0.16$ and 0.20.

TABLE 4.10: Required sample size for a pre-specified level of the probability of an Indeterminate decision.

P(Indeterminate)	Sample size per arm	
	$\Delta_T = 0.16$	$\Delta_T = 0.20$
0%	286	286
5%	252	223
10%	220	179
15%	190	144
20%	161	117
25%	135	94
30%	110	74
35%	88	57
40%	67	43

It is easy to verify that, when $\Delta_T = \Delta_{TV}$, the sample size per trial arm can be computed using the following simple formula:

$$ n = \frac{2 \left[z_{1-\tau_I - \tau_{TV}} \sqrt{\hat{\sigma}^2_{TV}} + z_{1-\tau_{LRV}} \sqrt{\hat{\sigma}^2_{LRV}} \right]^2}{(\Delta_{TV} - \Delta_{LRV})^2}. $$

It is important to note that the iterative and closed-form solutions for computing the sample size based on a target value of the probability of an Indeterminate decision are generalizable to other types of clinical endpoint. For example, if the primary endpoint is a time-to-event endpoint, the Bernoulli variance estimates of $\bar{\theta}_{LRV}(1 - \bar{\theta}_{LRV})$ and $\bar{\theta}_{TV}(1 - \bar{\theta}_{TV})$ are replaced by the variance quantities relevant to this type of endpoints. For example, $\sigma^2 = 1$ for the log-hazard ratio, which leads for the iterative formula for computing the number of events in a trial:

$$ m_i = \frac{4 \left[\Phi^{-1} \left(\Phi \left((\Delta_{TV} - \Delta_T) \sqrt{\frac{m_{i-1}}{2}} + z_{\tau_{TV}} \right) + \tau_I \right) + z_{\tau_{LRV}} \right]^2}{(\Delta_T - \Delta_{LRV})^2}. $$

If $\Delta_T = \Delta_{TV}$, the required number of events is computed from

$$ m = \frac{4 [z_{1-\tau_I - \tau_{TV}} + z_{1-\tau_{LRV}}]^2}{(\Delta_{TV} - \Delta_{LRV})^2}, $$

where Δ_{TV} and Δ_{LRV} are the TPP-specified log-hazard ratios. The events may not be evenly distributed between the two trial arms even though the patients are equally allocated.

Similarly, if the primary endpoint is normally distributed, $\sigma^2 = \sigma_0^2$. The required sample size per arm is estimated by

$$ n_i = \frac{2\sigma_0^2 \left[\Phi^{-1} \left(\Phi \left((\Delta_{TV} - \Delta_T) \sqrt{\frac{n_{i-1}}{2\sigma_0^2}} + z_{\tau_{TV}} \right) + \tau_I \right) + z_{\tau_{LRV}} \right]^2}{(\Delta_T - \Delta_{LRV})^2} $$

or, with $\Delta_T = \Delta_{TV}$,

$$n = \frac{2\sigma_0^2[z_{1-\tau_I-\tau_{TV}} + z_{1-\tau_{LRV}}]^2}{(\Delta_{TV} - \Delta_{LRV})^2},$$

where τ_V and Δ_{LRV} are the TPP-specified mean treatment differences.

Finally, if no analytical formula exists, the trial's sponsor may simply generate operating characteristics of the Bayesian decision criteria introduced above for a range of sample sizes and empirically select the data model that results in the desired Indeterminate zone probability.

4.4.5 Software implementation

Listing 4.4 provides the R code to estimate decision probabilities of the Bayesian decision criterion introduced in this case study, e.g., the operating characteristics shown in Table 4.7. An example of the function call corresponding to Data model 2 with 109 patients per trial arm and true treatment difference of 15% is provided at the end of this listing.

LISTING 4.4: Operating characteristics of Bayesian decision criteria with a non-informative prior

```
OpCharNonInf  = function(TV=0.2,LRV=0.1,pbo.rate=0.2,n,delta
   , seed=12345,iter.n=100000) {
  # TV = Target value
  # LRV = Lower reference value
  # prob.rate = True placebo response rate
  # delta = True treatment difference
  # iter.n = Number of simulation runs
  n0 = 2; a0 = c(1,1); b0 = n0-a0
  set.seed(seed); pLTV = c(.8,.1)
  LTV = c(LRV,TV)
  p0i = rbinom(iter.n,n,pbo.rate)+a0[1]
  p1i = rbinom(iter.n,n,pbo.rate+delta)+a0[2]
  b0i = n-p0i+n0; b1i = n-p1i+n0
  nmean = p1i/(n+n0)-p0i/(n+n0)
  nsd = sqrt(p1i*b1i/(n+n0)^2/(n+n0+1)+p0i*b0i/(n+n0)^2/(n+
    n0+1))
  pb.t = 1-pnorm(LTV[2],nmean,nsd)
  pb.m = pnorm(LTV[1],nmean,nsd)
  dec.GO = (pb.t>pLTV[2])&(pb.m<(1-pLTV[1]))
  dec.NG = (pb.t<=pLTV[2])
  dec.CO = !(dec.GO|dec.NG)
  dec.Pr = round(t(c(mean(dec.GO),mean(dec.CO),mean(dec.NG)
    )),3)
  colnames(dec.Pr) = c("Pr.GO","Pr.Indeterminate","Pr.NoGO"
    )
  dec.Pr
  }
```

```
OpCharNonInf (n=109,delta=0.15)
```

In addition to the R code provided in Listing 4.4, exact computation of the posterior distribution for risk differences, risk ratios and odds ratios is available via the R code provided in Sverdlov et al. (2014).

R code for computing operating characteristics of Bayesian decision criteria with an informative prior is provided in Listing 4.5.

LISTING 4.5: Operating characteristics of Bayesian decision criteria with an informative prior

```
OpCharInf =
function(n,hist.n,true.t,hist.t,pbo.r=0.2,h.pbo.r=pbo.r,TV
    =0.2,LRV=0.1,seed=12345,iter.n=100000) {
  # n = Sample size per arm in the current trial
  # hist.n = Equivalent size of historical data
  # true.t = True treatment difference in the current trial
  # hist.t = True treatment difference in historical data
  # pro.r = True placebo response rate in the current trial
  # hi.pbo.r = True placebo response rate in historical
      data
  # TV = Target value
  # LRV = Lower reference value
  # iter.n = Number of simulation runs
  set.seed(seed)
  n0 = hist.n; a0 =(h.pbo.r+(0:1*hist.t))*n0
  b0 = n0-a0; pLTV = c(.8,.1); LTV = c(LRV,TV)
  p0i = rbinom(iter.n,n,pbo.r)+a0[1]
  p1i = rbinom(iter.n,n,pbo.r+true.t)+a0[2]
  b0i = n-p0i+n0; b1i = n-p1i+n0
  nmean = p1i/(n+n0)-p0i/(n+n0)
  nsd = sqrt(p1i*b1i/(n+n0)^2/(n+n0+1)+p0i*b0i/(n+n0)^2/(n+
    n0+1))
  pb.t = 1-pnorm(LTV[2],nmean,nsd)
  pb.m = pnorm(LTV[1],nmean,nsd)
  dec.GO = (pb.t>pLTV[2])&(pb.m<(1-pLTV[1]))
  dec.NG = (pb.t<=pLTV[2])
  dec.CO = !(dec.GO|dec.NG)
  dec.Pr = t(c(mean(dec.GO),mean(dec.CO),mean(dec.NG)))
  colnames(dec.Pr) = c("Pr.GO","Pr.Indeterminate","Pr.NoGO"
    )
  round(dec.Pr,3)
  }
```

The following function call computes the decision probabilities presented in Table 4.9 under Data model 2 with 109 patients per arm.

```
OpCharInf(n=109,hist.n=40,true.t=.20,hist.t=.10,LRV=.10)
```

Sample size calculations in a clinical trial with a binary endpoint based on the iterative algorithm can be performed using the R code shown in Listing 4.6.

LISTING 4.6: Sample size calculations in a clinical trial with a binary endpoint

```
SSi = function(n0,true.t,TV,LRV,s2,z.TV,z.LRV,pr.indet) {
  (sqrt(s2[1])*qnorm(pnorm((TV-true.t)*sqrt(n0/s2[1])-z.TV)
    +pr.indet)-sqrt(s2[2])*z.LRV)^2/(LRV-true.t)^2
  }
SSGNGBinom = function(pr.indet,true.t=0.2,TV=0.2,LRV=0.12,
    tau.TV=0.1,tau.LRV=0.2,p0=o.2)  {
  # pr.indet = Probability of an Indeterminate decision
  # true.t = True treatment difference
  # TV = Target value
  # LRV = Lower reference value
  # tau.TV = Risk threshold for a false No-Go decision
  # tau.LRV = Risk threshold for a false Go decision
  # p0 = True placebo response rate

  p.bar = p0+c(TV,LRV)/2; T.bar=p0+true.t/2
  s2 = 2*p.bar*(1-p.bar)
  z.TV = qnorm(1-tau.TV)
  z.LRV = qnorm(1-tau.LRV)
  z.TV.con = qnorm(1-tau.TV-pr.indet)
  ni = c()
  ni[1:2]=sum(c(z.TV.con,z.LRV)*sqrt(s2))^2/(TV-LRV)^2
  for (i in 3:99) {
  ni[i]=SSi(mean(ni[i-1:2]), true.t,TV,LRV,s2,z.TV,z.LRV,pr
    .indet) }
  list(n.per.arm.for.GNG=ceiling(mean(tail(ni,2))))
  }
```

The sample size corresponding to the probability of an Indeterminate decision of 30% and true treatment difference of 16% is calculated as follows:

```
SSGNGBinom(pr.indet=0.3, true.t=0.16)
```

The R code in Listing 4.7 can be used to calculate the sample size in a trial with a normally distributed endpoint.

LISTING 4.7: Sample size calculations in a clinical trial with a normally distributed endpoint

```
SSGNGNorm =function(pr.indet,true.t=.2,s2=1,TV=true.t,LRV=
    TV/2,tau.TV=.1,tau.LRV=.2,p0=.2){
 # pr.indet = probability of Indeterminate decision
 # true.t = treatment effect
 # s2 = variance of treatment difference
 # TV = target value
 # LRV = lower reference value
 # tau.TV = risk threshold for false No-Go decision
 # tau.LRV = risk threshold for false Go decision
 # p0 = placebo response rate

 p.bar = p0+c(TV,LRV)/2; T.bar=p0+true.t/2
 z.TV = qnorm(1-tau.TV)
 z.LRV = qnorm(1-tau.LRV)
 z.TV.con = qnorm(1-tau.TV-pr.indet)
 ni = c(); s2=2*c(s2,s2)
 ni[1:2]=sum(c(z.TV.con,z.LRV)*sqrt(s2))^2/(TV-LRV)^2
 for (i in 3:99)
   ni[i]=SSi(mean(ni[i-1:2]),true.t,TV,LRV,s2,z.TV,z.LRV,
   pr.indet)
 list(n.per.arm.for.GNG=ceiling(mean(tail(ni,2))))
 }
```

The total number of events required in a clinical trial with a time-to-event endpoint can be estimated using the following R code (note that the treatment effect is measured on a hazard ratio scale):

```
SSGNGNorm(pr.indet=.3,true.t=log(.7),s2=1,TV=log(.7),LRV=
    log(.85))$n
```

4.4.6   Conclusions and extensions

In this case study, a general Bayesian framework for the GNG decision-making process was introduced. This framework applies to one set of criteria based on a TPP with two levels of efficacy-informing decision making and mitigates the inability of the traditional frequentist strategies to inform the TPP. It was shown how the choice of different data model parameters influences decision making for a given set of target and minimum reference values of the TPP and pre-determined level of acceptable risks associated with incorrect decisions. Given the pre-specified risk thresholds, the proposed Bayesian decision criteria can be used to optimally select the sample size in a proof-of-concept trial to facilitate GNG decision making. The need for a careful sample size determination that helps clinical development beyond just ensuring statistical significance was emphasized. The content of a TPP and the parameters involved in the GNG decision-making process differ among various sponsors

TABLE 4.11: GNG decision rules based on the significance and relevance criteria.

Decision	Posterior probability-based criteria	
	Criterion 1 (significance)	Criterion 2 (relevance)
Go	$P_\Delta(\Delta > 0 \mid x) > 0.9$	$P_\Delta(\Delta > \Delta_{\mathrm{TD}} \mid x) > 0.5$
No-Go	$P_\Delta(\Delta > 0 \mid x) < 0.9$	$P_\Delta(\Delta > \Delta_{\mathrm{TD}} \mid x) < 0.5$
Indeterminate	Otherwise	

and also for different compounds within a sponsor. The Bayesian framework proposed can be adopted to implement a unified decision-making process by properly linking the TPP and the results of a proof-of-concept trial.

4.5 Case study 4.2: Bayesian Go/No-Go evaluation using an alternative decision criterion

Recently, Fisch et al. (2015) developed a Bayesian formulation for Go/No-Go decision making in the presence of a single target level of efficacy. In this section, we will examine their proposed methods using the CSE framework.

4.5.1 Clinical trial

This case study will use the same clinical trial example as in Case study 4.1.

Data model

The data model for this case study will be identical to that utilized in Case study 4.1 (see Section 4.3.1).

Analysis model

Instead of specifying Δ_{LRV} and Δ_{TV} in a TPP, Fisch et al. (2015) considered a single target treatment effect, denoted by Δ_{TD}, such that efficacy below this target is not worth pursuing and efficacy above the target is of interest. The resulting decision rules are jointly based on a "significance criterion" and a "relevance criterion." While the significance criterion ensures, with high confidence, that a positive treatment effect exists, the relevance criterion establishes, with moderate confidence, that the treatment effect is at least Δ_{TD}. The probability thresholds for these two criteria are set at 0.9 and 0.5, respectively, and may be set by the trial's sponsor as shown in Table 4.11.

TABLE 4.12: Operating characteristics of the alternative Bayesian decision criterion with $\Delta_{TD} = 10\%$ under the three data models.

Δ_T	Data model 1	Data model 2	Data model 3
		P(Go)	
0%	5%	3%	8%
5%	9%	16%	24%
10%	48%	46%	49%
15%	88%	77%	73%
20%	99%	94%	89%
		P(Indeterminate)	
0%	10%	7%	2%
5%	41%	18%	3%
10%	40%	20%	1%
15%	11%	12%	0%
20%	1%	4%	0%
		P(No-Go)	
0%	90%	90%	90%
5%	50%	66%	73%
10%	11%	34%	49%
15%	1%	11%	26%
20%	0%	2%	11%

Evaluation model

These decision rules improve upon the frequentist criterion based on statistical significance by incorporating a dependence on the target value. An evaluation of the operating characteristics is provided in Tables 4.12 and 4.13 by applying the full simulation approach described in Section 4.4.1. The decision probabilities were calculated for different levels of efficacy relative to the target treatment effects of $\Delta_{TD} = 10\%$ and 20%. The data models used in these tables were defined in Section 4.3 (see Table 4.3).

Examining Tables 4.12 and 4.13, it is interesting to note that for efficacy in the middle of the TPP (15%), uncertainty increases with sample size. This is due to the fact that, as the sample size increases, the significance criterion becomes much more likely to be met, shifting the probability from a No-Go decision to an Indeterminate decision. In this example, larger sample sizes did not drive the sponsor to more certainty regarding the Go and No-Go decisions but instead drove the decision to the absence of a No-Go. For underlying efficacy equal to Δ_{TD}, driving the sample size to infinity would result in the significance criterion always being met and the relevance criteria being met 50% of the time resulting in a 50% probability of a Go decision and a 50% probability of an Indeterminate decision as the ultimate operating characteristics. This can be seen from Data model 1 in Tables 4.13 with $\Delta_{TD} = 20\%$. In addition, when Δ_{TD} is true, the maximal value of the probability of a Go decision is 50%. This behavior is driven by the choice

TABLE 4.13: Operating characteristics of the alternative Bayesian decision criterion with $\Delta_{TD} = 20\%$ under the three data models.

Δ_T	Data model 1	Data model 2	Data model 3
		P(Go)	
0%	0%	0%	0%
5%	0%	0%	1%
10%	1%	3%	7%
15%	10%	17%	22%
20%	49%	46%	45%
		P(Indeterminate)	
0%	10%	10%	10%
5%	50%	34%	25%
10%	88%	63%	43%
15%	89%	72%	52%
20%	51%	52%	45%
		P(No-Go)	
0%	90%	90%	90%
5%	50%	66%	73%
10%	11%	34%	49%
15%	1%	11%	26%
20%	0%	2%	11%

of the decision thresholds for this example and the simplification of having only one value Δ_{TD} delineating the TPP. Other thresholds would alter the distribution of the probability across the Go and Indeterminate options for large sample sizes.

4.5.2 Software implementation

The R code shown in Listing 4.8 can be used to calculate the operating characteristics of the alternative Bayesian decision examined in this case study similar to those summarized in Tables 4.12 and 4.13. The function call at the end shows how to perform calculations for Data model 2 with 109 patients per arm.

LISTING 4.8: Operating characteristics of the alternative Bayesian decision criteria

```
OpCharF = function(n,delta,TD=delta,prob.0=0.9, prob.TD
    =0.5, pbo.rate=0.2, seed=12345,iter.n=100000) {
  # n = Sample size per arm
  # delta = True treatment difference
  # TD = Target treatment effect
  # prob.0 = Posterior probability of the treatment effect
    greater than 0
```

```
# prob.TD = Posterior probability of the treatment effect
    greater than TD
# pbo.rate = True placebo response rate
# iter.n = Number of simulation runs

        set.seed(seed);
p0i = rbinom(iter.n,n,pbo.rate)
p1i = rbinom(iter.n,n,pbo.rate+delta)
nmi = (p1i+1)/(n+2)-(p0i+1)/(n+2)
nv0i = (p0i+1)*(-p0i+n+1)/(n+2)^2/(n+3)
nvi = (p1i+1)*(-p1i+n+1)/(n+2)^2/(n+3)+nv0i
go0 = ((1-pnorm(0,nmi,sqrt(nvi))) >prob.0)
goTD = ((1-pnorm(TD,nmi,sqrt(nvi)))>prob.TD)
GO = go0&goTD; NG = !go0&!goTD
dec.Pr = t(c(mean(GO),mean(!(GO|NG)),mean(NG)))
colnames(dec.Pr) = c("Pr.GO","Pr.Indeterminate","Pr.NoGO"
    )
round(dec.Pr,3)
}
OpCharF(n=109,delta=0.10)
```

4.5.3   Conclusions and extensions

In this case study, the Go/No-Go criteria developed by Fisch et al. (2015) were examined. This framework applies to a single threshold TPP in contrast to the criteria applicable to multi-level TPP developed in Case study 4.1. It was shown how the choice of Δ_{TD} and sample size impact the probabilities of Go or other decisions. For the true treatment effect greater or equal to Δ_{TD}, dominated by the relevance criterion, the Fisch approach performs well preserving the probability of a Go decision at least 50% approximately. However, an increase in the sample size results in an increase in the probability of an Indeterminate decision by reducing the probability of a No-Go decision. This behavior was not present in the criteria proposed in Case study 4.1. Nevertheless, the Fisch method supplements the evidence of beneficial treatment effect via the relevance criterion that the frequentist approach fails to achieve.

4.6   Case study 4.3: Bayesian Go/No-Go evaluation in a trial with an interim analysis

Interim assessments with futility stopping rules are often used in clinical trials, especially in late-phase trials with a larger sample size. In the setting of a mid-stage trial, the sponsor may wish to terminate a trial for futility if it becomes apparent that the TPP is highly unlikely. Similar to the comparison to the frequentist approach that relies on hypothesis testing which may stop a trial for futility if conditional or predictive power is low at an interim analysis, the methodology proposed in this case study would lead to futility stopping if the evidence for not meeting the TPP is sufficiently high based on the interim data. The Bayesian methodology naturally incorporates the learning of early data to reassess the evidence relative to the TPP in real time.

4.6.1 Clinical trial

The section will use the clinical trial example based on the proof-of-concept trial in SLE patients introduced in Section 4.3.1.

Data model

The data model is equivalent to that used in Case study 4.1.

Analysis model

The analysis model used in this case study will be identical to the one described in Case study 4.1 but will include an interim futility analysis. The operating characteristics of interest are related to the probability of terminating the trial at this interim analysis across various levels of efficacy in the TPP (including no effect), and the resulting impact on the probability of declaring a No-Go decision. This increase in the probability of a No-Go decision is similar to power loss in trials that employ frequentist futility stopping rules. The proposed Bayesian approach requires specification of a *futility threshold*, denoted by τ_{TV}^{ia}, at the interim analysis such that the trial continues to the final analysis if $P_\Delta(\mathbf{T} \mid \mathbf{x}) > \tau_{TV}^{ia}$. Given this additional threshold, the trial's sponsor may evaluate the operating characteristics around futility stopping as well as decision making at a study level.

Evaluation model

Table 4.14 provides a summary of the probability of a No-Go decision for Data models 1, 2 and 3 introduced in Section 4.3 with several values of τ_{TV}^{ia} and $\tau_{TV} = 10\%$. The interim analysis is carried out after 50% patients complete the trial. The upper block in this table provides the probability of stopping for futility (declaring No-Go) at the interim analysis and the values are approximately τ_{TV}^{ia} at the target efficacy of 20%. The lower block provides the probability of a No-Go decision at an overall study level. The criterion for a No-Go decision remains the same, i.e., a No-Go decision is adopted if $P_\Delta(\mathbf{T} \mid \mathbf{x}) \leq \tau_{TV}$ at the final analysis or $P_\Delta(\mathbf{T} \mid \mathbf{x}) \leq \tau_{TV}^{ia}$ at the interim analysis. The impact of the interim analysis is clear in that, for the 0% treatment effect, reasonable probabilities to declare futility were observed under all three data models. The tradeoff is an increase in the study-level false

TABLE 4.14: Operating characteristics of the Bayesian futility stopping rule under the three data models ($\tau_{TV}^{ia} = 0\%$ if there is no interim futility analysis).

Δ_T	Futility threshold τ_{TV}^{ia}								
	$0\%^a$	5%	10%	0%	5%	10%	0%	5%	10%
	Data model 1			Data model 2			Data model 3		
	Stopping at the interim analysis								
0%	0%	99%	100%	0%	84%	92%	0%	67%	78%
5%	0%	87%	94%	0%	62%	75%	0%	46%	60%
10%	0%	57%	71%	0%	35%	50%	0%	27%	40%
15%	0%	23%	36%	0%	16%	27%	0%	14%	23%
20%	0%	5%	11%	0%	6%	11%	0%	6%	11%
	Stopping at the interim analysis or final analysis								
0%	100%	100%	100%	99%	99%	99%	95%	95%	96%
5%	100%	100%	100%	93%	93%	94%	79%	81%	83%
10%	90%	91%	92%	69%	71%	73%	54%	57%	60%
15%	50%	52%	56%	35%	38%	42%	28%	31%	36%
20%	11%	13%	16%	11%	13%	17%	11%	13%	17%

negative rate which is induced due to the presence of the futility analysis. Under Data model 2, one can see how empirically this error increased from 11% to 13% to 17% as the futility threshold τ_{TV}^{ia} increased. False stopping for an underlying value of 15% which may certainly be of commercial interest increased as well. It is important to evaluate the operating characteristics of this futility stopping rule across the full range of the TPP as well as at zero or other undesirable values.

Another important consideration in Phase II futility trials is that the trial's sponsor must be prepared to stop learning at the interim analysis. For example, other endpoints that may be of interest, or patient selection subgroup analysis to generate further hypotheses, may be limited by not finishing the trial. If another clinical trial is to be planned, it may suffer from a lack of data due to the failure to complete the initial trial. As a result, futility in mid-stage trials should be considered very carefully.

It is worth noting that this case study largely focused on futility assessments but the alternative decision to initiate Phase III trial activities at risk based on an accelerated Go decision is possible as well. Operating characteristics of the associated decision criteria could be evaluated in a similar fashion. One important point, however, is that if the sponsor chose to start Phase III trial(s) based on an interim analysis, the current trial would not be stopped. As a result, the final data set would still be available (in most cases prior to the Phase III trials) to facilitate final decision making. This approach differs from futility assessments where no final trial result would exist.

4.6.2 Software implementation

The R code to calculate the operating characteristics of the proposed Bayesian futility stopping rule, similar to the characteristics presented in Table 4.14, is presented below. The function call at the end shows how to perform calculations of No-Go probabilities under Data model 3 with 64 patients per arm at the final analysis and selected values of the true treatment difference.

LISTING 4.9: Calculation of No-Go probabilities at the interim analysis and at study level

```
FutilityProb = function(n,true.t=c(TV,LRV),tau.ia=c
    (0,0.05,0.1),TV=0.2,LRV=0.1, tau.TV=0.1,p0=0.2,seed
    =23451,iter.n=100000) {
  # n = Sample size per arm
  # true.t = Treatment effect assumptions
  # tau.ia = Futility threshold
  # TV = Target value
  # LRV = Lower reference value
  # tau.TV = Risk threshold for the probability of false No
    -Go decision
  # p0 = True placebo response rate

  t1=c(true.t,0);t1.n=length(t1);p0=0.2
  n1=ceiling(n/2); n2=n-n1
  f.GO.n=length(tau.ia);I4=rep(1,t1.n)
  set.seed(seed)

  p0i=array(rbinom(iter.n,n1,p0),c(1,iter.n))[I4,]
  p0f=p0i+array(rbinom(iter.n,n2,p0),c(1,iter.n))[I4,]
  p1i=array(rbinom(t1.n*iter.n,n1,p0+t1),c(t1.n,iter.n))
  p1f=p1i+array(rbinom(t1.n*iter.n,n2,p0+t1),
      c(t1.n,iter.n))

  nmi=(p1i-p0i)/(n1+2); nmf=(p1f-p0f)/(n+2)
  nvi =((p0i+1)*(-p0i+n1+1)+(p1i+1)*(-p1i+n1+1))/(n1+2)^2/(
    n1+3)
  nvf =((p0f+1)*(-p0f+n+1)+(p1f+1)*(-p1f+n+1))/(n+2)^2/(n
    +3)

  pr0.TV=1-pnorm(TV,nmi[1,],sqrt(nvi[1,]))
  fi.GO=quantile(pr0.TV,tau.ia); if (tau.ia[1]==0) fi.GO
    [1]=0
          fi.GO=tau.ia
  pri.TV=1-pnorm(TV,nmi,sqrt(nvi))
  NGi =array(pri.TV,c(t1.n,iter.n,f.GO.n))<rep(fi.GO,each=
    t1.n*iter.n)
  prf.TV =1-pnorm(TV,nmf,sqrt(nvf))
  NGf =(prf.TV<tau.TV)
  I.NG=round(apply(NGi,c(1,3),mean)[t1.n:1,],2)
```

```
F.NG=apply(NGi|array(NGf,c(t1.n,iter.n,f.GO.n)),c(1,3),
  mean)[t1.n:1,]
rownames(I.NG)=rownames(F.NG)=paste(round(100*rev(t1),0),
  "% effect",sep="")
colnames(I.NG)=colnames(F.NG)=paste("Pr(stop|TV)=",tau.ia
  ,sep="")
list(Pr.NOGO.at.interim=I.NG,Pr.NOGO.at.interm.or.final=
  round(F.NG,2))
}
FutilityProb(n=64, true.t=c(0.20,0.15,0.10,0.05))
```

4.6.3   Conclusions and extensions

A strategy to evaluate futility at an interim analysis in an ongoing clinical trial or potentially evaluate further clinical development at the end of a trial was outlined in this case study. An additional parameter (τ_{TV}^{ia}) was introduced to modulate the degree of futility assessment. Higher values of this threshold result in a higher hurdle to continue with the current trial or further evaluation. The proposed framework is particularly useful when interim results are contrasted directly with the pre-specified multi-level TPP.

4.7   Case study 4.4: Decision criteria in Phase II trials based on Probability of Success

4.7.1   Clinical trial

Consider a two arm Phase II trial which is designed to provide key information for GNG decisions for an experimental treatment compared to placebo. For concreteness, the primary endpoint in the trial is assumed to be binary, i.e., represents an improvement rate. If a Go decision is made at the end of this Phase II trial, a Phase III program would consist of two trials of the same design as required for a potential regulatory approval of the experimental treatment and the primary endpoint in the Phase III trials would be the same as the Phase II trial. In designing the Phase II trial, it is in the sponsor's best interest to understand what Phase II results would predict a high probability of a positive Phase III program. An approach that relies on Probability of Success (POS) introduced in Section 4.2.3 will be employed in this case study.

Data model

A simple data model with a binary outcome variable will be considered. The true response rates in the treatment and placebo arms will be denoted by p_1

and p_2, respectively. A higher value of the response rate indicates a beneficial effect.

Analysis model

The primary objective of the Phase II trial is to test the null hypothesis of no effect, i.e., $H_0 : p_1 - p_2 \leq 0$, against the alternative $H_a : p_1 - p_2 > 0$. In applying POS to predict for the end of Phase II GNG decisions, the Phase II trial results will be first summarized using a Bayesian approach. Assume beta priors for the true response rates p_1 and p_2. The resulting posterior distributions for p_1 and p_2, denoted by $\pi(p_i)$, $i = 1, 2$, are also Beta distributed. The posterior distributions are then used to define the design prior, $\pi(\theta) = \pi(p_1)\pi(p_2)$, using the notation defined in Section 4.2.3, for the prediction of the POS in the Phase III trials. Within each Phase III trial, an appropriate two-sided test will be conducted for testing if the response rate in the treatment arm (p_1) is greater than that in the placebo arm (p_2) at a significance level of 0.05.

Evaluation model

In this particular setting, the experimental treatment will be considered commercially viable if it provides a significantly higher response rate and, in addition, the difference in the response rate exceeds a pre-defined threshold denoted by δ ($\delta > 0$). Given the design prior computed from the Phase II trial, the POS of the Phase III program can be computed using the following simulation-based algorithm which serves as an extension of the mixed Bayesian-frequentist algorithm defined in Section 4.2.3.

1. Sample Phase III response rates from $\pi(\theta)$.
2. Simulate two Phase III trials based on these response rates.
3. Assess if the pre-defined success criteria are met, i.e., (1) the difference between p_1 and p_2 is statistically significant and (2) the difference in the observed response rates is greater than δ.
4. Repeat Steps 1 to 3 a large number of times. The POS is estimated by the proportion of runs where the success criteria are met.

Now consider the case that another treatment for the same indication disclosed its registration trial results and is expected to be approved and this treatment will be used as a commercial benchmark. This alternative treatment showed 20% and 30% response rates in the placebo and active treatment arms in its key Phase III trial. It is believed that, to be commercially viable, the new treatment would need to demonstrate an 8% higher response rate compared to placebo to be considered non-inferior through indirect comparison to the commercial benchmark. Furthermore, the clinical development plan specifies that 60 patients per arm would be enrolled in the Phase II trial

TABLE 4.15: Probability of Success in the
Phase III trial predicted from the Phase II data
assuming uniform priors.

Observed Phase II response rates		Phase III POS
Placebo	Treatment	
20%	30%	0.42
20%	32%	0.50
20%	34%	0.58
20%	36%	0.66
20%	38%	0.73
20%	40%	0.79
20%	42%	0.85

and 180 patients per arm in each of the Phase III trials. Before starting the Phase II trial, the sponsor may want to estimate the POS for the Phase III program under different Phase II outcome scenarios to determine whether a high enough Phase III POS is attainable with the current program.

As an illustration, Table 4.15 presents the Phase III POS predictions for several Phase II outcome scenarios in this setting. The Phase II primary response data are summarized with uniform priors for the response rates. Using this prediction, the sponsor may realize that obtaining a Phase II outcome scenario sufficient to predict a high enough POS in the Phase III program, e.g., 60%, is unlikely. As a result, the sponsor may decide to abort further development of the compound early. If the Phase II trial already started, the sponsor could conduct an interim prediction in the ongoing trial and include other GNG decision points before the end of this Phase II trial. Finally, the complete Phase II data would provide the end of Phase II GNG decisions possibly according to a paradigm outlined earlier and complemented by POS information.

Of note, the joint POS of two or more Phase III trials is not a simple product of POSs for the individual trials. Zhang et al. (2013) showed that the probabilities of success of future Phase III trials are stochastically correlated when the successes are predicted based on the same observed data. The joint POS can be appropriately evaluated using the closed-form formulas provided in Zhang et al. (2013) or by a Monte Carlo approximation.

4.7.2   Software implementation

The R code for evaluating POS in Phase III trials is shown in Listing 4.10.

LISTING 4.10: POS evaluation

```
EOP2=function(n2, n3, p1, p2, delta, t, K)
{
  # n2 = Sample size per arm in the Phase II trial
  # n3 = Sample size per arm in each Phase III trial
```

```
# p1 = Observed treatment response rate in the Phase II
  trial
# p2 = Observed placebo response rate in the Phase II
  trial
# delta = Superiority margin
# t = Two-sided significance level in each Phase III
  trial
# K = Number of situation runs

tc.p=rbeta(K,(1+n2*p1),(1+n2*(1-p1)))
pb.p=rbeta(K,(1+n2*p2),(1+n2*(1-p2)))
count=0
for (i in 1:K){
 tc_1=rbinom(1,n3,tc.p[i])
 pb_1=rbinom(1,n3,pb.p[i])
 sc1_1=((tc_1-pb_1)/n3)>delta
 sc2_1=t.test(c(rep(0,(n3-pb_1)),rep(1,pb_1)),c(rep(0,(n3
 -tc_1)),rep(1,tc_1)),mu=0,alternative='two.sided')$p.
 value<t
 tc_2=rbinom(1,n3,tc.p[i])
 pb_2=rbinom(1,n3,pb.p[i])
 sc1_2=((tc_2-pb_2)/n3)>delta
 sc2_2=t.test(c(rep(0,(n3-pb_2)),rep(1,pb_2)),c(rep(0,(n3
 -tc_2)),rep(1,tc_2)),mu=0,alternative='two.sided')$p.
 value<0.05
 count=count+sc1_1*sc2_1*sc1_2*sc2_2
}
cat("PrSS=", count/K, "\n")
}
```

The following function call performs POS calculations under the assumptions used in Table 4.15.

```
EOP2(n2=60, n3=180, p1=0.46, p2=0.2, delta=0.08, t=0.05, K
  =10000)
```

4.7.3 Conclusions and extensions

In this case study, a Bayesian formulation of POS was applied to evaluate decisions to progress from a Phase II trial to a Phase III development program. This technique can be helpful to optimally re-allocate the sponsor's internal resources to other promising programs if a sufficiently high level of POS is unlikely to be achieved in a clinical development program and thereby reducing the failure rate in Phase III trials.

4.8   Case study 4.5: Updating POS using interim or external information

In addition to the problems of POS calculations based on the results of earlier clinical trials considered in Case study 4.4, trial sponsors are often interested in updating POS predictions during the execution of a trial using interim or external information. If POS needs to be updated based on new external information only, POS is easily re-calculated using the same algorithm that was used in the original POS calculations. The only difference is that a design prior computed from the updated external information needs to be utilized. Note that typically there would be no reason to unblind the ongoing trial for such POS re-calculation.

It is more challenging to update POS using the interim trial data, which would have more direct bearing on the ongoing trial than external information. As such, any updates would need to explicitly consider the impact on the Type I error rate and power (as with any interim analysis), and any use of unblinded decision making would need to be coordinated with regulatory agencies. Using a non-Bayesian solution, the conditional power approach (Lan et al., 1982) mentioned in Section 4.2.3 could be applied to predict future outcomes from the observed outcomes and then update the frequentist power calculations performed at the trial's design stage. From the Bayesian arsenal, the predictive power (mixed Bayesian-frequentist) and Bayesian predictive (fully Bayesian) approaches (Dmitrienko and Wang, 2006; Wang, 2007) could be considered to perform interim POS re-calculation. The differentiating step is to predict the unobserved outcomes using the outcomes observed at the interim analysis and then include both in POS re-calculation. In predicting the unobserved outcomes, the interim data can replace the original design prior, combined with the original design prior or merged with a revised design prior based on the updated external data to form an *updated design prior* for POS re-calculation.

The following simulation-based algorithm can be applied to update POS based on the predictive power approach:

1. Use the observed trial data, with or without external information, to form an updated design prior $\tilde{\pi}(\theta)$, where θ is the true treatment difference, in place of the original design prior $\pi(\theta)$ to predict the future data.

2. Sample a value of θ from $\tilde{\pi}(\theta)$.

3. Given the value of θ, simulate the future observations from $f(\mathbf{x}|\theta)$.

4. Given the observed and simulated future observations, define success as $T_0(\mathbf{x}) > t_\alpha$, where $\mathbf{x}$ comprises both the observed and predicted future observations at the final analysis, T_0 is the relevant

test statistic and t_α is the appropriate quantile of its null distribution.

5. Repeat the above steps a large number of times. The proportion of successes is an estimate of POS.

To update the fully Bayesian POS by the Bayesian predictive approach, the following simulation-based algorithm can be applied:

1. Use the observed trial data, with or without external information, to form an updated design prior $\tilde{\pi}(\theta)$ in place of the original design prior $\pi(\theta)$ to predict the future data.

2. Sample a value of θ from $\tilde{\pi}(\theta)$.

3. Given the value of θ, simulate the future observations from $f(\mathbf{x}|\theta)$.

4. Given the observed and simulated observations as well as the analysis prior $\pi^\star(\theta)$, calculate the posterior probability $P(\theta \in H_\alpha|\mathbf{x})$ and examine if it is greater than η to define success.

5. Repeat the above steps a large number of times. The proportion of successes is an estimate of POS.

Although POS can be updated using interim trial data and/or revised external information in a blinded or unblinded manner, the trial's sponsor needs to be careful about modifying the original trial design, e.g., the predefined sample size, since it may affect the integrity of the trial. The general approach defined above is more appropriate for non-registration trials, e.g., proof-of-concept or Phase II trials.

4.8.1 Clinical trial

As an illustration, a clinical trial example introduced in Dmitrienko and Wang (2006) will be re-visited. This example deals with a proof-of-concept trial for the treatment of generalized anxiety disorder and incorporates several interim analyses. Patients were enrolled to receive either an experimental treatment or placebo for 6 weeks. The primary endpoint was improvement in the Hamilton anxiety rating scale (HAMA) as a continuous variable. The null hypothesis of interest was formulated in terms of the difference between the mean changes in the HAMA score between the treatment and placebo arms. Assuming normally distributed responses with equal variances in the two trial arms, the total projected sample size per arm was 41 patients (note that this sample size calculation was not informed by the POS approach). Three unblinded interim analyses were performed by an internal assessment committee to support futility stopping decisions using the predictive power and fully Bayesian approaches, with the results summarized in Tables I and III of Dmitrienko and Wang (2006).

Data model

Consider an adaptive design in the proof-of-concept trial introduced above with an unblinded sample size re-assessment which will be performed using the POS approach at the second interim analysis after 20 patients complete the trial in each trial arm. Improvement in the HAMA score is assumed normally distributed. The mean change from baseline follows $N(\mu_1, \sigma^2)$ in the treatment arm and $N(\mu_2, \sigma^2)$ in the placebo arm.

Analysis model

The prima analysis in the trial focuses on testing the null hypothesis of no treatment effect $(H_0 : \mu_1 \leq \mu_2)$ versus an alternative hypothesis of a beneficial treatment effect $(H_a : \mu_1 > \mu_2)$.

This case study will illustrate an application of the fully Bayesian approach to updating POS at an interim analysis. For the Bayesian analysis, let the standard deviation of the primary endpoint in both trial arms be fixed as σ^2 as was done in Dmitrienko and Wang (2006). Note that this assumption can be relaxed using a prior distribution assumed in Case study 4.4 or the one considered in Wang (2007). To simplify the presentation of formulas, the treatment index i, $i = 1, 2$, will be suppressed. Let the design prior for the mean response in a trial arm utilized at the interim analysis be denoted by $\pi(\mu) \sim N(\mu^*, (\sigma^*)^2)$, which can be the original design prior (if the trial was sized using the POS approach), updated information about the experimental treatment or placebo, other extraneous information, or a combination of the above. The interim data from n patients in a trial arm can be summarized using $(\overline{X}_{(n)}, S^2_{(n)})$. Then the updated design prior $\tilde{\pi}(\mu)$ for predicting outcomes of the future patients is normally distributed with the mean and variance given by

$$\mu_{(n)} = \sigma^2_{(n)} \left(\frac{\mu^*}{(\sigma^*)^2} + \frac{n\overline{X}_{(n)}}{\sigma^2} \right), \ \sigma^2_{(n)} = \left(\frac{1}{(\sigma^*)^2} + \frac{n}{\sigma^2} \right)^{-1}.$$

Note that the sample variance $S^2_{(n)}$ is not utilized in these formulas since σ^2 is assumed to be fixed.

Evaluation model

Given the updated design prior, the interim POS can be re-calculated using Steps 2-5 of the algorithm outlined earlier. First, consider the scenario when the POS update is to be completely driven by the observed data. If the trial was sized using the POS approach with an informative prior, the design prior would be reset as a non-informative for the interim POS re-assessment. This is achieved by setting $(\sigma^*)^2 \cong \infty$ that results in $\mu_{(n)} = \overline{X}_{(n)}$ and $\sigma^2_{(n)} = \sigma^2/n$. Continuing the illustration by updating the fully Bayesian POS, the

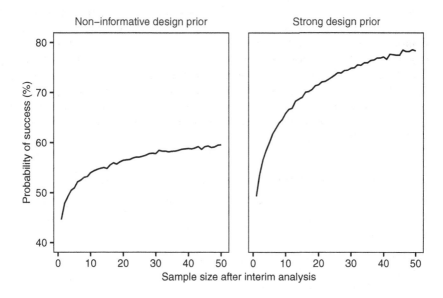

FIGURE 4.7: Fully Bayesian POS as a function of the post-interim sample size with non-informative and strong design priors for the treatment means in Case study 4.5.

analysis prior would also be assumed non-informative to maintain a more objective approach to conducting the trial. In addition, let the test significance threshold be set to $\eta = 0.7$. Suppose that the mean HAMA improvement and (standard deviation) observed at the second interim analysis were 9.4 (6.7) and 8.1 (6.9) in the treatment and placebo arms, respectively, as given in Table II of Dmitrienko and Wang (2006). Then the updated design prior $\tilde{\pi}(\theta)$ to simulate future patients' outcomes in the first step of the simulation-based algorithm is composed of $N(9.4, 6.7^2/20)$ and $N(8.1, 6.9^2/20)$ for the means in the treatment and placebo arms, respectively. Figure 4.7 presents the resulting POS as a function of the post-interim sample size. It follows from the left-hand panel of the figure that, with a non-informative prior, the POS function increased slowly up to about 60% with 50 additional patients per trial arm. And, bounded by the updated design prior, the POS can go up to 69% with an infinite sample size; see the discussion in Wang (2007).

Use of a more informative design prior is also possible, particularly in situations where a large amount of data has been accumulated before the trial in question. For example, using the cumulative information on the experimental treatment up to date, the strong design priors of $N(12, 2^2)$ and $N(8, 2^2)$ in the treatment and placebo arms can be considered, as assumed in Dmitrienko and Wang (2006). Then, according to the formula given above, the updated design priors for the mean are calculated to be of $N(10.6, 1.4^2)$ and $N(8.1, 1.4^2)$ in the two arms. As can be expected, the fully Bayesian POS is increased when a strong prior is assumed, as shown in the right-hand panel of Figure 4.7. Compared to the non-informative setting in the left-hand panel, it would be easier to make a decision concerning mid-course sample size adaptation with this or similar strong prior. For instance, if a POS of 70% was desired, then about 20 additional patients per arm would need to be enrolled after the interim analysis. Again, the POS is capped by the updated design prior at 91% in this particular scenario. Moreover, the frequentist test-based POS can be updated in a similar manner.

4.8.2 Software implementation

The R code for updating POS at an interim analysis using the full Bayesian approach based on both prior information and interim data is provided in Listing 4.11.

LISTING 4.11: Updating POS based on interim information

```
POSUpdate=function(n1, n2, n, m1, sd1, m2, sd2, pm1, pm2,
    psd1, psd2, sd, eta, K) {
  # n1 = Interim sample size in the treatment arm
  # n2 = Interim sample size in the placebo arm
  # n = Common post-interim sample size in both trial arms
  # m1 = Interim observed mean in the treatment arm
  # sd1 = Interim observed standard deviation in the
    treatment arm
  # m2 = Interim observed mean in the placebo arm
  # sd2 = Interim observed standard deviation in the
    placebo arm
  # pm1 = Prior mean for the mean response in the treatment
    arm
  # pm2 = Prior mean for the  mean response in the placebo
    arm
  # psd1 = Prior standard deviation for the mean response
    in the treatment arm
  # psd2 = Prior standard deviation for the mean response
    in the placebo arm
  # sd = Assumed fixed standard deviation of responses in
    both arms
  # eta = Threshold for the probability for success
  # K = Number of simulation runs

  qsd1=sqrt(1/(1/psd1^2+n1/sd^2))
  qsd2=sqrt(1/(1/psd2^2+n2/sd^2))
  qm1=qsd1^2*(pm1/psd1^2+n1*m1/sd^2)
  qm2=qsd2^2*(pm2/psd1^2+n2*m2/sd^2)
  count=0
  for (i in 1:K){
    sm1=rnorm(1,qm1,qsd1)
```

```
    sm2=rnorm(1,qm2,qsd2)
    mv1=rnorm(m,sm1,sd)
    mv2=rnorm(m,sm2,sd)
    pm1=mean(c(mv1, rep(m1,n1)))
    pm2=mean(c(mv2, rep(m2,n2)))
    count=count+sum((1-pnorm(0,(pm1-pm2),sqrt(sd^2/(n1+n)+
    sd^2/(n2+n))))>eta)
  }
  cat("POS=", count/K, "\n")
}
```

The following function call performs POS re-calculation using a flat prior with very large prior standard deviations for the mean responses in the treatment and placebo arms (psd1 and psd2):

```
POSUpdate(n1=20, n2=20, n=30, m1=9.4, sd1=6.7, m2=8.1, sd2
    =6.9, pm1=12, pm2=8, psd1=100000, psd2=100000, sd=8.5,
    eta=0.7, K=100000)
```

A strong prior is considered in this call:

```
POSUpdate(n1=20, n2=20, n=30, m1=9.4, sd1=6.7, m2=8.1, sd2
    =6.9, pm1=12, pm2=8, psd1=2, psd2=2, sd=8.5, eta=0.7, K
    =100000)
```

Bibliography

[1] Alosh, M., Bretz, F., Huque, M. (2014). Advanced multiplicity adjustment methods in clinical trials. *Statistics in Medicine*. 33, 693–713.

[2] Alosh, M., Huque, M.F., Bretz, F., D'Agostino, R.B. (2017). Tutorial on statistical considerations on subgroup analysis in confirmatory clinical trials. *Statistics in Medicine*. 36, 1334–1360.

[3] Amado, R.G., Wolf, M., Peeters, M., Cutsem, E.V., Siena, S., Freeman, D.J., Juan, T., Sikorski, R., Suggs, S., Radinsky, R., Patterson, S.D., Chang, D.D. (2008). Wild-type KRAS is required for panitumumab efficacy in patients with metastatic colorectal cancer. *Journal of Clinical Oncology*. 26, 1626–1634.

[4] Arrowsmith, J., Miller, P. (2013). Trial Watch: Phase II and Phase III attrition rates 2011–2012. *Nature Reviews Drug Discovery*. 12, 569.

[5] Atkinson, A.C. (2008). DT-optimum designs for model discrimination and parameter estimation. *Journal of Statistical Planning and Inference*. 138, 56–64.

[6] Atkinson, A.C., Donev, A.N. (1992). *Optimum Experimental Designs*. Clarendon Press, Oxford.

[7] Beer, T.M., Armstrong, A.J., Rathkopf, D.E., Loriot, Y., Sternberg, C.N., Higano, C.S., Iversen, P., Bhattacharya, S., Carles, J., Chowdhury, S., Davis, I.D., de Bono, J.S., Evans, C.P., Fizazi, K., Joshua, A.M., Kim, C.S., Kimura, G., Mainwaring, P., Mansbach, H., Miller, K., Noonberg, S.B., Perabo, F., Phung, D., Saad, F., Scher, H.I., Taplin, M.E., Venner, P.M., Tombal, B. (2014). Enzalutamide in metastatic prostate cancer before chemotherapy. *New England Journal of Medicine*. 371, 424–433.

[8] Benda, N., Branson, M., Maurer, W., Friede, T. (2010). Aspects of modernizing drug development using clinical scenario planning and evaluation. *Drug Information Journal*. 44, 299–315.

[9] Brechenmacher, T., Xu, J., Dmitrienko, A., Tamhane, A. C. (2011). A mixture gatekeeping procedure based on the Hommel test for clinical trial applications. *Journal of Biopharmaceutical Statistics*. 21, 748–767.

[10] Brutti, P., De Santis, F., Gubbiotti, S. (2008). Robust Bayesian sample size determination in clinical trials. *Statistics in Medicine*. 27, 2290–2306.

[11] Cappuzzo, F., Ciuleanu, T., Stelmakh, L., Cicenas, S., Szczesna, A., Juhasz, E., Esteban, E., Molinier, O., Brugger, W., Melezinek, I., Klingelschmitt, G., Klughammer, B., Giaccone, G. (2010). Erlotinib as maintenance treatment in advanced non-small-cell lung cancer: A multicentre, randomised, placebo-controlled phase 3 study. *Lancet Oncology.* 11, 521–529.

[12] Chuang-Stein, C. (2006). Sample size and the probability of a successful trial. *Pharmaceutical Statistics.* 5, 305–309.

[13] Chuang-Stein, C., Kirby, S., French, J., Kowalski, K., Marshall, S., Smith, M.K., Bycott, P., Beltangady, M. (2011). A quantitative approach for making Go/No-Go decisions in drug development. *Pharmaceutical Statistics.* 45, 187–202.

[14] Chuang-Stein, C., Kirby, S. (2014). The shrinking or disappearing observed treatment effect. *Pharmaceutical Statistics.* 13, 277–280.

[15] Cohen, A.T., Harrington, R., Goldhaber, S.Z., Hull, R., Gibson, C.M., Hernandez, A.F., Kitt, M.M., Lorenz, T.J. (2014). The design and rationale for the acute medically ill venous thromboembolism prevention with extended duration betrixaban (APEX) study. *American Heart Journal.* 167, 335–341.

[16] Cohen, A.T., Spiro, T.E., Buller, H.R., Haskell, L., Hu, D., Hull, R., Mebazaa, A., Merli, G., Schellong, S., Spyropoulos, A.C., Tapson, V. (2013). Rivaroxaban for thromboprophylaxis in acutely ill medical patients. *New England Journal of Medicine.* 368, 513–523.

[17] Correll, C.U., Skuban, A., Ouyang, J., Hobart, M., Pfister, S., McQuade, R.D., Nyilas, M., Carson, W.H., Sanchez, R., Eriksson, H. (2015). Efficacy and safety of brexpiprazole for the treatment of acute schizophrenia: A 6-week randomized, double-blind, placebo-controlled trial. *The American Journal of Psychiatry.* 172, 870–880.

[18] Dmitrienko, A., D'Agostino, R.B. (2013). Tutorial in Biostatistics: Traditional multiplicity adjustment methods in clinical trials. *Statistics in Medicine.* 32, 5172–5218.

[19] Dmitrienko, A., D'Agostino, R.B., Huque, M.F. (2013). Key multiplicity issues in clinical drug development. *Statistics in Medicine.* 32, 1079–1111.

[20] Dmitrienko, A., Kordzakhia, G., Brechenmacher, T. (2016). Mixture-based gatekeeping procedures for multiplicity problems with multiple sequences of hypotheses. *Journal of Biopharmaceutical Statistics.* 26, 758–780.

[21] Dmitrienko, A., Millen, B., Lipkovich, I. (2017). Statistical and regulatory considerations in subgroup analysis. *Statistics in Medicine.* To appear.

[22] Dmitrienko, A., Millen, B.A., Brechenmacher, T., Paux, G. (2011). Development of gatekeeping strategies in confirmatory clinical trials. *Biometrical Journal.* 53, 875–893.

[23] Dmitrienko, A., Muysers, C., Fritsch, A., Lipkovich, I. (2016). General guidance on exploratory and confirmatory subgroup analysis in late-stage clinical trials. *Journal of Biopharmaceutical Statistics.* 26, 71–98.

[24] Dmitrienko, A., Paux, G., Brechenmacher, T. (2015). Power calculations in clinical trials with complex clinical objectives. *Journal of the Japanese Society of Computational Statistics.* 28, 15–50.

[25] Dmitrienko, A., Paux, G., Pulkstenis, E., Zhang, J. (2016). Tradeoff-based optimization criteria in clinical trials with multiple objectives and adaptive designs. *Journal of Biopharmaceutical Statistics.* 26, 120–140.

[26] Dmitrienko, A., Tamhane, A., Wiens, B. (2008). General multistage gatekeeping procedures. *Biometrical Journal.* 50, 667–677.

[27] Dmitrienko, A., Tamhane, A.C. (2011). Mixtures of multiple testing procedures for gatekeeping applications in clinical trials. *Statistics in Medicine.* 30, 1473–1488.

[28] Dmitrienko, A., Tamhane, A.C. (2013). General theory of mixture procedures for gatekeeping. *Biometrical Journal.* 55, 402–419.

[29] Dmitrienko, A., Tamhane, A.C., Bretz, F. (editors). (2009). *Multiple Testing Problems in Pharmaceutical Statistics.* Chapman and Hall/CRC Press: New York.

[30] Dmitrienko, A., Wang, M. (2006). Bayesian predictive approach to interim monitoring in clinical trials. *Statistics in Medicine.* 25, 2178–2195.

[31] Edwards, A. W. F. (1992). *Likelihood: Expanded Edition.* Johns Hopkins University Press, Baltimore.

[32] Efron, B. (2012). Bayesian inference and the parametric bootstrap. *The Annals of Applied Statistics.* 6, 1971–1997.

[33] EMA. (2002). *Points to consider on multiplicity issues in clinical trials.* European Medicines Agency/Committee for Medicinal Products for Human Use. EMA/EWP/908/99.

[34] EMA. (2014). *Guideline on the investigation of subgroups in confirmatory clinical trials.* European Medicines Agency/Committee for Medicinal Products for Human Use. EMA/CHMP/539146/2013.

[35] EMA. (2017). *Guideline on multiplicity issues in clinical trials.* European Medicines Agency/Committee for Human Medicinal Products. EMA/CHMP/44762/2017.

[36] FDA. (2012). *Enrichment strategies for clinical trials to support approval of human drugs and biological products.* U.S. Food and Drug Administration.

[37] FDA. (2017). *Multiplicity endpoints in clinical trials.* U.S. Food and Drug Administration.

[38] Fisch, R., Jones, I., Jones, J., Kerman, J., Rosenkranz, G.K., Schmidli, H. (2015). Bayesian design of proof-of-concept trials. *Therapeutic Innovation and Regulatory Science.* 49, 155–162.

[39] Frewer, P., Mitchell, P., Watkins, C., Matcham, J. (2016). Decision making in early clinical drug development. *Pharmaceutical Statistics.* 15, 255–263.

[40] Friede, T., Nicholas, R., Stallard, N., Todd, S., Parsons, N.R., Valdes-Marquez, E., Chataway, J. (2010). Refinement of the clinical scenario evaluation framework for assessment of competing development strategies with an application to multiple sclerosis. *Drug Information Journal.* 44, 713–718.

[41] Gan, H.K., You, B., Pond, G.R., Chen, E.X. (2012). Assumptions of expected benefits in randomized Phase III trials evaluating systemic treatments for cancer. *Journal of the National Cancer Institute.* 104, 590–598.

[42] Graf, A.C., Posch, M., Koenig, F. (2015). Adaptive designs for subpopulation analysis optimizing utility functions. *Biometrical Journal.* 57, 76–89.

[43] Grouin, J.M., Coste, M., Lewis, J. (2005). Subgroup analyses in randomized clinical trials: Statistical and regulatory issues. *Journal of Biopharmaceutical Statistics.* 15, 869–882.

[44] Hee, S.W., Stallard, N. (2012). Designing a series of decision-theoretic Phase II trials in a small population. *Statistics in Medicine.* 31, 4337–4351.

[45] Herson, J. (1979). Predictive probability early termination plans for Phase II clinical trials. *Biometrics.* 35, 775–783.

[46] Hung, J., Wang, S.J. (2009). Some controversial multiple testing problems in regulatory applications. *Journal of Biopharmaceutical Statistics.* 19, 1–11.

[47] Keystone, E.C, Kavanaugh, A.F., Sharp, J.T., Tannenbaum, H., Hua, Y., Teoh, L.S., Fischkoff, S.A., Chartash, E.K. (2004). Radiographic, clinical, and functional outcomes of treatment with adalimumab (a human anti-tumor necrosis factor monoclonal antibody) in patients with active rheumatoid arthritis receiving concomitant methotrexate therapy. *Arthritis and Rheumatism.* 50, 1400–1411.

[48] Kirby, S., Burke, J., Chuang-Stein, C., Sin, C. (2012) Discounting Phase II results when planning Phase III clinical trials. *Pharmaceutical Statistics.* 11, 373–385.

[49] Kola, I., Landis, J. (2004). Can the pharmaceutical industry reduce attrition rates? *Nature Reviews Drug Discovery.* 3, 711–715.

[50] Krisam, J., Kieser, M. (2015). Optimal decision rules for biomarker-based subgroup selection for a targeted therapy in oncology. *International Journal of Molecular Sciences.* 16, 10354–10375.

[51] Lalonde, R.L., Kowalski, K.G., Hutmacher, M.M., Ewy, W., Nichols, D.J., Milligan, P.A., Corrigan, B.W., Lockwood, P.A., Marshall, S.A., Benincosa, L.J., Tensfeldt, T.G., Parivar, K., Amantea, M., Glue, P., Koide, H., Miller, R. (2007). Model-based drug development. *Clinical Pharmacology and Therapeutics.* 82, 21–32.

[52] Lan, K.K.G., Simon, R., Halperin, M. (1982). Stochastically curtailed tests in long-term clinical terms. *Communications in Statistics: Sequential Analysis.* 1, 207–219.

[53] Lewis, R.J., Viele, K., Broglio, K., Berry, S.M., Jones, A.E. (2013). An adaptive Phase II dose-finding clinical trial design to evaluate L-carnitine in the treatment of septic shock based on efficacy and predictive probability of subsequent Phase III success. *Critical Care Medicine.* 47, 1674–1678.

[54] Lipkovich, I., Dmitrienko, A., D'Agostino, R.B. (2017). Tutorial in Biostatistics: Data-driven subgroup identification and analysis in clinical trials. *Statistics in Medicine.* 36, 136–196.

[55] Mallinckrodt, C., Lipkovich, I. (2017). *Analyzing Longitudinal Clinical Trial Data. A Practical Guide.* Chapman and Hall/CRC Press: New York.

[56] Mandrekar, S.J., Sargent, D.J. (2009). Clinical trial designs for predictive biomarker validation: Theoretical considerations and practical challenges. *Journal of Clinical Oncology.* 27, 4027–4034.

[57] Meltzer, H.Y., Cucchiaro, J., Silva, R., Ogasa, M., Phillips, D., Xu, J., Kalali, A.H., Schweizer, E., Pikalov, A., Loebel, A. (2011). Lurasidone in the treatment of schizophrenia: A randomized, double-blind, placebo- and olanzapine-controlled study. *American Journal of Psychiatry.* 168, 957–967.

[58] Millen, B., Dmitrienko, A., Mandrekar, S., Zhang, Z., Williams, D. (2014). Multi-population tailoring clinical trials: Design, analysis and inference considerations. *Therapeutic Innovation and Regulatory Science.* 48, 453–462.

[59] Millen, B., Dmitrienko, A., Ruberg, S., Shen, L. (2012). A statistical framework for decision making in confirmatory multipopulation tailoring clinical trials. *Drug Information Journal.* 46, 647–656.

[60] Millen, B., Dmitrienko, A., Song G. (2014). Bayesian assessment of the influence and interaction conditions in multi-population tailoring clinical trials. *Journal of Biopharmaceutical Statistics.* 24, 94–109.

[61] Millen, B.A., Dmitrienko, A. (2011). Chain procedures: A class of flexible closed testing procedures with clinical trial applications. *Statistics in Biopharmaceutical Research.* 3, 14–30.

[62] Nasrallah, H.A., Silva, R., Phillips, D., Cucchiaro, J., Hsu, J., Xu, J., Loebel, A. (2013). Lurasidone for the treatment of acutely psychotic patients with schizophrenia: A 6-week, randomized, placebo-controlled study. *Journal of Psychiatric Research.* 47, 670–677.

[63] O'Hagan, A., Stevens, J.W., Campbell, M.J. (2005). Assurance in clinical trial design. *Pharmaceutical Statistics.* 4, 187–201.

[64] Ondra, T., Dmitrienko, A., Friede, T., Graf, A., Miller, F., Stallard, N., Posch, M. (2016). Methods for identification and confirmation of targeted subgroups in clinical trials: A systematic review. *Journal of Biopharmaceutical Statistics.* 26, 99–119.

[65] Ondra, T., Jobjörnsson, S., Beckman, R.A., Burman, C.F., König, F., Stallard, N., Posch, M. (2016). Optimizing trial designs for targeted therapies. *PLoS ONE.* 11, e0163726.

[66] O'Neill, R.T. (1997). Secondary endpoints can not be validly analyzed if the primary endpoint does not demonstrate clear statistical significance. *Controlled Clinical Trials.* 18, 550–556.

[67] Paul, S.M., Mytelko, D.S., Dunwiddie, C.T., Persinger, C.C., Munos, B.H., Linborg, S.R., Schacht, A.L. (2010). How to improve R&D productivity: The pharmaceutical industry's grand challenge. *Nature Reviews.* 9, 203–214.

[68] Paux, G., Dmitrienko, A. (2016). **Mediana**: Clinical Trial Simulations. R package version 1.0.4. Available at `http://gpaux.github.io/Mediana/`.

[69] Pulkstenis, E., Patra, K., Zhang, J. (2017). A Bayesian paradigm for decision making in proof of concept trials. *Journal of Biopharmaceutical Statistics.* 27, 442–456.

[70] Rothmann, M.D., Zhang, J.J., Lu, L., Fleming, T. R. (2012). Testing in a pre-specified subgroup and the intent-to-treat population. *Drug Information Journal.* 46, 175–179.

[71] Sabin, T., Matcham, J., Bray, S., Copas, A., Parmar, M.K.B. (2014). A quantitative process for enhancing end of Phase II decisions. *Statistics in Biopharmaceutical Research.* 6, 67–77.

[72] Sarkar, S. (1998). Some probability inequalities for censored MTP2 random variables: A proof of the Simes conjecture. *The Annals of Statistics.* 26, 494–504.

[73] Sarkar, S. (2008). On the Simes inequality and its generalization. *Beyond Parametrics in Interdisciplinary Research: Festschrift in Honor of Professor Pranab K. Sen.* Balakrishnan, N., Pena, E.A., Silvapulle, M.J. (editors). Institute of Mathematical Statistics, Beachwood, Ohio. 231–242.

[74] Sarkar, S., Chang, C.K. (1997) Simes' method for multiple hypothesis testing with positively dependent test statistics. *Journal of the American Statistical Association.* 92, 1601–1608.

[75] Schlömer, P., Brannath, W. (2013). Group sequential designs for three-arm 'gold standard' non-inferiority trials with fixed margin. *Statistics in Medicine.* 32, 4875–4889.

[76] Simon, R. (1989). Optimal two-stage designs for clinical trials. *Controlled Clinical Trials.* 10, 1–10.

[77] Spiegelhalter, D.J., Abrams, K.R., Myles, J.P. (2004). *Bayesian Approaches to Clinical Trials and Health-care Evaluation.* Wiley, London.

[78] Stucke, K., Kieser, M. (2012). A general approach for sample size calculation for the three-arm 'gold standard' non-inferiority design. *Statistics in Medicine.* 31, 3579–3596.

[79] Sverdlov, O., Ryeznik, Y., Wu, S. (2014). Exact Bayesian inference comparing binomial proportions, with application to proof-of-concept trials. *Therapeutic Innovation and Regulatory Science.* 49, 163–174.

[80] Van Cutsem, E., Keohne, C.H., Hitre, E., Zaluski, J., Chang Chien, C.R., Makhson, A., D'Haens, G., Pinter, T., Lim, R., Bodoky, G., Roh, J.K., Folprecht, G., Ruff, P., Stroh, C., Tejpar, S., Schlichting, M., Nippgen, J., Rougier, P. (2009). Cetuximab and chemotherapy as initial treatment for metastatic colorectal cancer. *New England Journal of Medicine.* 360, 1408–1417.

[81] Wang, D., Li, Y., Wang, X., Liu, X., Fu, B., Lin, Y., Larsen, L., Offen, W. (2015). Overview of multiple testing methodology and recent development in clinical trials. *Contemporary Clinical Trials.* 45, 13–20.

[82] Wang, M.D. (2007). Sample size re-estimation by Bayesian prediction. *Biometrical Journal.* 49, 365–377.

[83] Wang, M.D. (2015). Applications of probability of study success in clinical drug development. *Selected Papers from 2013 ICSA/ISBS Joint Statistical Meetings.* 4, 185–196.

[84] Wang, S.J., Hung, H.M. (2014). A regulatory perspective on essential considerations in design and analysis of subgroups correctly classified. *Journal of Biopharmaceutical Statistics.* 24, 19–41.

[85] Wang, Y., Fu, H., Kulkarni, P., Kaiser, C. (2013). Evaluating and utilizing probability of study success in clinical development. *Clinical Trials.* 10, 407–413.

[86] Wasserstein R. L., Lazar N. A. (2016). The ASA's statement on p-values: context, process, and purpose. *The American Statistician.* 70, 129–133.

[87] Westfall, P.H., Tsai, K., Ogenstad, S., Tomoiaga, A., Moseley, S., Lu, Y. (2008). Clinical trials simulation: A statistical approach. *Journal of Biopharmaceutical Statistics.* 18, 611–630.

[88] Zhang, J., Zhang, J.J. (2013). Joint probability of statistical success of multiple Phase III trials. *Pharmaceutical Statistics.* 12, 358–365.

Index

Adaptive design, 5
Adaptive design clinical trial (case
        study), 59–67
Additive tradeoff-based criterion,
        64–65
Additive weighting scheme, 97
Adjusted critical value, 66
Adjusted significance level, 66,
        129–130
α-allocation, 78, 79, 151
Alternative Bayesian Go/No-Go
        decision criterion (case
        study), 283–286
    clinical trial, 283–286
    conclusions and extensions, 286
    software implementation,
        285–286
Analysis, defines AnalysisMode
        object, 15
AnalysisModel, 5
AnalysisModel.object, 10, 11, 12,
        151, 152
Analysis model(s)
    in clinical development decision
        making, 254–255, 269–270,
        283–284, 287–288, 291, 296
    in clinical trial optimization,
        9–13, 38–42, 59–67
    description of, 3, 9–11
    in multiple objectives clinical
        trials, 93–95, 116–117,
        124–130, 150–152, 156–159,
        169–170
    specification of, 17–18, 24–26
    in subgroup analysis, 178–179,
        189–191, 210–213, 225, 230,
        246

APEX trial, 1
Assumptions, 2, *see also* Data models
Assurance R package, 263–264

Bayesian approach
    fully Bayesian approach, 261,
        263
    mixed Bayesian-frequentist
        approach, 259–261, 263
Bayesian formulation, of influence
        condition, 217
Bayesian framework, 37
Bayesian Go/No-Go decision criteria
        (case study), 269–283
    clinical trial, 269–271
    conclusions and extensions,
        282–283
    general sensitivity assessments,
        271–274
    with informative priors, 274–276
    sample size consideration,
        276–279
    software implementation,
        279–282
Bayesian Go/No-Go in interim
        analysis trial (case study),
        286–290
    clinical trial, 290
    conclusions and extensions, 290
    software implementation,
        289–290
Bayesian inferences, 49
Beta prior distribution, 48
Biased success criterion, 180
Binary classifier, 39
Biomarkers, 11, 174, 176, 189–213,
        see also Predictive

biomarkers; Prognostic
   biomarker
Bivariate criterion, 65, 68
Bivariate normal distribution, 149
Bivariate optimization algorithm,
   238
Bivariate outcome distribution, 122
Bonferroni-based chain procedure,
   125–130
Bonferroni-based corrections, 72, 78,
   85
Bonferroni-based procedure, 172
Bonferroni procedure, 191
   chain procedure and, 81
   decision rules used in, 79
   disjunctive power for, 194–195
   multiple adjustments and, 94
   null hypothesis and, 182
   weighted power for, 197
Bonferroni tests, 159
Bootstrap-based perturbations, 37
Bootstrap algorithm, parametric, 37,
   45–46, 108–109
Bootstrap-based marginal
   probabilities, 51
Bootstrap-based sensitivity, 48
Bootstrap-based weighted power, 207
Bootstrap data models, 36–37,
   46–47, 108, 148, 204
Broad claim, 180, 181, 185, 192, 193,
   198, 216, 218–219, 220–221,
   231–233, 238

Case study(ies)
   adaptive design clinical trial,
      59–67
   alternative Bayesian Go/No-Go
      decision criterion, 283–286
   Bayesian Go/No-Go decision
      criteria, 269–283
   Bayesian Go/No-Go in interim
      analysis trial, 286–290
   direct selection of optimal
      procedure parameters,
      121–156

multiplicity adjustment optimal
   selection, 91–120, 188–214
normally distributed endpoint
   clinical trial, 16–20
phase II trials decision criteria
   based on POS, 290–293
three potential claims decision
   rules, 228–250
tradeoff-based selection of
   optimal procedure
   parameters, 156–172
two patient populations clinical
   trial, 38–42
two potential claims decision
   rules, 215–228
two-time-to-event endpoints
   clinical trial, 20–27
updating POS using interim or
   external information,
   294–299
Clinically meaningful evaluation
   criterion, 180
Clinical scenario evaluation (CSE)
   in clinical development decision
      making, 251–298
   and clinical trial optimization,
      1–69
   components of, 2–4
   in confirmatory subgroup
      analysis, 176–188
   framework, 73–91
   function, 15
   introduction to, 1–2
   in multiple objectives clinical
      trials, 71–172
   in multiplicity adjustment,
      188–214
   multiplicity issues and, 72
   software implementation, 4–15
   subgroup analysis in clinical
      trials and, 173–250
Clinical trial optimization, *see also*
   Direct optimization
   definition and basic principles
      of, 28–30

direct optimization, 30–31
optimization algorithm, 31,
    33–34
sensitivity assessments, 29,
    34–35
tradeoff-based optimization,
    31–33
Clinical trial(s), *see also* Clinical
    trial optimization
    with adaptive design, 59–67
    in clinical development decision
        making, 265–268, 269–271,
        283–284, 287–288, 290, 295
    designing, CSE-based approach
        to, 1–2
    with multiple objectives, 92–99,
        121–133, 156–161
    with normally distributed
        endpoint, 16–20
    subgroup analysis in, 189–194,
        215, 228–233
    with two patient populations,
        38–59
    with two time-to-event
        endpoints, 20–27
Cochran-Mantel-Haenszel (CHM)
    method, 40
Cochran-Mantel-Haenszel test, 93
Competing goals, 160
Component procedure, 85, 157
Component.procedure, 169
Compound criterion, 31
Conditional power, 62
Conditional power approach,
    260–261
Confidence interval, 33, 50, 56, 134
Confidence region, 33
Confirmatory subgroup analysis, 174
Conjunctive criterion, 87
Constrained optimization algorithms,
    31, 220, 222–224
Correlation coefficients, 9
Criteria based on multiplicity
    penalties, 89–91
Criterion function, 67

Criterion object, 13–14, 19, 117–118,
    211
CRYSTAL trial, 186
CSE, *see also* Clinical Scenario
    Evaluation (CSE)
CSE approach, 15
Custom criterion, 117

data, defines DataModel object, 15
data.model, 5, 16
DataModel, 5, 116
DataModel object, 6, 9, 15, 16, 116,
    209
Data model(s)
    in clinical development decision
        making, 253–254, 269, 283,
        287, 290–291, 296
    in clinical trial optimization,
        38–42, 59–67
    defined, 3, 5–6
    focus and steps of, 5–6
    main, 34–35, 40, 50, 163
    in multiple objectives clinical
        trials, 74, 92–93, 115–116,
        122–123, 149–150, 156, 169
    specification of, 16–17, 21–24
    in subgroup analysis, 176–177,
        189–190, 208–209, 215,
        229–230, 244–245
D-dimer levels, 38, 39
Decision-making framework, 184–185
Decision rules, 125–126, 129–130,
    183, 187–188, 193
Design object, 8–9
Design parameter sets, 8
Design prior, 261
Design stage, 94
DiffMeanStat statistic, 18
Disjunctive criterion, 42, 53–56, 58,
    86, *see also* Subset
    disjunctive criterion
Disjunctive power criterion, 179, 193
Direct optimization
    based on disjunctive power,
        194–195

based on weighted power,
196–198
conclusions and extensions,
154–156
qualitative sensitivity
assessments, 35–36
quantitative sensitivity
assessments, 36–37
strategies, 29, 30–31
target parameter, 53–59
target parameter in Procedure
B1, 133–140
target parameter in Procedure
B2, 140–154
two patient populations clinical
trial, 38 42
Direct selection of optimal procedure
parameters (case study),
121–156
clinical trial, 121–133
conclusions and extensions,
154–156
sensitivity assessments, 145–148
software implementation,
149–154
target parameter in Procedure
B1, 133–140
target parameter in Procedure
B2, 140–145
Disjunctive criterion, 86, 117, 131,
160, 165–166
Disjunctive power, 43
direct optimization based on,
194–195
evaluation criteria based on, 42,
95–96
as function of target parameter,
162–164
for the Holm procedure, 46–47
and related criteria, 86–87
sensitivity assessment based on,
100–103, 109–111
DisjunctivePower method, 117, 211
Distributional information, in
multiplicity adjustments, 77

Dropout parameters, 115
Dunnett-adjusted significance, 66
Dunnett procedure, 66, 82–83, 94,
183

Effect sizes, 122–123
Efficacy claims (broad, restricted,
and enhanced claims), 181,
185, 187
EMA, *see* European Medicines
Agency (EMA)
Enhanced claim, 181, 185, 187,
231–233, 236, 238
Enrichment ratio, 214
Error rate, 217–218, 234, 242, 243,
see also Influence error rate;
Interaction error rate
European Medicines Agency (EMA),
71, 173
evaluation, defines EvaluationModel
object, 15
EvaluationModel, 5
EvaluationModel object, 152–153
Evaluation model(s)
in clinical development decision
making, 255–258, 270–271,
284–285, 287–288, 291–292,
296–298
in clinical trial optimization,
13–14, 38–42, 59–67
description of, 3, 13–14
in multiple objectives clinical
trials, 85–91, 95–99,
117–119, 131–133, 152–154,
159–161, 170–171
in optimal procedure parameters
direct selection, 131–133,
152–154
specification of, 18–19, 26–27
in subgroup analysis, 179–181,
192–194, 211–213, 215,
225–227, 230–233, 246–249
Event-driven designs, 5
Event object, 6
Event rate, 39–40, 50

Exceedence-based evaluation criteria, 95, 97, 100
Exceedence criteria, 85
α-exhaustive procedure, 78
Expectation criteria, 85, 97, 100

False Go risk, 255
False No-Go risk, 255
Family, 169
Familywise error rate, 75, 82, 84
FDA, *see* U.S. Food and Drug Administration (FDA)
First source of multiplicity, 121
Fixed designs, 5, 17
FixedSeqAdj method, 25, 117
Fixed-sequence procedure, 21, 25–26, 77, 78, 80–81, 94, 95, *see also* Multiplicity adjustment procedure (MultAdjProc)
Fixed-sequence testing method, 101, 105
Frequentist approach, mixed Bayesian, 259–261
Frequentist confidence interval approach, 255
Frequentist decision criterion, 267
Frequentist decision rule, 267, 268
Frequentist method, 254, 267
Fully Bayesian approach, 261, 263
Futility rule, 61–62, 69

Gama, 169
Gatekeeping procedures, 76, 84–85, 125
General gatekeepers, 84
General sensitivity assessment, in Bayesian Go/No-Go decision criteria, 271–274
GNG, *see* Go/No-Go
Go/No-Go decision criteria, in clinical development decision making, 255–258

Hazard rates, 22, 229–230, 232, 244, 250
Hazard ratio, 22, 23, 187

High-confidence setting, 48
High-uncertainty setting, 49
HochbergAdj method, 117
Hochberg and Hommel procedures, 81–82, 85, 94, 183
Hochberg-based keeping procedure, specification of, 169–170
Hochberg-based multiplicity adjustment, 104, 230, 234
Hochberg procedure, 157–158, 191, 239
Holm procedure
decision rules used in, 79
disjunctive power for, 194–195
multiplicity adjustments and, 41–42, 43, 45, 78, 80, 94
testing algorithm, 81, 182
weighted power for, 197
Hommel-based gatekeeping procedure, 172

Influence and interaction thresholds, optimal selection of, 238–244
Influence condition, 215–216, 231–232
Influence error rate, 217, 222–223, 234, 240–241
Influence threshold, optimal selection of, 219–220
Influence threshold, 217, 226, 248
Interaction condition, 187, 231–232, 233–238
Interaction error rate, 234, 236, 241
interaction threshold, 248

Joint optimal regions, 144–145

Key data model parameters, 47
Key secondary endpoint, 121, 122
KRAS subgroup, 186

label, in Criterion object, 14
Linear interpolation, 235
Local control, 159
Locally optimal model, 29

Local optimization approach, 146
Logical restrictions, 125–126, 157
Lower reference value (LRV), 253,
        254, 265
Low-uncertainty setting, 48
LRV, *see* Lower reference value
        (LRV)

Main data model, 34–35, 40, 50, 163
MarginalPower method, 211
Marginal probability of restricted
        claim, custom function for,
        212
Marginal probability of success, 52
Marker-negative, 39
Marker-status, 39
Mediana package, R code based on,
        26
    descriptive statistics supported
        in, 12
    introduction of, 4–5
    multiplicity adjustment
        procedures supported in, 13
    multiplicity adjustments in,
        114–116
    patient dropout models and, 8
    trial endpoints supported by, 7
Medium-uncertainty setting, 49
method
    in Criterion object, 13
    in Statistic object, 11
    in Test object, 10
Metrics, 2, *see also* Evaluation
        models
Mixed Bayesian-frequentist
        approach, 259–261, 263
Mixture-based gatekeeping
        procedures, 85
Mixture method, 85
Monotonicity assumption, 101
Monte Carlo approximations, 33
MultAdjProc, *see* Multiplicity
        adjustment procedure
        (MultAdjProc)
MultAdjProc object, 11–13, 25

MultAdProc, 10
MultiAdjProc object, 11–13,
        116–117, 169, 210
Multiple objectives clinical trials
    clinical scenario evaluation
        framework, 73–91
    direct selection of optimal
        procedure parameters,
        121–156
    introduction, 71–73
    multiplicity adjustment
        selection, 91–120
    tradeoff-based selection of
        optimal procedure
        parameters, 156–172
MultipleSequenceGatekeepingAdj
        method, 169
Multiple-sequence gatekeeping
        procedures, 172
Multiple testing procedures, 183
    classification of, 76–77
    multiplicity penalty of, 97
    in Procedure H, 172
Multiplicity adjustment framework,
        general, 83
Multiplicity adjustment optimal
        selection, 91–120
Multiplicity adjustment optimal
        selection (case studies),
        91–120, 188–214
    clinical trial, 92–99, 189–194
    conclusions and extensions, 120,
        213–214
    direct optimization based on
        disjunctive power, 194–195
    direct optimization based on
        weighted power, 196–198
    introduction, 91–92
    qualitative sensitivity
        assessment, 99–107,
        199–203
    quantitative sensitivity
        assessment, 107–114,
        203–207

software implementation, 114–120, 208–213

Multiplicity adjustment procedure (MultAdjProc), 10, 12–13, 25

Multiplicity adjustment procedure object (MultAdjProc), *see* MultAdjProc object

Multiplicity adjustment procedures set (MultAdj), 10

Multiplicity adjustments
  based on Bonferroni and Hochberg procedures, 194–195
  based on semiparametric procedures, 82
  Bonferroni-based chain procedures, 151
  clinical trial, 1
  evaluating, 43
  Holm procedure, 41, 42, 45, 47, 52, 53, 55
  in multiplicity problems in confirmatory subgroup analysis, 181–184
  multi-population clinical trials and, 216
  selecting, 42, 53

Multiplicity adjustment set, 12

Multiplicity-based calibration, 66

Multiplicity penalties, 86, 98
  criteria based, 89–91
  sensitivity assessments based on, 103–107, 111–113

Multiplicity penalty matrix, 97–98, 104

Multiplicity problems, in multiple objectives clinical trials, 74–76

Multi-population tailoring designs, 173

MVNormalDist method, 149

Nonparametric chain procedures, 78

Nonparametric multiple testing procedures, 77, 78–81, 83, 84

Nonparametric procedures, 182, 191

Non-separable procedure, 157

Normally distributed endpoint clinical trial (case study), 16–20

Optimal analysis models, 29

Optimal interval, 33, 55, 134, 138–140, 166–168, 224

Optimal region, 33–34

Optimism bias, 43

Optimization algorithms, 31, 33–34, 121, 134, 140, 192, 194–198, 240–243

Optimization criterion, 193, 221

Optimization strategies, 30–33, 220–224

Options, 2, *see also* Analysis models

OutcomeDist, 6

OutcomeDist object, 7–8, 116, 149, 209, 245

Outcome distribution parameters, 122

Outcome parameter sets, 9

Parallel gatekeepers, 84

Parametric bootstrap algorithm, 37, 45–46, 108–109

Parametric bootstrap approach, 147–148

Parametric chain procedures, 77, 78, 80, 81

Parametric multiple testing procedures, 77, 82–83, 84

Parametric procedures, 183–184

Partition-based weighted criteria, 88, 95–97, 100–103, 132, 134, 136, 137–139, 142–143, 181, 200

Partition-based weighted power, 148, 180, 192, 223

Performance functions, 32, 63–64

Performance loss evaluations,

multiplicity adjustments
and, 113–114
Permutation-based approach, to
sensitivity assessments,
52–53
Perturbation-based assessments, 35,
44, 50, 52–53
PFS, 229, 230
Phase II trials, 59–60, 252, 263–264,
271, 288
Phase II trials decision criteria based
on POS (case study),
290–293
clinical trial, 290
conclusions and extensions, 293
software implementation,
292–293
Pivoting-based assessments, 34, 43,
see also Quantitative
sensitivity assessment
Placebo Bio Neg, 210
Placebo Bio Pos, 210
POC trial, *see* Proof-of-concept
(POC) trial
Point estimate, 134, 138
POS, *see* Probability of success
(POS)
Power gain, 67
Pre-defined marker, 38
Predicted probability of success, 62
Predictive biomarkers, 57, 176–178
Predictive power approach, 260
PREVAIL trial, 1
prevalence.pos, 244
Primary endpoint, 9, 121, 122, 176,
189
Probability of success (POS), 252,
254, 255, 258–264, 262
Prognostic biomarker, 176–178
Proof-of-concept (POC) trial,
264–269
clinical trial, 265–268
vs. Go/No-Go approaches,
262–263

software implementation,
268–269
α-propagation rules, 78, 79, 151
PropTest method, 116
p-values, 217

Qualitative assessments, 34–35
Qualitative or pivoting-based
approach, 99
Qualitative sensitivity assessment
based on supportive data model
parameter, 147–148
clinical trial optimization,
199–203
conducting, 43–44
goal in optimization, 35–36
in multiplicity adjustment
selection, 199–203
selecting optimal analysis
model, 99
Quantitative assessments, 34–35, 43
Quantitative sensitivity assessment
based o key data model
parameters, 146–147
evaluating multiple testing
procedures, 107–109
framework for, 44–53
goal in optimization, 36–37
in multiplicity adjustment
selection, 203–207
tradeoff-based optimization, 168

RatioEffectSizeEventStat method,
246
R code based on Mediana package,
11–15, 26, 114–120
Rejection rules, 80, 185
Relevant loss, 51
Relevant performance loss,
multiplicity adjustments
and, 113–114
Restricted claim, 180, 181, 185, 192,
216, 218–219, 220–221,
231–233, 238
Robustness profiles
of analysis model, 52

of optimal analysis model, 35
  sensitivity assessment and, 43
R package (Mediana), 4–5, 7

Sample object, 9, 150
samples
  in Statistic object, 11
  in Test object, 10
Sample size, in Bayesian Go/No-Go
    decision criteria, 276–279
Semiparametric multiple testing
    procedures, 77, 81–82, 83,
    84, 159
Semiparametric procedures,
    Bonferroni procedure and,
    183
Sensitivity assessments, *see also*
    Qualitative sensitivity
    assessments; Quantitative
    sensitivity assessments
  based on disjunctive and
    weighted power, 100–103,
    109–111
  based on multiplicity penalties,
    103–107, 111–113
  in clinical trial optimization, 29,
    34–35
  in joint optimal interval, 146
Sequentially rejective, 142
Sequentially rejective algorithm, 80
Sequential Organ Failure Assessment
    (SOFA), 60–61
Serial gatekeepers, 84
Several sources of multiplicity, 75
Simes test, 81, 82
SimParameters, 5
SimParameters object, 14
Simple and partition-based power,
    134–138
Simple and partition-based weighted
    power, 141–144
Simple weighted criterion, 87,
    136–137, 142, 161, 166–167
Simple weighted power, as function

of target parameter,
    164–165
simulation, defines SimParameters
    object, 15
Simulation-based algorithm, 262,
    270–271, 291, 294–295
Simulation-based clinical scenario
    evaluation, 14–15
Simulation-based POS calculations,
    262
Simulation-based results, 20
Simulation results
  in multiple objectives clinical
    trials, 119–120, 154, 155,
    171–172
  in multiplicity adjustment
    selection, 213, 214
  in normally distributed
    endpointclinical trial, 20
  three claims decision rules, 249
  two claims decision rules, 227
Single source of multiplicity, 75
Single-step Dunnett procedures, 183
SLEDAI Responder Index-4 (SRI-4),
    265
SLE Disease Activity Index by 4, 265
SOFA, *see* Sequential Organ Failure
    Assessment (SOFA)
Software implementation
  in clinical development decision
    making, 268–269, 279–282,
    285–286, 289–290, 292–293,
    298–299
  in multiple objectives clinical
    trials, 114–120, 149–154,
    168–172
  in subgroup analysis clinical
    trials, 208–213, 225–227,
    244–249
α-splitting methods, 182
Statistic object, 11, 18, 19, 118, 211,
    225, 246
statistic.result, 211, 225, 247
statistics, in Criterion object, 13
Step-down algorithm, 81

Step-down Dunnett procedure, 183
Step-up algorithm, 82
study.duration, 8
subgroup.cs2.BroadClaimPower, 226
subgroup.cs2.RestrictedClaimPower,
226
subgroup.cs1.WeightedPower, 211
subgroup.cs3.WeightedPower, 247
subgroup.cs3.WeightedPower
function, 247
Subset disjunctive criterion, 85, 87,
131, 134–135, 136, 140–141
Subset disjunctive power, 131, 134,
140–141

Tailored or restricted claim, 180
Target parameter, 29
direct optimization approach,
53–59
optimal values of, 224
tradeoff-based optimization
approach, 67–69
Target parameter optimal selection
direct optimization approach,
53–59
in Procedure H, 161–168
tradeoff-based optimization
approach, 67–69
Target product profile (TPP),
253–254, 268
Target value (TV), 253–254, 265
Testing algorithm, 126–127
Test object, 10–11, 211
test.result, 211
tests
in Criterion object, 13
in MultAdjProc object, 12
Test statistics, 94
Three potential claims selection
(case study), 228–249
clinical trial, 228–233
conclusions and extensions,
249–250
influence and interaction

thresholds selection,
238–244
interaction condition, 233–238
software implementation,
244–249
TPP, *see* Target product profile
(TPP)
Tradeoff-based algorithm, 160, 164
Tradeoff-based criterion, 160, 161,
165–166
Tradeoff-based disjunctive criterion,
162–163, 164
Tradeoff-based optimization, 29,
31–33
adaptive design clinical trial,
59–67
target parameter optimal
selection, 67–69
Tradeoff-based optimization
algorithm, 156, 220–221
Tradeoff-based selection of optimal
procedure parameters (case
study), 156–172
clinical trial, 156–161
conclusions and extensions, 172
software implementation,
168–172
target parameter selection of
Procedure H, 161–167
Transition parameters, 78
Treatment arm, 5, 6, 9, 11, 16,
176–178, 189
Treatment-by-biomarker interaction
test, 187
Treatment effect
biomarker-positive subset and,
191, 231
Bootstrap-based probabilities
and, 47
disjunctive power and, 43
in MCC clinical trial, 22
in normally disturbed endpoint
trial, 16–17
optimal analysis models and, 29,
35

test, 40–41, 178

Treatment effect test, in proof-of-concept trial, 265–266

Treatment event rate, 49

Trial designs, 5

Truncated Hochberg procedure, 159

truncation parameter, 157, 158–159

TTest method, 210

TV, *see* Target value (TV)

Two potential claims decision criteria (case study), 215–228
clinical trial, 215
conclusions and extensions, 228
influence condition, 215–219
influence threshold optimal selection, 219–224
software implementation, 225–227

Two-time-to-event endpoints clinical trial, 20–27

Type I error gate, 19, 20, 21, 31, 41, 71, 72, 75, 78, 95

Type II error rate, 63–64, 124, 127, 159, 182, 216

Uncertainty parameter, 37, 46, 48–50, 108

Updating POS using interim or external information (case study), 294–299
clinical trial, 295
software implementation, 298–299

U.S. Food and Drug Administration (FDA), 71, 173

Utility-based approach, based on weighted power, 192, 194

Weighted criterion, 165–166, 197, 205–207, 233

Weighted power, *see also* Partition-based weighted power
Bootstrap-based, 207

custom function for computing, 212
direct optimization based, 196–198
distribution of, 205–206
evaluation criteria and, 96
as function of influence threshold and interaction threshold, 240–243
as function of target parameter, 224
as function of total number of events, 234–236
sensitivity assessment based on, 100–103, 109–111
in three potential claims decision rules, 247
in two potential claims decision rules, 226
utility-based approach based on, 192, 194

Weighted power criterion, 87–89, 96–97, 179, 180–181, 193, 233, 239

WeightedPower method, 117

weight parameter, 12

Printed in the United States
by Baker & Taylor Publisher Services